Extraordinary
Disorders of
Human Behavior

CRITICAL ISSUES IN PSYCHIATRY
An Educational Series for Residents and Clinicians

Series Editor: Sherwyn M. Woods, M.D., Ph.D.
University of Southern California School of Medicine
Los Angeles, California

A RESIDENT'S GUIDE TO PSYCHIATRIC EDUCATION
Edited by Michael G. G. Thompson, M.D.

STATES OF MIND: Analysis of Change in Psychotherapy
Mardi J. Horowitz, M.D.

DRUG AND ALCOHOL ABUSE: A Clinical Guide to
Diagnosis and Treatment
Marc A. Schuckit, M.D.

THE INTERFACE BETWEEN THE PSYCHODYNAMIC AND
BEHAVIORAL THERAPIES
Edited by Judd Marmor, M.D., and Sherwyn M. Woods, M.D., Ph.D.

LAW IN THE PRACTICE OF PSYCHIATRY
Seymour L. Halleck, M.D.

NEUROPSYCHIATRIC FEATURES OF MEDICAL DISORDERS
James W. Jefferson, M.D., and John R. Marshall, M.D.

ADULT DEVELOPMENT: A New Dimension in Psychodynamic Theory
and Practice
Calvin A. Colarusso, M.D., and Robert A. Nemiroff, M.D.

SCHIZOPHRENIA
John S. Strauss, M.D., and William T. Carpenter, Jr., M.D.

EXTRAORDINARY DISORDERS OF HUMAN BEHAVIOR
Edited by Claude T. H. Friedmann, M.D., and Robert A. Faguet, M.D.

MARITAL THERAPY: A Combined Psychodynamic–Behavioral Approach
Edited by R. Taylor Segraves, M.D.

TREATMENT INTERVENTIONS IN HUMAN SEXUALITY
Edited by Carol C. Nadelson, M.D., and David B. Marcotte, M.D.

A Continuation Order Plan is available for this series. A continuation order will bring
delivery of each new volume immediately upon publication. Volumes are billed only
upon actual shipment. For further information please contact the publisher.

Extraordinary Disorders of Human Behavior

Edited by

CLAUDE T. H. FRIEDMANN, M. D.

University of California at Irvine
Medical Center
Orange, California

and

ROBERT A. FAGUET, M. D.

University of California at Los Angeles School of Medicine
Los Angeles, California

PLENUM PRESS · NEW YORK AND LONDON

Library of Congress Cataloging in Publication Data

Main entry under title:

Extraordinary disorders of human behavior.

(Critical issues in psychiatry)
Bibliography: p.
Includes index.
1. Psychology, Pathological—Addresses, essays, lectures. I. Friedmann,
Claude T. H. II. Faguet, Robert Andrew. III. Series. [DNLM: 1. Mental disorders.
WM 100 E965]
RC454.4.E925 1982   616.89   82-12286
ISBN 0-306-40875-9

© 1982 Plenum Press, New York
A Division of Plenum Publishing Corporation
233 Spring Street, New York, N.Y. 10013

Printed in the United States of America

Contributors

FARUK S. ABUZZAHAB, SR., M.D., Ph.D. • Associate Clinical Professor of Psychiatry, University of Minnesota, 606 South 24th Avenue, #818, Minneapolis MN 55454

RANSOM J. ARTHUR, M.D. • Dean, School of Medicine, The Oregon Health Sciences University 3181 S.W. Sam Jackson Park Road, Portland, OR 97201

DANIEL B. AUERBACH, M.D. • Adjunct Assistant Professor of Psychiatry, University of California at Los Angeles, 15760 Ventura Boulevard, #1929, Encino CA 91436

BURTON G. BURTON-BRADLEY, M.D. • Honorary Professor of Psychiatry, University of New Zealand; Mental Health Services, P.O. Box 1239, Boroko, Papua New Guinea

HARRY D. EASTWELL, M.D. • Senior Lecturer in Psychiatry, Royal Brisbane Hospital, Brisbane, Queensland 4029, Australia

KAY F. FAGUET, Ph.D. • Assistant Clinical Professor of Psychiatry (Psychology), University of California at Los Angeles, Neuropsychiatric Institute, 760 Westwood Plaza, Los Angeles CA 90024

ROBERT A. FAGUET, M.D. • Assistant Clinical Professor of Psychiatry, University of California at Los Angeles, 11665 W. Olympic Boulevard, Suite 410, Los Angeles, CA 90064

CHARLES V. FORD, M.D. • Professor of Psychiatry, Vanderbilt University School of Medicine, Nashville TN 37232

CLAUDE T. H. FRIEDMANN, M.D. • Assistant Professor of Psychiatry, University of California at Irvine, 101 City Drive South, Orange, CA 92668

JAMES S. GROTSTEIN, M.D. • Clinical Professor of Psychiatry, University of California at Los Angeles, 9777 Wilshire Boulevard, Los Angeles CA 90212

KAY REDFIELD JAMISON, Ph.D. • Assistant Professor of Psychiatry (Psychology) and Director, University of California at Los Angeles, Affective Disorders Clinic, Los Angeles CA 90024

IRA M. LESSER, M.D. • Assistant Professor of Psychiatry, University of California at Los Angeles, Harbor General-UCLA Medical Center, Building D-5, Psychiatry, 1000 West Carson Street, Torrance CA 90509

E. MANSELL PATTISON, M.D. • Chairman and Professor, Department of Psychiatry and Health Behavior, Medical College of Georgia, Augusta, GA 30901

ROBERT F. REBAL, JR., M.D. • Assistant Professor of Psychiatry, University of Southern California School of Medicine, 1934 Hospital Place, Los Angeles CA 90033

ROBERT T. RUBIN, M.D., Ph.D. • Professor of Psychiatry, University of California at Los Angeles, Harbor General-UCLA Medical Center, Building B-4, 1000 West Carson Street, Torrance CA 90509

DAVID RUDNICK, M.D., Ph.D. • Assistant Clinical Professor of Psychiatry, University of California at Los Angeles-Neuropsychiatric Institute, 19144-9 Hamlin Street, Reseda CA 91335

JOSEPH WESTERMEYER, M.D., Ph.D. • Professor of Psychiatry, University of Minnesota, Department of Psychiatry, University Hospitals, Box 393, Mayo Memorial Building, Minneapolis, MN 55455

SHERWYN WOODS, M.D., Ph.D. • Professor of Psychiatry, University of Southern California, 1934 Hospital Place, Los Angeles CA 90033

Foreword

Clinicians have long been fascinated by the rare and exotic in medicine. Similarly, psychiatrists and mental health professionals have been intrigued by the uncommon and extraordinary syndromes which, despite their rarity, have much to teach us about the limitless forms of human adaptation. Of particular interest is the fact that fragments and partial expressions of these rare disorders are often encountered in the dreams and fantasies of the "ordinary" patient. For this reason, the understanding and insights collected in this volume are likely to have clinical usefulness far beyond those rare occasions when we encounter the exotic in its fully developed form.

These disorders demonstrate the complex interplay between intrapsychic dynamic forces and the cultural influences which act to shape overt symptomatology. The section on extraordinary syndromes from non-Western cultures demonstrates the universality of the psychodynamic roots of human suffering, despite the seemingly strange forms in which this suffering is expressed. As clinicians we are too often restricted by ethnocentric attitudes and culturally determined stereotypes. This volume provides a stimulating and enjoyable opportunity to reach beyond those limitations.

Sherwyn M. Woods
Series Editor

Preface

Human personality, the most complex organization known, has evolved a staggering variety of adaptive mechanisms. Its plasticity is described by Kolb (1977):

> Since adaptation is the very essence of life, it is not strange that man, the most highly developed species, has evolved not only anatomical adjustments, which protect him structurally or physiologically in respect to his environment, but also psychological devices, which assist him in dealing with emotional needs and stresses. These devices help meet the needs for affection, personal security, personal significance, and defense against perturbing affects. (p. 11)

There are a number of disorders, however, that represent atypical adaptations in that they do not easily conform to standard diagnostic frameworks (neither in Kraepelin's time nor in the modern era of DSM-III). These entities have usually been termed uncommon, rare, exotic, esoteric, extraordinary, and unclassifiable.

These "fragments," as Lehmann (1975) calls them, are scattered widely over the literature. We have attempted to contemporize and update them in one clinically relevant volume. It is our impression that even though the general psychiatrist may encounter only one or two such disorders in his lifetime, he will most certainly see their innumerable partial and fragmentary expressions in his patients' dreams, fantasies, and behaviors. An interest in, and familiarity with, these syndromes will therefore assist him, we hope, in understanding and treating his patients.

We hope, too, that new interest will be stimulated in these disorders; not only do we find them individually fascinating but we recognize that the study of unusual syndromes often helps elucidate the more common disorders.

Finally, in accordance with the current trend in American psychiatry to revise diagnostic criteria and improve the reliability of diagnostic judgments (Spitzer, 1978), we wonder: Will these syndromes continue to stand apart as ungrouped entities or will they be seen in the future as "typical" variants of the more common psychiatric disorders?

In addition to the sections on rare syndromes and extraordinary presentations of common syndromes, we are including a section on extraordinary syndromes from non-Western cultures. These entities are further illustrations of the extraordinary evolution of psychological self-preservation and underscore the notion that what is extraordinary in one culture may not be so in another. Human behavior is in part culturally determined and must always be judged in context.

C.T.H.F.
R.A.F.

REFERENCES

Kolb, L. C., 1977, "Modern Clinical Psychiatry," W. B. Saunders, Philadelphia.
Lehmann, H. E., 1975, Unusual psychiatric disorders and atypical psychoses, in "Comprehensive Textbook of Psychiatry II" (A. Freedman, H. Kaplan, and B. Sadock, eds.), pp. 1724–1736, Williams and Wilkins, Baltimore.
Spitzer, R. L., 1978, Foreword, in "DSM-III: Diagnostic Criteria Draft," Task Force on Nomenclature and Statistics, American Psychiatric Association.

Contents

Etiology and Classification   41
Conclusion   45
References   45

4   Psychiatric Symptoms in Prisoner of War and
    Concentration Camp Survivors   47
    Ransom J. Arthur

    Examination of Stressors   50
    Methods of Coping   53
    Subsequent Course of Illness   54
    The Vietnam War   56
    Genesis of Syndrome   59
    Treatment of Syndrome   60
    References   61

5   Autoscopic Phenomena   65
    James S. Grotstein

    Epidemiology   67
    Review of the Literature on Causation   67
    Case Examples   71
    Discussion   73
    Summary   75
    References   76

6   Gilles de La Tourette Syndrome or Multiple Tic
    Disorder   79
    Faruk S. Abuzzahab, Sr.

    Definition   79
    History   81
    Epidemiology   84
    Symptoms   85
    Experimental and Laboratory Information   86
    Differential Diagnosis   87
    Treatment   89

Tourette Syndrome Association, Inc.   93
Conclusion   93
References   93

7   The Paranoid-Erotic Syndromes   99
    F. David Rudnick

    The Capgras Syndrome   99
    Syndrome of Fregoli 111
    The Intermetamorphosis Syndrome 112
    Cotard's Syndrome 113
    De Clerambault's Syndrome 113
    References 117

8   Unusual Sexual Syndromes 121
    Ronald F. Rebal, Jr., Robert A. Faguet,
    and Sherwyn M. Woods

    Necrophilia 121
    Vampirism 126
    Zoophilia 128
    Autoerotic Asphyxia 132
    Coprophilia and Related Paraphilias 136
    Incest 139
    Hypersexuality 146
    References 151

9   Koro (Shook Yang): A Culture-Bound Psychogenic
    Syndrome 155
    Robert T. Rubin

    Introduction 155
    The 1967 Singapore Koro Epidemic 164
    Koro and Koro-like Cases in Westerners 167
    Psychodynamics, Diagnostics and Treatment of Koro . . 170
    References 172

La Folie à Deux

ROBERT A. FAGUET and KAY F. FAGUET

> It is certain my Conviction gains infinitely, the moment another soul will believe in it.
>
> *Novalis*

Folie à deux, a syndrome characterized by the sharing of delusional ideas and/or bizarre behavior between closely associated people, was so named over a hundred years ago by Lasègue and Falret (1877/1964).* However, according to Gralnick (1942), similar syndromes were described even earlier ("infectiousness of insanity," Ideler, 1838; "psychic infection," Hoffbauer, 1846) and later by other eponyms ("contagious insanity," Seguin; "reciprocal insanity," Parsons; "psychosis of association," Gralnick; "insanity by contagion," Carrier; "double insanity," Tuke; "collective insanity," Ireland; "conjugal insanity," Rhein; "influenced psychosis," Gordon; "mystic paranoia," Pike).

---

*Their paper is at once a fine example of traditional descriptive psychiatry and a pioneering work in modern dynamic psychiatry. In Speck's (1964) view, Lasègue and Falret's psychological sophistication is seen in their attention to intrafamilial and interpersonal problems, in their discussion of such concepts as disordered communication and symbiosis, and in their anticipation of certain contemporary ideas like that of the "schizophrenogenic mother" (Fromm-Reichmann, 1948).

Lasègue and Falret's characterization of folie à deux (literally "psychosis of two") was made on the basis of seven case observations, the first one of which is reproduced below.

Observation I. Two elderly spinsters were given sole custody by one of their sisters of a small, frail, and slow-witted 8-year-old orphan girl. Financial conditions among the three were poor. With the death of one sister and the subsequent lowered income, the economic difficulties increased. The remaining sister developed a common delusion of persecution, of a senile type. She felt the neighborhood to be leagued against her, heard

---

ROBERT A. FAGUET • Department of Psychiatry, University of California at Los Angeles, California.   KAY F. FAGUET • Department of Psychiatry, University of California at Los Angeles, California.

Sometimes a psychosis is induced in more than one person. For example, Sims *et al.* (1977) reported folie à quatre, Goduco-Agular and Wintrob (1964) described folie à sept, and Waltzer (1963) contributed a case of folie à douze.

In discussing the special conditions in which the "contagion of insanity" may take place, Lasègue and Falret (1877/1964) stated:

> In "folie à deux," one individual is the active element; being more intelligent than the other he creates the delusion and gradually imposes it upon the second or passive one; little by little the latter resists the pressure of his associate, continuously reacting to correct, modify, and coordinate the delusional material. The delusion soon becomes their common cause to be repeated to all in almost identical fashion. (p. 18)

Of course, in ordinary circumstances a healthy person does not become delusional when exposed to an insane individual. Lasègue and Falret explained:

> To allow this intellectual process to take place in two different minds, it is necessary for both individuals to have lived a very close-knit existence in

---

insulting voices and different noises which she considered to be threatening. The mental deterioration increased gradually and after four years grew to such an extent that other occupants in the house became alarmed.

The aunt constantly remained behind locked doors and allowed the child to go out only when absolutely necessary. Questioning the girl, we were told that someone had tried to poison her and her aunt. Both had experienced serious accidents; kidnappers had tried to break into the house to seize the child. To all questions the orphan replied with the poise peculiar to children raised exclusively among elderly people. These statements, reflecting the delusion of the sick aunt, when attenuated and pruned by the niece, who was not mentally ill, seemed plausible.

On many occasions we have been struck by the fact that delusional ideas when modified and expressed by a half-sane intelligence seem more reasonable than when originally conceived in the psychotic mind.The listener now more readily accepts the "stories" since the child has omitted those ideas which seem impossible and retained those with a modicum of validity. The experiment conforms to the rule previously stated: the less preposterous the insanity, the easier it becomes communicable.

The neighbors consider the welfare of the child. They call the authorities, imagining a fairy tale to be the source of the pretended persecutions. Inquiry and examination would lead anyone to conclude as much, without a doubt. The spinster was placed in a mental institution and the child in an orphanage where she is no longer troubled by the parasitic illness of her former guardian. The people of her neighborhood, however, hold on to their suspicions and still doubt the girl's sanity.

In some other cases, the environment participates more actively, welcomes as well as stimulates confidences, and passes on the story gradually polished or amplified. The child finds himself between two currents; one, that of the insane person who has provoked the conceptions; the other, that of the bystanders, who minimize the unlikely aspects and modify the acceptable sides to fit their own wishes. Misled by the one, corrected by others, the child finally believes and convinces others of his secondhand inventions.

the same environment for a long period of time, sharing the same feelings, the same interests, the same apprehensions and the same hopes, and be completely isolated from any outside influences.

. . . the delusion should be kept within the limits of the possible, based on past events, an apprehension or hope in the future. This condition of probability itself makes it communicable from one individual to another and allows the conviction of one to take root in the mind of the other. (p. 18)

Three conditions, then, are prerequisite for the diagnosis of folie à deux (Dewhurst and Todd, 1956): (1) There must be definite evidence that the partners have been intimately associated. (2) The content and motif of the delusional idea must be identical in both partners. (3) The evidence must be unequivocal that the partners accept, share, and support each other's delusions.

Similarly, folie à deux, also called a "shared paranoid disorder" in the DSM-III, is described as a paranoid delusional system that develops as a result of a close relationship with another person who already has an established paranoid psychosis, with the delusions at least partly shared.

CASE EXAMPLES

Case 1. To illustrate the sharing of a delusion, a portion of an interview of a husband–wife folie à deux is given (by permission of NPI/UCLA Media Laboratory). In this case, the husband, who appeared to be more dominant, probably originated the paranoid ideas and passed them on to his wife.

MR. A: Why, she'd shake hell out of me and I'd be groggy. I wouldn't know what was going on for a few minutes. And she'd get me outside; I've done the same with her. And I've dragged the dog outside too. I would just grab her by a leg and take her out because we knew that it could finish us if we didn't. And we'd get clear out and get some air and get clear away from the buildings or the camper or the apartment or the house.

DR.: This must have seemed very frightening.

MR. A.: Here, Doctor, is the psychological thing about it—it's a gas—it seemed to be a gas. We knew that from the beginning. It had an odor and there was a petroleum distillate mixed with it. We could detect that much in some cases, in other cases not. It appeared to be more a gas and such an insidious thing. You get so full of it, you can't smell it, and you don't know where it's at. You find stains. You don't know whether they are just ordinary dirty stains, or something else, you know? And you're just full of it. You can't smell it. Why, I try to clean these places up as much as possible on account of both of us, and I couldn't smell it because it saturated my tissues. My nasal passages were saturated with it, and I'd have to wet my finger and wipe across it and I knocked myself out sometimes.

Dr.: But you could still smell it, eh?

Mrs. A.: Yes.

Mr. A.: The dog can smell better than either one of us. She used to go around the house and smell these spots.

Mrs. A.: Well, could I say something?

Mr. A.: Yes.

Mrs. A.: That's what scared me in the beginning. It was put around where we live, down there at P.B. Why, at the home in S. he'd go around tasting stuff and he'd get sick and I got so that I'd have to watch him.

Dr.: Now, let me get this straight. He was getting sick on the food which wasn't making you sick.

Mrs. A.: No, I didn't say food.

Dr.: Oh, he was tasting . . .

Mr. A.: She was saying the stuff that was put around, that we found.

Dr.: I see.

Mr. A.: See, we found this in a number of different forms as a colorless powder. Our Sparkletts water had it. When we came back from Dr. T.'s office that night, the house was reeking. It was in the furnace. The furnace was blowing and it was reeking all through the house. She thought her water tasted funny, sorta sweet, you know, and so I got the flashlight and I looked inside. I took the bottle off and there was a clear white crystal floating on top. Now, what it was, I don't know. And so I told her she'd better use tap water, even though it is alkaline.

Dr.: You suspected it might be insecticide?

Mr. A.: Well, I don't know what it was. I was afraid it might be some toxic material. I can't say what it was, except that it was a more or less colorless crystal—flat, crystal, flakelike.

Dr.: But possibly toxic was your thought?

Mr. A.: But possibly toxic. The point is, Doctor, when you have been subject to this so much . . .

Dr.: You don't—it's better not to take any chances. And the tap water, I don't see how they could get to it. It's possible to get it into that, but I don't see how they could. Let me get back to the effects on your health. Now, we get the passing out. The other day you told me about your cough.

Mrs. A.: Yes. Like I've told you from the beginning, it has affected both of our chests. It cuts your breathing off.

Mr. A.: You feel like your muscles in your chest—I do at least—are more or less partially paralyzed. And in order to inhale, you have to put the pressure on. In asthma, you have trouble getting your air in but you can get rid of it. In bronchitis, it's the opposite. In this case, it's both ways.

Dr.: Which one of you got these chest symptoms first?
Mrs. A.: Well, I'd ... we'd ...
Mr. A.: About the same time, Doctor.
Dr.: Do you agree with that? Did it seem to you to come on about the same time?
Mrs. A.: Well, we've had the chest problems, like I told you before, but this seemed to be different. It was just—it was so strong, we really got a strong dose of it.
Mr. A.: And afterwards, for several days afterwards, during the night especially when you've been asleep and quiet, you wake up coughing.
Mrs. A.: I tell you, we was both afraid to go to sleep. We'd take turns.
Mr. A.: Yes, we've done that.

Case 2. The delusions in folie à deux, Lasègue and Falret wrote, are "moderate" and "sentimental" and in "concordance with the temperament" of the person who adapts himself to them. They stressed that the delusions are kept within the limits of possibility and are based on past events, apprehensions, or common hopes in the future. Paranoid delusions are most frequent, followed by religious, grandiose, and depressive delusions and delusions of infidelity.*

The following letter, written jointly by a senile mother (R.) and a schizophrenic daughter (M.), is a typical paranoid delusion of folie à deux. Included is a laboratory report that they claimed supported their belief. It is easy to see how such evidence (whatever it means) may fortify a delusional system.

> Dear Doctor:
> M. and I send you affectionate greetings. I wish we could give them to you in person, finding that you are well, and able to carry on your work. We hope your family are all well, too, relieving you of that worry.
> There is much to tell you about us—not too good. I am afraid our neighbor, Mr. N. who homesteaded all the canyons (where we live)—and thereby became a multimillionaire, was murdered Christmas Eve by a man who entered his home through a hole they had made in his roof, robbed him and attacked him. Now it is thought advisable for us to have an armed guard. Also, something is pumped in our living room. It collects on beams, wooded furniture, a large tray, etc. We sent a specimen to H. in C. and the report came back that our specimen consisted of *eighteen* (18) different pesticides [see Figure 1]. We are told that those with criminal intent are trying to drive us out of our house! We keep getting offers for it, but we are not ready to leave yet.

*Pearce (1972) reported an interesting case that can be seen to represent the reverse of the delusion of infidelity: folie à deux associated with de Clerambault's syndrome (psychose passionelle). In this instance, a mother and daughter shared the delusional belief that the daughter was receiving telepathic messages from a man who wished to marry her.

Sample: 1 Sample Kleenex wipe for Paraquat, Delnav, and chlorinated hydrocarbon
               pesticides

Identification: Kleenex wipe taken from tray in living room 2/2/78—area = 8″ × 19″

               Paraquat   None detected
               Delnav   None detected
               Chlorinated hydrocarbons:
                  Dieldrin   0.06 ppm
                  DDE   0.02 ppm
                  p,p-DDT   0.10 ppm

Paraquat detection limit = 0.50 ppm
Delnav detection limit = 0.50 ppm
Chlorinated hydrocarbon pesticide detection limits (ppm):

α-BHC	0.01	Heptachlor epoxide	0.01	Methoxychlor	0.20
Lindane:	0.01	DDE	0.02	Chlordane	0.10
Heptachlor	0.01	o,p-DDT	0.02	Toxaphene	0.50
Aldrin	0.01	p,p-DDD	0.02	Dieldrin	0.01
Kelthane:	0.02	Hexachlorobenzene	0.01	Thiodan	0.01
Endrin	0.02	p,p-DDT	0.02		
Mirex	0.20				

FIGURE 1. Documentation of shared paranoid delusion provided by patients R. and M. (Case 2).

I must stop now so M. can mail this. We hope to hear from you soon. (please excuse the messy letter).

M. and I send our best to you,
Ever sincerely,
R.

Dear Doctor:
     Enclosed is a copy, Xerox, of the lab report about the stuff being pumped into our living room. The stuff looks just like mildew on the ceiling beams, furniture, the tray and other things. That's what people thought it was until this report came. It's damaged our dog's pancreas (she has to have Viocase now) and sometimes we feel sick. We're awfully glad to have this evidence and not be thought paranoid any more.
     Mother and I are taking golfing lessons. Our good doctor here thought we should have more exercise. With the heat outside this was not possible. Hope all is well with you and your family.

Affectionately,
M.

EPIDEMIOLOGY

Folie à deux is usually described as a rare psychiatric phenomenon, with incidence estimated as 1.7% of all psychiatric admissions (Gralnick, 1942). It is likely, however, that many cases are unrecognized or unreported.

In a majority of cases, the presenting picture is one in which a dominant person (principle, primary agent, inductor) "transmits" the delusion to the submissive partner (associate, secondary agent, inductee). The dominant person is always psychotic (Sims *et al.*, 1977), with the usual diagnoses being schizophrenia, paraphrenia, and affective and senile psychoses (Soni and Rockley, 1974). Oatman (1942) felt that most dominant partners in folie à deux suffered primarily from a form of affective disease; the systematic and plausible delusions that they communicated were, he believed, not the bizarre, primitive beliefs of schizophrenia.

The psychiatric status of the submissive partner is more controversial. He is usually seen as highly suggestible, dependent, more passive, socially deprived, of low intelligence, or disadvantaged physically—and not as deeply affected by the delusion as the dominant person. For example, Soni and Rockley (1974), after selectively reviewing the literature, found that, among the associated partners, personality disorders (marked dependency, hysterical features, paranoid personality), schizophrenia, and paraphrenia, along with disabilities like deafness, stroke, alcohol overindulgence, mental subnormality and language barriers, were frequently noted. The associate is usually viewed as "not really insane . . . but suffering from temporary moral pressure" (Lasègue and Falret, 1877/ 1964). Others disagree. Greenberg (1956), for example, after reviewing cases of crime in folie à deux, regarded the associate as psychotic by the very fact that he not only believed in the partner's delusions but *acted* upon them. He stated, "The inadequacy of regarding the 'passive' partner in a psychotically motivated crime simply as a credulous 'malade par reflet' is obvious when behavior so aberrant as murder is involved" (p. 773). Similarly, Layman and Cohen (1957) believed that both partners were psychotic, and that the associate, rather than being "pressured," eagerly adopted the delusional system because it fulfilled his own morbid psychic structure.

Folie à deux is identical in character among males and females—children, adults, and elderly. Tuke (1888) stated that a young person was more likely to adopt the delusions of an older person than vice versa, yet exceptions are not uncommon. Solomon *et al.* (1978) reported such an instance in a case in which a 9-year-old child acted as the dominant partner in a folie à deux with his mother, transferring to her the delusion that his father was sticking needles in him. Gralnick (1942) noted that, in a great majority of cases, there was a blood relationship. Most common were sister–sister combinations, followed by mother–child pairs. In the non-blood-related groups, husband–wife combinations were most frequent. Women seemed to be more often involved in folie à deux than men, and Gralnick explained this on the basis of women's more restricted roles and narrowed opportunities resulting in their readiness to identify with and depend upon a dominant person. According to Lehmann

(1975), folie à deux usually flourishes among those living in poverty and in economic distress, but the poverty of the afflicted persons is more likely to be the result of their illness than a causative factor.

SUBTYPES OF FOLIE À DEUX

At least four subgroups of folie à deux have been proposed, according to Dewhurst and Todd (1956).

1. *Folie imposée:* Delusions of a psychotic person are transferred to a mentally sound person, and the delusions tend to disappear after separation.
2. *Folie simultanée:* A paranoid, depressive psychosis simultaneously appears in two morbidly predisposed persons.
3. *Folie communiquée:* There is a contagion of ideas after the second person has resisted them for a long time. After finally adopting the delusions, the recipient maintains them despite separation from the inducer.
4. *Folie induite:* New delusions are acquired by one psychotic patient under the influence of another.

In reviewing the subgroups, Dewhurst and Todd pointed out that they are unnecessary and confusing, and of doubtful theoretical validity and practical value. They noted that the only difference between folie imposée and folie communiquée is whether or not the delusions disappear upon separation, a factor that could be an artifact of the duration of the folie à deux (with delusions becoming more fixed with time). Also criticized is the concept of a delusion "coincidentally" appearing in two people, as in the case of folie simultanée. Dewhurst and Todd maintained that it is improbable that one person did not develop the delusions first, and inconceivable that two persons could not have influenced one another. Such a diagnosis is thus likely to occur as a result of an inadequate history.

ETIOLOGY

The high incidence of blood relations in folie à deux raises the question of constitutional predisposition, and although some authors (Kallman and Mickey, 1946) tended to stress the genetic factor in consanguinous cases of folie à deux, most modern writers (Dewhurst and Todd, 1956; Anthony, 1969; Soni and Rockley, 1974) suggested that genetic makeup, personality style, and psychosocial factors play equally important roles in the genesis of the disorder. The family tree from Sims *et al.* (1977), shown in Figure 2, is a good example of the admixture of genetic and environmental factors in the psychosis of association. The authors believed that the three siblings, Ruby, George, and John, suffered from folie simultanée. Rose, in whom we see a strong predisposition to neuropsychiatric illness, on the other hand, is seen as the recipient of folie imposée from her husband, John.

Psychodynamic hypotheses for such associated psychoses have been offered by a number of writers. Lindner (1954) described his famous temporary folie à deux with a paranoid patient as self-deception in the service of "long dormant needs and desires" (p. 201). The following passage illustrates, phenomenologically, the gradual shaping of his shared delusional system.

> At this point, I find it necessary to assure the reader that, despite the foregoing, I was not myself psychotic either during the phase I have been

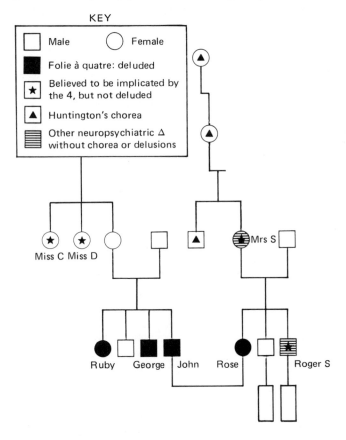

FIGURE 2. Family tree of four patients with folie à quatre (from Sims *et al.*, 1977).

describing or later when these strange manifestations increased in quantity and quality. My condition throughout was, rather, that of enchantment developing toward obsession. I never lost sight of the fact that the "trips" Kirk made into a far future to a remote, nonexistent galaxy were impossible. But, in my preoccupation with the fantasy as such, I found it convenient to overlook, so far as I was concerned, the manner in which its wonderful details were made available to me. This is to say, I omitted from my concern how Kirk collected "facts" and attended only to the "facts" themselves. That he employed the implausible vehicle of "teleportation" or some equally incredible and psychotic means to do what was required of him, I simply overlooked in my enthusiasm for the elaborate conceit.

As the days passed, however, the symptoms I have been writing about increased in number and intensity. They were all of an obsessional nature and, as such disturbances tend to do, they began to invade my thought and behavior to an ever greater degree. Whereas the fantasy and its delights had previously beckoned only when I was actually with Kirk or in spare time, it now intruded itself into moments when I was not fully engaged otherwise, and even, on occasion, when I was attending affairs far removed from Kirk and his delusion. I found myself, for example, translating certain words, terms and names into the "Olmayan" language. Phrases in this weird tongue, unannounced and unbidden, often came into my thoughts and remained there to plague consciousness annoyingly like a haunting melody until I set them down on paper and transposed them to English. At a startlingly rapid rate, it seems, larger and larger areas of my mind were being taken over by the fantasy. (pp. 200–201)

The mechanism of identification is recognized as playing a key role in the development of folie à deux (Gralnick, 1942; Pulver and Brunt, 1961; Oberndorf, 1934; Deutsch, 1938; Fliess, 1953; Bonnard, 1954; Waltzer, 1963). As Lehmann (1975) explained:

The primary focus of induced psychosis is usually a paranoid or paraphrenic schizophrenic whose special adjustment to the world is characterized not only by his persecutory and grandiose delusions but also by a deeply rooted relationship with another person, who is usually in the dependent position. The recipient or passive partner in this psychotic relationship has much in common with the dominant partner because of many shared life experiences, common needs and hopes, and most importantly, a deep emotional rapport with and concern for the partner. In order to relinquish his contact with reality to the extent of sharing the delusions of the other person, he must probably be very restricted in his ability to form relationships with other people. He is then faced with the choice of either losing the only person to whom he has been—and perhaps ever will be—very close, or joining this person in his pathological world in order to avoid the loss. Because of this strong emotional involvement, the folie à deux psychosis has been referred to as a transference phenomenon. (p. 726)

The development of folie à deux has been recognized as similar to the process of suggestion that occurs during hypnosis (Dewhurst and Todd, 1956) and psychotherapy (Orne, 1962; Victor, 1975). Waltzer (1963) found that the transfer of delusions from one person to another in folie à deux is very similar to brainwashing and suggested that each involves three phases. In the first phase, there is disorganization and regression. The breakdown of existing defenses and resistances is accomplished through relative sensory and ideational isolation. In the second phase, there is an identification with the aggressor, who is viewed as a rescuer. In the final phase, there is reindoctrination by constant monoideational stimulation. New ideas are eventually submissively incorporated and a closed community formed through isolation and denial of the healthy counterbalancing influences of the outside world.

Finally, the element of hostility in folie à deux is frequently discussed (Pulver and Brunt, 1961). It is obvious in Greenberg's (1956) discussion of crime and folie à deux, Tucker and Cornwall's (1977) report of attempted patricide by a mother–son folie à deux; and the Money and Werlwas (1976) description of folie à deux and child abuse masquerading as the shared delusion of devoted parenthood. (In the latter case, one parent initiated child abuse and the other condoned it. The children's victimization resulted in "reversible hyposomatotropinism" or "psychological dwarfism," in which removal from the pathological environment produced a catch-up in statural and mental growth, improvement in behavior, and reversal in growth hormone deficiency.)

DIFFERENTIAL DIAGNOSIS

The distinction between folie à deux, an induced psychosis, and "collective psychoses" or "psychotic epidemics" affecting larger groups of people is not always clear. The term *collective psychoses* may in fact be misleading, since these epidemics are believed to represent mass hysteria instead of true psychosis. A better name might be "collective mental disorders." As examples of such disorders, Lehmann (1975) described German dancing mania, hysterical epidemics of laughing and jumping, the Salem witch trials, and the aggressive behavior of lynchings and looting mobs. Similarly, Arieti and Meth (1959) cited various epidemics in Europe during the Middle Ages, such as those of the Flagellants, who attempted to atone for their sins by self-abuse, and the Palamites, who tried to touch the umbilicus with their heads in order to see Divine Glory. In addition, there were epidemics of St. Vitus's Dance; tarantulism (so called because those afflicted manifested generalized excitement and convulsions and were thought to have been bitten by the spider *Lycosa tarantula*); and lycanthropy, where those affected considered themselves transformed into animals, especially wolves. For contemporary examples of "collective mental disorders" we may look to the self-torturing *Los Hermanos Penitentes de Sangre de Christo* living in northern New Mexico and southern Colorado (Menninger, 1938) and, of course, the recent tragic collective suicide-murders of Jonestown, Guyana.

Arieti and Meth emphasized that these so-called collective psychoses are most likely manifestations of fanaticism and hysterical psychoneuroses induced in predisposed individuals. They stated: "The atmosphere of superstition, ignorance, and intense religiosity predispose(d) unstable individuals to this form of collective hypnosis" (p. 552). Zilboorg (1941) added that such epidemics, while definitely of a pathological order, are certainly psychosocial phenomena rather than manifestations of individual mental illness. The inaccurate terms applied to these phenomena, such as *mass hysteria* or *mass psychoses*, are merely descriptive literary phrases and not diagnostic terms, for the individuals who form a part of these mass reactions need not be and are not always mentally ill. To put it in the somewhat quaint language of an older writer, Zilboorg (1941): "There are epidemics of insanity which are met with among healthy people. The cause which produces these epidemics is moral contagion. The neuropathic, hysterical state which frequently manifests itself in such epidemics is not at all the cause of these epidemics; it is an epiphenomenon which is neither necessary nor always present. This hysterical state is the result of the influence which the mind or the emotions exercise on the nervous system" (pp. 141–142).

TREATMENT

Most modern-day treatment of folie à deux hinges on the original (1887) therapeutic recommendation of Lasègue and Falret to separate the passive partner from the sphere of influence of the dominant partner.* The dominant partner has to be treated like any other patient suffering from a functional psychosis.

Layman and Cohen (1957) cautioned that the belief that the delusional ideas are dropped by the recipient upon separation, though very widespread, does not appear to be substantiated in fact. These authors, in reviewing the literature, found only 1 case out of 140 in which separation of the two persons was followed by spontaneous recovery of the passive partner. Dewhurst and Todd (1956) believed that the stability of the psychosis in the passive partner depended on three factors: the duration of the folie à deux, the nature of the delusions (if these are of value to the weaker partner, i.e., satisfy a psychological need, he will cling

*B. B. Faguet (personal communication, 1979) pointed out an interesting medical counterpart of folie à deux and its treatment in a rare hypersensitivity disease known as sympathetic opthalmia (sympathetic uveitis). After a penetrating injury, a damaged eye (exciting eye) becomes inflamed and the fellow (sympathizing) eye follows. The cause of the "transfer" of inflammation from one eye to another is unknown, but recommended treatment is immediate enucleation of the severely injured eye to prevent blindness in the other.

tenaciously to the psychosis), and the suggestibility of the weaker partner. Soni and Rockley (1974) believed that the outcome is far less auspicious for an associate who becomes deluded against the background of his own "morbid endogenous psychosis (e.g., depression and schizophrenia)" than for the person with a less malignant condition such as low intelligence or inadequate personality. The prognosis also seems to be more favorable in the young.

Simonds and Glen (1976) suggested initial management of the passive partner in an intensive, supportive, and multidisciplinary setting with appropriate treatment of any serious preexisting illness. In this way, reality-testing and social skills are enhanced and new authority models are provided. Foster placement may be necessary in the case of young children, and, frequently, psychotropic medications are required to allay initial separation anxiety in both partners. Psychotherapy is recommended by Freedman *et al.* (1976) to work through the loss of the partner and to come to grips with a new reality. The clinician must also be aware of the dangers of treatment, as separation of a folie à deux pair may precipitate a life-threatening depression in one or both partners. Lehmann (1975) emphasized that particular attention must be paid to the existential separation trauma of an intensely symbiotic folie à deux pair. Only time, personal working through, and new, trusting relationships will help the individuals involved in a psychosis of association to overcome their separation and to achieve more open, independent, and fruitful lives.

REFERENCES

Anthony, E. J., 1969, A clinical evaluation of children with psychotic parents, *Am. J. Psychiatry* 126:177.

Arieti, S., and Meth, J., 1959, Rare, unclassifiable, collective, and exotic psychotic syndromes, *in* "American Handbook of Psychiatry"/I (S. Arieti, ed.), pp. 546–563, Basic Books, New York.

Bonnard, A., 1954, The metapsychology of the Russian trial confessions, *Int. J. Psycho-Anal.* 35:208.

Deutsch, H., 1938, Folie à deux, *Psychoanal. Q.* 7:307.

Dewhurst, K., and Todd, J., 1956, The psychosis of association—folie à deux, *J. Nerv. Ment. Dis.* 124:451.

Fliess, R., 1953, Countertransference and counteridentification, *J. Am. Psychoanal. Assoc.* 1:268.

Freedman, A. M., Kaplan, H. I., and Sadock, B. J., 1976, "Modern Synopsis of Comprehensive Textbook of Psychiatry"/II, pp. 848–849, Williams and Wilkins, Baltimore.

Fromm-Reichmann, F., 1948, Notes on the development of treatment of schizophrenics by psychoanalytic psychotherapy, *Psychiatry* 2:263.

Goduco-Agular, C., and Wintrob, R., 1964, Folie à famille in the Philippines, *Psychiatr. Q.* 38:278.

Gralnick, A., 1942, Folie à deux—The psychosis of association, *Psychiatr. Q.* 16:230.

Greenberg, H. P., 1956, Crime and folie à deux: Review and case history, *J. Ment. Sci.* 102:772.

Kallman, F. J., and Mickey, J. S., 1946, Genetic concepts of folie à deux—Reexamination of induced insanity in the family units, *J. Hered.* 37:298.

Lasègue, C., and Falret, J., 1964, La Folie à deux (ou folie communiquée), *Am. J. Psychiatry (Suppl.)* 121:1. (Originally published, 1877, *Ann. Med.-Psychol.* 18:321.)

Layman, W. A., and Cohen, L., 1957, Modern concept of folie à deux, *J. Nerv. Ment. Dis.* 125:412.

Lehmann, H., 1975, Unusual psychiatric disorders and atypical psychoses, in "Comprehensive Textbook of Psychiatry"/II (A. Freedman, H. Kaplan, and B. Sadock, eds.), pp. 1724–1736, Williams and Wilkins, Baltimore.

Lindner, R., 1954, "The Fifty-Minute Hour," Bantam Books, New York.

Menninger, K. A., 1938, "Man Against Himself," Harcourt, Brace & World, New York.

Money, J., and Werlwas, J., 1976, Folie à deux in the parents of psychosocial dwarfs: Two cases, *Bull. Am. Acad. Psychiatr. Law* 4:351.

Oatman, J. G., 1942, Folie à deux—Report of a case in identical twins, *Am. J. Psychiatry* 98:842.

Oberndorf, C. P., 1934, Folie à deux, *Int. J. Psycho-Anal.* 15:14.

Orne, M. T., 1962, Implications for psychotherapy derived from current research on the nature of hypnosis, *Am. J. Psychiatry* 118:1097.

Pearce, A., 1972, De Clerambault's syndrome associated with folie à deux (Letter), *Br. J. Psychiatry* 121:116.

Pulver, S. E., and Brunt, M. Y., 1961, Deflection of hostility in folie à deux, *Arch. Gen. Psychiatry* 5:257.

Simonds, J. F., and Glenn, T., 1976, Folie à deux in a child, *J. Autism Child. Schizophr.* 6:61.

Sims, A., Salmons, P., and Humphreys, P., 1977, Folie à quatre, *Br. J. Psychiatry* 130:134.

Solomon, J. G., Fernando, T. G., and Solomon, S. M., 1978, Mother–son folie à deux: A case report, *J. Clin. Psychiatry* 39:819.

Soni, S. D., and Rockley, G. J., 1974, Socio-clinical substrates of folie à deux, *Br. J. Psychiatry* 125:230.

Speck, R. V., 1964, Some remarks on the present day significance of Lasègue and Falret's paper, "La Folie à Deux," *Am. J. Psychiatry (Suppl.)* 121:1.

Tucker, L. S., and Cornwall, T. P., 1977, Mother–son folie à deux: A case of attempted patricide, *Am. J. Psychiatry* 134:1146.

Tuke, D., 1888, Folie à deux, *Brain* 10:408.

Victor, G., 1975, Sybil: Grande hysterie or folie à deux? (Letter), *Am. J. Psychiatry* 132:202.

Waltzer, H., 1963, A psychotic family—folie à douze, *J. Nerv. Ment. Dis.* 137:67.

Zilboorg, G., 1941, "A History of Medical Psychology," W. W. Norton, New York.

2

Munchausen Syndrome

CHARLES V. FORD

INTRODUCTION

A syndrome of malingering, pseudologia fantastica, and peregrination was first described by Asher (1951) and subsequently confirmed by case reports from all over the world (Chapman, 1957; York, 1960; Blackwell, 1965; Chugh, 1966; Ireland *et al.*, 1967). Asher dedicated the syndrome to the Baron von Münchhausen, an infamous storyteller of 18th-century Germany. Despite objections in the literature that the eponym is inappropriate and inaccurate, it has persisted, probably because of its whimsical nature. Alternative names for the syndrome such as peregrinating problem patients (Chapman, 1957), hospital hoboes (Clark and Melnick, 1958), and hospital addicts (Barker, 1962) have fallen by the wayside.

Each year the number of reported cases grows and the number of etiologic explanations for the syndrome increases. Physicians appear to respond to "Can you top this?" One particularly colorful patient, the "Indiana Cyclone," has been reported numerous times (Chapman, 1957; Cramer *et al.*, 1971), including once in verse (Bean, 1959). With the number of carefully detailed cases now available, certain patterns appear to be emerging and there is progressively greater understanding of this fascinating but perplexing behavioral syndrome.

HISTORICAL ORIGINS OF THE MUNCHAUSEN STORIES

Hieronymus Carl Friedrich von Münchhausen (1720–1797), a German cavalry officer, retired to his estate in Bodenwerder (near Hameln) following military service that included campaigns against the Turks in Russia and the Swedes. He enjoyed country life and was a well-known

CHARLES V. FORD • Department of Psychiatry, Vanderbilt University School of Medicine, Nashville, Tennessee.

raconteur whose tall tales served only to entertain his friends (Sakula, 1978).

The published Munchausen stories *The Singular Travels, Campaigns and Adventures of Baron Munchausen* (Raspe, 1948) were actually anonymously written by Rudolph Eric Raspe (1737–1794), a highly intelligent, well-educated man with questionable morals (Carswell, 1950). Born in Hanover, Raspe was frequently forced to move to keep ahead of his creditors. Although Raspe might have actually met the baron, it is certain that he at least knew of him as they were from the same area, Hanover-Cassel. Raspe eventually arrived in England, where he was able to use his skill as a geologist before falling upon hard times.

The motivation for writing the Munchausen stories is unknown. Apparently it was not for financial gain. Perhaps it was anger at a society that had rejected him. Raspe's biographer regards the stories as an exaggerated projection of himself (Carswell, 1950).

Whatever the circumstances surrounding the creation of the Munchausen stories, they proved to be enormously successful. There have been innumerable editions and translations in the nearly 200 years since the first publication in London, 1785. In fact, an early translation into German caused Baron Münchhausen considerable grief. He felt humiliated and his privacy was violated as flocks of sightseers trespassed onto his estate in an effort to catch a glimpse of him. He died a morose and embittered recluse, the innocent victim of another man's whimsy.

CASE REPORTS

The following unreported brief case reports illustrate some of the characteristics of Munchausen patients. These cases are not as dramatic as many of those previously reported, but in the respect of being more ordinary, they may also be more typical.

Case 1. A 24-year-old Caucasian man presented to the emergency room of a metropolitan teaching hospital stating that he had fallen from a porch and struck the back of his head. He had evidence of both horizontal and vertical nystagmus and was admitted to the neurology service for further studies. There he complained of memory disturbance and told his physician that he was a psychologist and the director of a mental health clinic in another county. When pressed for details, however, he became vague and complained of memory difficulties. Following an extensive neurological diagnostic evaluation, he was presented to a neurology case conference, when he was recognized by a resident visiting from another teaching hospital. It was learned that he had previously received a complete evaluation at that hospital but, following discharge, had failed to keep scheduled outpatient visits. The patient was confronted with this information and offered psychiatric help. He responded with anger and left against medical advice. The discharge diagnosis was congenital nystagmus and Munchausen syndrome.

Case 2. A 21-year-old Caucasian woman was admitted to the medical service of a metropolitan county hospital stating she had had previous hospitalizations elsewhere with a diagnosis of ulcerative colitis. She claimed approximately 20 bloody bowel movements per day and, indeed, stool samples were positive for blood. Suspicions were raised, however, when she failed to lose weight despite her continued complaints of almost hourly diarrhea. Requests for further stool samples resulted in repeated excuses that she had forgotten and "flushed" the toilet. Further studies failed to substantiate the presumptive diagnosis of ulcerative colitis, and it was assumed, but not proven, that the blood in the first samples was of factitious origin.

Seen in psychiatric consultation, she stated that she lived with her mother in an apartment and was intimate with an international news correspondent. There was no evidence of a thought disorder. She was not confronted with the staff's suspicions, but the psychiatrist did offer to see her as an outpatient as soon as she was medically discharged. She kept several appointments with him, continuing to offer the same, almost stereotyped, stories about her boyfriend. For example, she said that he routinely flew in from places like Vietnam or Paris to take her to dinner. These stories of "international sophistication" contrasted sharply with her somewhat dirty and unkempt appearance, poor grooming, and moderate obesity. She continued (despite the lack of any apparent weight loss) to complain of approximately 20 bowel movements per day. The therapist listened in a supportive, nonconfronting way. His request for permission to contact her mother, however, precipitated the patient's disappearance. All efforts to contact either the patient or her mother were unsuccessful, and there was never an answer to the telephone number that had been given to the hospital admitting clerk.

PHENOMENOLOGY OF THE SYNDROME

The original description of the Munchausen syndrome by Asher (1951) emphasized these patients' dramatic and untruthful symptoms and histories. Asher was quick to point out, however, that the stories were a "matrix of fantasy and falsehood in which fragments of complete truth are surprisingly imbedded." Similarly, he noted that not all of the patients' symptoms are entirely false and the "patients are often quite ill although their illness is shrouded by duplicity and distortion."

In the many case reports in the literature, the term *Munchausen syndrome* is used quite freely and inconsistently. While there are no "official" diagnostic criteria, those features that seem most characteristic of the syndrome are pseudologia fantastica (pathological lying), peregrination (wandering), and simulated or factitious disease. Interestingly, Munchausen patients often do have genuine organic illness or "hard" physical examination findings, which facilitate their capacity for dramatic presentations in hospital emergency rooms.

It must be recognized that the Munchausen syndrome is a spectrum of patient behavior rather than a specific disease. Therefore, both the classic cases and the variants of the syndrome (Chertok, 1972) are helpful in understanding the complex tissues of malingering and factitious illness.

Presenting Symptoms

Asher originally described three symptomatic subtypes of the syndrome: the acute abdominal type, the hemorrhagic type, and the neurologic type. Presenting symptoms from these three categories continue to be the most common, but other symptom groups have also been described, including hyperpyrexia and fevers of unknown origin (Michaels et al., 1964; Ford, 1973; Ferguson and Maki, 1978), chest pain (Bagan, 1962; Bursten, 1965; Puzzuoli, 1978; Mayer, 1978), hypoglycemia (Moore et al., 1973), tuberculosis (Griffith, 1961), and caisson disease (Kemp and Munro, 1969). More recently, there have even been patients with simulated psychiatric symptoms (Gelenberg, 1977; Cheng and Hummel, 1978; Snowdon et al., 1978). Patients with symptoms of renal colic are considered as having a variant of the acute abdominal type syndrome (Carrodus and Earlom, 1971; Atkinson and Earll, 1974; Jones et al., 1978). According to a recent report (Hollender et al., 1978), one patient got more than she bargained for: Using a mydriatic to simulate neurological disease, the patient absorbed a sufficient amount of the eye-drop preparation to develop a full-blown anticholinergic delirium!

In general, the choice of symptoms does not seem to be specific and therefore of no particular symbolic significance. Many patients use varying symptoms and simulate illnesses of different organ systems (Bagan, 1962; von Mauer et al., 1973; Yassa, 1978). One possible exception to this lack of specificity is those patients who use bleeding as the major presenting symptom. Bleeding disorders are a common choice of symptoms for Munchausen patients (Steinbeck, 1961; Hale, 1966; Chugh, 1966; Victor, 1972; Abram and Hollender, 1974; Carrodus and Earlom, 1971; Fries et al., 1977), probably because of their dramatic nature and possibly because of their symbolic significance. Most patients with factitious bleeding have been women, and Agle *et al.* (1970) report that the child-hood histories of these patients often include beatings with bruising or bleeding, a parent with a bleeding problem, and/or a remembered association of bleeding with sexual trauma.

The second major feature of the Munchausen patients is their use of pseudologia fantastica. Their capacity to tell apparently feasible but prevaricated stories is remarkable. These stories inevitably have such characteristics as to make the patient seem more important or to make the physician more interested in the patient. For example, a patient may present himself as the president of a foreign university (Jones *et al.*, 1978), a National Football League player (Ford, 1973), the fiancee of a recently deceased ambassador (Ford, 1973), or, as in the first case report above, a mental health clinic director. The stories that the patients tell have a plastic, elusive quality to them. The patients cannot fill in the specific details, claim memory problem, and often modify these stories when pressed for details.

The third major feature of the Munchausen syndrome is that of peregrination. The patients have multiple hospitalizations, often widely separated geographically. They almost invariably withhold information about the extent of prior hospital admissions, particularly the most recent, and it is therefore difficult to have an accurate picture of how much they travel. To date, the record for the largest number of hospital admissions appears to be held by the patient reported by von Mauer *et al.* (1973). This particular patient, whose *modus operandi* is to appear at hospital emergency rooms with complaints of epigastric pain and hematemesis or with seizures (he has an abnormal EEG), has been hospitalized 423 times! He has had at least 102 upper GI series!

The primary reason for the amount of traveling done by these patients may be fairly overt: One patient, previously reported by the author (Ford, 1973), when asked why he traveled so widely, simply stated, "You can only snow people for so long." Other less obvious factors related to these patients' travels may be their discomfort with intimacy or depression (Stengel, 1939).

Childhood Histories

Detailed, accurate histories are difficult to obtain from these prevaricating patients. However, frequently we learn from auxiliary sources that the Munchausen patient has had an emotionally deprived childhood. Often the patient was physically abused or otherwise mistreated (Hoyer, 1959; Barker, 1962; Cramer *et al.*, 1971; Ford, 1973; Gelenberg, 1977; Stone, 1977; Cheng and Hummel, 1978; Friedmann, 1978), one or both parents had serious illnesses or died (Hoyer, 1959; Steinbeck, 1961;

Bursten, 1965; George and Cheatham, 1965; Cramer *et al.*, 1971; Ford, 1973; Cheng and Hummel, 1978; Friedmann, 1978), institutionalization in orphanages or other settings was required (Barker, 1962; Bursten, 1965; George and Cheatham, 1965; Cramer *et al.*, 1971; Ford, 1973; Friedmann, 1978), and there was reported delinquency or bizarre behavioral patterns (Hoyer, 1959; Barker, 1962; Bursten, 1965; George and Cheatham, 1965; Ford, 1973; Stone, 1977). Not infrequently a person in the medical profession was important to the Munchausen patient during childhood (Cramer *et al.*, 1971).

Adult Adjustment

The patients, despite their self-reported exploits and grandiose self-descriptions, have, on the whole, failed to make mature adult adjustments. Work histories are poor. If the patient has worked at all, it is likely that it has been in some area of health services (Hoyer, 1959; Blackwell, 1965; Cramer *et al.*, 1971; Ford, 1973; Wise and Shuttleworth, 1978). Marriages, if there have been any, have been brief and/or turbulent (Victor, 1972; Ford, 1973; Stone, 1977). The patients frequently have run afoul of the law, particularly in the area of narcotics offenses (Steinbeck, 1961; Barker, 1962; Blackwell, 1965; Cramer *et al.*, 1971; Ananth, 1977; Cheng and Hummel, 1978; Friedmann, 1978). A history of one or more psychiatric hospitalizations is common, as well as a history of suicide attempts (Hoyer, 1959; Barker, 1962; Blackwell, 1965; Bursten, 1965; George and Cheatham, 1965; Cramer *et al.*, 1971; Ford, 1973; Stone, 1977; Cheng and Hummel, 1978). In summary, a pattern of repetitive maladjustive behavior has been the rule during adult life.

Psychiatric Diagnoses

Too often psychiatrists have had insufficient information to make well-considered psychiatric diagnoses. Among those diagnostic labels most commonly applied to patients exhibiting the Munchausen syndrome are psychopathic (sociopathic) personality disorder, schizophrenia, borderline personality, inadequate personality, and hysterical personality. It would appear that a constellation of certain psychodynamic factors in a person predisposed with major ego deficits is more important than a specific diagnostic category.

ETIOLOGIC HYPOTHESES OF THE SYNDROME

It is probable that there is no single explanation of the motivations, both conscious and unconscious, of these patients. Rather, for a particular patient, there may be a number of different motivations, which may even vary during his lifetime. The following section critically explores some of the proposed etiologies of the syndrome.

A Desire for Free Board and Lodging

This most obvious explanation may be the least probable. Although board and room may be obtained in the bargain, the price, in terms of painful procedures, seems rather high. In addition, most derelicts have little difficulty obtaining more comfortable accommodations at organizations such as the Salvation Army.

An Effort to Escape from the Police and/or Incarceration

It is more understandable that someone might subject himself to hospitalization to avoid jail, but there is little evidence that this is a common motivation. Some reports do, however, suggest that in individual cases this may be a significant etiologic factor (Vail, 1962; Bursten, 1965; Friedmann and Weinstein, 1976; Ananth, 1977).

Narcotic Addiction

Manufacturing symptoms in order to obtain access to narcotics is an apparently reasonable explanation for the syndrome. Although withdrawal symptoms have not been described in these patients, with the possible exception of the case reported by Puzzuoli (1978), Mendel (1974) has stressed that a large number of these patients are narcotic users. He believes that the Munchausen behavior should be considered a syndrome of drug abuse. The personal experience of this author, however, does not support the idea that these patients, on the whole, are addicts. Rather, their surreptitious efforts to obtain narcotics may be more important in terms of their need to deceive physicians.

A Desire to Be the Center of Attention

This explanation, described in the initial report by Asher (1951), suggested that patients may be engaged in a reversal of the "Walter Mitty" syndrome. Instead of playing the dramatic role of the surgeon, they submit to the equally dramatic role of the patient. Asher does not speculate as to whether this may be a conscious or unconscious motivation. Certainly these patients do manipulate staff in such a manner that they become either the "star" patient or the focus of anxious concern.

Psychodynamic Explanations

The masochistic nature of the Munchausen syndrome has been emphasized by Spiro (1967), who employed the concepts of masochism as described by Berliner (1947) and Menaker (1953) to understand these patients. In Spiro's formulation, the hospital serves to dual role of providing for dependency needs while also representing a place of fear and pain. This situation may be analogous to the patients' childhood circumstance, where the mother (or surrogates) mixed love with beatings. Bursten (1965), also stressing masochistic themes, sees the Munchausen patient as engaged in a kind of reversal. Aggressive impulses once directed outward are now projected into another person (the physician) only to be then redirected back toward the patient.

Cramer et al. (1971) have stressed the Munchausen patients' prior relationships to physicians. This observation has certainly been confirmed in many other case reports, both in the Munchausen patients' personal relationships and in their efforts to seek employment in areas of health service. Cramer et al. believe that physicians are selected objects toward whom love and anger are acted out.

Bursten (1965) suggests that defenses are also important components of the syndrome. He believes that the Munchausen patient seeks out that which he fears most. By "playing" the sick role, he rises above his fear of illness and death and obtains mastery of the situation. Thus, he defends against castration anxiety by seeking repeated operations (Cramer et al., 1971).

Imposture as a significant factor in the psychodynamics of these patients has been mentioned by a number of authors (Bursten, 1965; Spiro, 1967; Cramer et al., 1971; Ford, 1973). Imposture may be an attempt to reduce conflict between the impostor's exaggerated ego ideals and the devalued and guilt-laden aspect of his ego (Deutsch, 1955). Persons who have failed to establish a sense of self-identity may use imposture to "create" such an identity (Greenacre, 1958). Imposture as an attempt to master prior trauma has been suggested by Grinker (1961) and Spiro (1967), and Ford (1973) posits that imposture serves to master current feelings of helplessness in response to separation anxiety.

A Synthesis of Etiologic Hypotheses

Although the secondary gains of hospitalization (i.e., room and board, procurement of narcotics) may be contributing factors to the behavior of Munchausen patients, it appears much more probable that significant and serious psychiatric disorders underlie this syndrome. Such a disorder is best described in terms of character pathology. These patients have minimal ego strengths and are unable to deal with relatively minor stresses, and the syndrome may be regarded as a defense against overwhelming anxiety and/or psychotic decompensation. Diagnostically, they might be termed inadequate or "borderline" personalities. The choice of illness simulation as a response to stress is probably tied to prior experience in their lives with illness, physicians, and/or institutions. In the process of defending against the fear of being helpless, they become important persons commanding the attention of "physician-parents"; yet they feel superior because they have rendered the physicians impotent by virtue of having deceived them.

TREATMENT AND MANAGEMENT

Attempts to treat patients with the Munchausen syndrome, as well as factitious illness in general, have generally been unsuccessful. This is not surprising, considering the paradoxical situation in which a physician attempts to establish a therapeutic relationship with a patient whose symptoms are predicated upon deceiving the physician. Most physicians who have attempted treatment with these patients have found that although the patient may accept help temporarily, he often leaves the hospital against medical advice or simply disappears, as in case 2 above. Thus, despite the fact that these patients seek close relationships with physicians (or other members of the health professions), the intimacy they seek is obviously too frightening (Ford, 1973; Gelenberg, 1977).

Early reports of the syndrome emphasized the need to recognize these kinds of patients and prevent their abuse of hospital facilities. The patients were seen primarily as miscreants who were exploiting the medical profession for the purpose of obtaining free lodging and/or narcotics. Blacklists or circulating descriptions were among the methods suggested for coping with Munchausen patients (Birch, 1951; Williams, 1951). Published letters to the editor of various medical journals served to alert other physicians and hospitals and, more recently, "informational letters" have been used to warn of professional patients "working" in an area (Mayer, 1978).

Psychotherapeutically, what is the first step? How do we confront these patients with our knowledge that their illness is factitious? Hollender and Hersh (1970) suggest that the referring physician confront the patient, so that the psychiatrist can serve as an ally instead of an inquisitor. Wise and Shuttleworth (1978) believe that the patient should be confronted and that it be made clear that the patient's need to emphasize his distress is recognized. Direct confrontation of the patient should be approached with caution. Ford (1973) has hypothesized that the syndrome may serve as a defense against psychotic decompensation. To suddenly withdraw the defense could result in a psychotic reaction, increased factitial behavior, or the likelihood of immediate rehospitalization elsewhere.

When such help is accepted, there are occasionally good results. Jamieson *et al.* (1979) have described two-therapist treatment of a Munchausen patient. One therapist acted as a confronter while the other (seen separately) was much more supportive. Treatment appeared successful for several months until the patient became separated from her therapist. Using techniques expounded by Crabtree (1967), namely, an emphasis on the therapeutic relationship with little attention to the acquisition of insight, Fras and Coughlin (1971) reported success with seven-month follow-up of a patient with severe factitial renal disease.

On the other hand, Stone (1977) expresses the opinion that successful treatment "will only come about through timely, vigorous and repeated confrontation about the true nature of the patient's illness and about his vengeful exploitative and antisocial attitudes." However, he recognizes the risky nature of this course and feels it should be reserved for hospitalized patients who possess sufficient ego strengths. In the case reported by Stone, the patient, after vigorous confrontation, left treatment angrily but was later able to request help from him and then resumed treatment with another therapist. The follow-up period was only ten months, but at least there was some room for optimism regarding continued remission of symptoms.

In one reported instance of successful treatment of Munchausen syndrome, there were unique circumstances (Yassa, 1978). In this case, the patient was committed to a psychiatric hospital from which she would elope, only to seek admission to other hospitals with simulated physical disease. Over a 3-year period, the patient was treated with a combination of supportive psychotherapy and behavioral modification. She was rehabilitated to the extent that she was able to leave the hospital and obtain employment. Although there can be little argument with the treatment plan described, the legal environment of most localities does not permit the extended involuntary hospitalizations required to pursue such a program.

In summary, one must conclude the treatment attempts with these patients have not been encouraging. A few isolated patients have been helped transiently, but the overwhelming majority of patients have rejected therapeutic efforts. At our present level of understanding, it seems most important to quickly recognize these patients both to spare them unnecessary and dangerous diagnostic and surgical procedures and to save valuable hospital dollars (Hyatt, 1959; Mayer, 1978). Munchausen patients must be approached with a therapeutic posture that appreciates the extent of their underlying psychiatric disorder(s). Stone (1977) believes that Munchausen patients can best be helped by psychotherapy with those modifications required for treatment of the borderline personality. Psychiatric hospitalization may be required for the acute reactive situation following the patient's confrontation with the factitious nature of his disease.

CONCLUSIONS AND SUMMARY

Munchausen syndrome, a fascinating collection of symptoms involving simulation of disease, pathological lying, and wandering, has now been reported numerous times all over the world. Explanations for this perplexing behavior have varied, but it appears to be much more complex than the simple seeking of room and bed. In recent years the syndrome has been increasingly viewed as defensive in nature. Thus, these patients who use the Munchausen symptoms to defend against severe anxiety and/or psychosis are seen as having severe ego deficits. Treatment is extremely difficult because of the Munchausen patients' need to deceive and because of their discomfort with intimacy. Long-term psychiatric hospitalization combined with a modified psychotherapeutic approach is most likely the ideal treatment approach, but unfortunately it is often not a practical option.

REFERENCES

Abram, H. S., and Hollender, M. H., 1974, Factitious blood disease, *South. Med. J.* 67:691.
Agle, D. P., Ratnoff, O. D., and Spring, G. K., 1970, The anticoagulant malingerer, *Ann. Intern. Med.* 73:67.
Ananth, J., 1977, Munchausen syndrome: Problematic diagnosis, *N.Y. State J. Med.* 77:115.
Asher, R., 1951, Munchausen syndrome, *Lancet* 1:339.
Atkinson, R. L., and Earll, J. M., 1974, Munchausen syndrome with renal stones, *J. Am. Med. Assoc.* 230:89.
Bagan, M., 1962, Munchausen's syndrome: A case and review of the literature, *Boston Med. Q.* 13:113.
Barker, J. C., 1962, The syndrome of hospital addiction (Munchausen's syndrome), *J. Ment. Sci.* 108:167.
Berliner, B., 1947, On some psychodynamics of masochism, *Psychoanal. Q.* 16:459.
Bean, W. B., 1959, The Munchausen syndrome, *Perspect. Biol. Med.* 2:247.
Birch, C. A., 1951, Munchausen's syndrome, *Lancet* 1:412.
Blackwell, P., 1965, Munchausen at Guy's, *Guy's Hosp. Rep.* 114:257.
Bursten, B., 1965, On Munchausen's syndrome, *Arch. Gen. Psychiatry* 13:261.
Carrodus, A. L., and Earlom, M. S. S., 1971, Haematuria as a feature of the Munchausen syndrome: Report of a case, *Aust. N. Z. J. Surg.* 40:365.
Carswell, J., 1950, "The Romantic Rogue," Fulton, New York.
Chapman, J., 1957, Peregrinating problem patients: Munchausen's syndrome, *J. Am. Med. Assoc.* 165:927.

Cheng, L., and Hummel, L., 1978, The Munchausen syndrome as a psychiatric condition, *Br. J. Psychiatry* 133:20.
Chertok, L., 1972, Mania operativa: Surgical addiction, *Psychiatry Med.* 3:105.
Chugh, K. S., 1966, Haemorrhagica histrionica: The bleeding Munchausen syndrome, *J. Indian Med. Assoc.* 46:90.
Clark, E., and Melnick, S. C., 1958, The Munchausen syndrome or the problem of hospital hoboes, *Am. J. Med.* 25:6.
Crabtree, J. H., Jr., 1967, A psychotherapeutic encounter with a self-mutilating patient, *Psychiatry* 30:91.
Cramer, B., Gershberg, M. R., and Stein, M., 1971, Munchausen syndrome: Its relationship to malingering hysteria and the physician–patient relationship, *Arch. Gen. Psychiatry* 24:573.
Deutsch, H., 1955, The impostor: Contribution to ego psychology of a type of psychopath, *Psychoanal. Q.* 24:483.
Ferguson, E. E., and Maki, D. G., 1978, A baffling hyperpyrexia, *Hosp. Pract.* 13:111.
Ford, C. V., 1973, The Munchausen syndrome: A report of four new cases and a review of psychodynamic considerations, *Psychiatry Med.* 4:31.
Fras, I., and Coughlin, B. E., 1971, The treatment of factitious disease, *Psychosomatics* 12:117.
Friedmann, C. T. H., 1978, Munchausen's syndrome: The consultant's dilemma, in "Contemporary Models in Liaison Psychiatry" (R. A. Faguet, F. I. Fawzy, D. K. Wellisch, and R. O. Pasnau, eds.), pp. 79–86, Spectrum, New York.
Friedmann, C. T. H., and Weinstein, M. H., 1976, Munchausen's syndrome: Report of a case, *Am. Surg.* 42:611.
Fries, H., Norlen, B. J., and Danielson, B. G., 1977, Self-inflicted haematuria and the syndrome of hospital addiction, *Scand. J. Urol. Nephrol.* 11:309.
Gelenberg, A. J., 1977, Munchausen's syndrome with a psychiatric presentation, *Dis. Nerv. Syst.* 38:378.
George, M. D., and Cheatham, J. S., 1965, Munchausen's syndrome: A case report and a brief discussion, *J. Iowa Med. Soc.* 60:20.
Greenacre, P., 1958, The impostor, *Psychoanal. Q.* 27:359.
Griffith, A. H., 1961, A case of pulmonary tuberculosis with Munchausen syndrome, *Tubercle (London)* 42:512.
Grinker, R. R., Jr., 1961, Imposture as a form of mastery, *Arch. Gen. Psychiatry* 5:449.
Hale, P., 1966, The background of a "Munchausen" patient (hospital addict), *Postgrad. Med. J.* 42:791.
Hollender, M. H., and Hersh, S. P., 1970, Impossible consultation made possible, *Arch. Gen. Psychiatry* 23:343.
Hollender, M. H., Jamieson, R. C., McKee, E. A., and Roback, H. B., 1978, Anticholinergic delirium in a case of Munchausen syndrome, *Am. J. Psychiatry* 135:1407.
Hoyer, T. V., 1959, Pseudologia fantastica, *Psychiatr. Q.* 33:203.
Hyatt, I., 1959, The Munchausen syndrome, *Sinai Hosp. J.* 8:167.
Ireland, P., Sapira, J. D., and Templeton, B., 1967, Munchausen's syndrome: Review and report of an additional case, *Am. J. Med.* 43:579.
Jamieson, R., McKee, E., and Roback, H., 1979, Munchausen's syndrome: An unusual case, *Am. J. Psychother.* 33:616.
Jones, W. A., Cooper, T. P., and Kiviat, M. D., 1978, Munchausen syndrome presenting as urolithiasis, *West. J. Med.* 128:185.
Kemp, J. H., and Munro, J. G., 1969, Munchausen's syndrome simulating caisson disease, *Br. J. Ind. Med.* 26:81.
Mayer, N., 1978, The Baron revisited: A case report, *J.A.C.E.P.* 7:276.

Menaker, E., 1953, Masochism: A defense reaction of the ego, *Psychoanal. Q.* 22:205.

Mendel, J. G., 1974, Munchausen's syndrome: A syndrome of drug dependence, *Compr. Psychiatry* 15:59.

Michaels, A. D., Domino, E. G., and Moore, R. A., 1964, The case of the feverish impostor: A psychiatric and neurologic puzzle, *J. Neuropsychiatry* 5:213.

Moore, G. L., McBurney, P. L., and Service, F. S., 1973, Self-induced hypoglycemia: A review of psychiatric aspects and report of three cases, *Psychiatry Med.* 4:301.

Puzzuoli, G., 1978, Munchausen's syndrome: A case report, *W. Va. Med. J.* 74:12.

Raspe, R. E., 1948, "The Singular Travels, Campaigns and Adventures of Baron Munchausen," Cresset Press, London.

Sakula, A., 1978, Munchausen: Fact and fiction, *J. R. Coll. Physicians London* 12:286.

Snowdon, J., Solomons, R., and Deuce, H., 1978, Feigned bereavement: Twelve cases, *Br. J. Psychiatry* 133:15.

Spiro, H., 1967, Chronic factitious illness, *Arch. Gen. Psychiatry* 18:569.

Steinbeck, A. W., 1961, Haemorrhagica histrionica: The bleeding Munchausen syndrome, *Med. J. Aust.* 1:451.

Stengel, E., 1939, Studies on the psychopathology of compulsive wandering, *Br. J. Med. Psychol.* 18:250.

Stone, M. H., 1977, Factitious illness: Psychological findings and treatment recommendations, *Bull. Menninger Clin.* 41:239.

Vail, D. J., 1962, Munchausen returns, *Psychiatr. Q.* 36:317.

Victor, R. G., 1972, Self-induced phlebotomy as a cause of factitious illness, *Am. J. Psychother.* 36:425.

von Mauer, K., Wasson, K. R., Deford, J. W., and Caranasos, G. J., 1973, Munchausen's syndrome: A thirty year history of peregrination *par excellence, South. Med. J.* 66:629.

Williams, B., 1951, Munchausen's syndrome, *Lancet* 1:527.

Wise, G. R., and Shuttleworth, E. C., 1978, Munchausen's disorder: A case of a factitious neurological emergency, *J. Clin. Psychiatry* 39:353.

Yassa, R., 1978, Munchausen's syndrome: A successfully treated case, *Psychosomatics* 19:242.

York, J. R., 1960, A case of Munchausen syndrome with an unusual presenting symptom, *Med. J. Aust.* 47:538.

3

The Ganser Syndrome

DANIEL B. AUERBACH

In 1897 Dr. Sigbert J. M. Ganser delivered a lecture reporting upon "A Peculiar Hysterical State." In this lecture and its subsequent publication (Ganser, 1898/1965) he attached clinical significance to a constellation of symptoms and signs that came to bear his name. Since his report, the Ganser syndrome has become one of a group of "rare" psychiatric illnesses, and it is discussed, or referred to in passing, in most psychiatric textbooks (Sim, 1968; Curran and Partridge, 1963; Kolb, 1977; Meyer-Gross et al., 1960; Lehmann, 1975; Arieti and Bemporad, 1974).

Ganser initially reported four cases with common features that could be grouped together as a distinct entity. The major symptom was the "inability" of his patients to "answer correctly the simplest questions which were asked of them, even though by many of their answers they have grasped, in a large part, the sense of the question, and in their answers they betray at once a baffling ignorance and a surprising lack of knowledge which they most assuredly once possessed or still possess." For example, his patients were unable to count in sequence correctly but, based upon the examples given, were never far wrong. He also gave examples of incorrect, silly, and absurd answers to the simplest questions, such as: "Have you eyes? I have no eyes. How many fingers do you have? Eleven. How many legs does a horse have? Three. (Glancing at the eagle stamped upon a coin) I don't know that person; is it Kaiser Wilhelm?"

Ganser noted that "we cannot fail to recognize how in the choice of answers the patient appears to pass over deliberately the indicated correct answer and to select a false one which any child could easily recognize as such." Ganser's patients would intersperse in their responses

DANIEL B. AUERBACH • Department of Psychiatry, University of California at Los Angeles and Psychosomatic-Liaison Service, Veterans Administration Medical Center, Sepulveda, California.

correct answers to the same types of questions to which they gave incorrect and silly answers during the same interview. Further, Ganser considered it significant that in no case did his patients volunteer approximate answers, but gave them only when questioned, and appeared troubled by repeated examinations.

He was quite certain that this manner of answering questions was not "crude malingering" but rather was a genuine symptom "which frequently makes its appearance in a certain kind of illness, as a part of the total picture of the disease."

In addition, Ganser's cases had these features in common: All of his patients were prisoners. He did not state whether they were awaiting trial or already convicted. They presented with the picture of "acute hallucinatory delirium" (a term not further defined by Ganser), consisting of strong evidence of auditory and visual hallucinations. All were disoriented, with recent memory loss, and some evidenced catalepsy of a dramatic degree. Ganser felt that patients could be placed on a continuum of clouded consciousness ranging from an essentially clear sensorium to stupefaction. They "showed strongly pronounced hysterical stigmata throughout their illness," including wide areas of analgesia so complete that the deepest pinprick elicited no pain. Furthermore, and most significant to Ganser, in every case the symptoms would suddenly subside completely. The patients experienced total amnesia for the episode, were suprised at being in the hospital, and were "astonished" when their behavior was described. They then answered all questions correctly, and all hysterical disturbance disappeared. However, in most of his cases, the return to normal did not last, and the symptoms returned. In each case there was a history of trauma, which Ganser considered a "strongly operative precipitating factor." In one, severe typhus preceded the episode; in two others, head injury with loss of consciousness and shock preceded the illness. Ganser did not further specify the temporal relationship between the injury or illness and the episode.

In summary, Ganser described a number of symptoms and signs that he felt could be grouped together as a *clinical* syndrome. He ultimately reported 20 such patients (Ganser, 1898/1965, 1904). Even though all of his cases were prisoners, he in no way suggested that the clinical syndrome was specific to prisoners. The symptoms and signs included (1) a peculiar way of answering questions, never volunteered, in which the correct answer appeared to be deliberately passed by and an incorrect one given. In answer to other questions, irrelevant, silly, and absurd answers were given; (2) auditory and visual hallucinations, or behavior in response to hallucinations, called by Ganser "acute hallucinatory delirium"; (3) disorientation, memory loss, catalepsy; (4) clouding of consciousness of a varying degree from slight to profound; (5) clear-cut hysterical symptoms, such as analgesia; (6) sudden and complete clearing, with amnesia for the entire episode but with the return of normal memory for all events before the episode.

THE SYMPTOM OF APPROXIMATE ANSWERS

Even though Ganser clearly described a syndrome, it was the peculiar way of answering questions that intrigued subsequent investigators. Indeed, it is this symptom that many authors feel distinguishes Ganser's syndrome from other psychiatric disorders and that thus became for them the *sine qua non* for the diagnosis. The symptom is generally referred to by the German word *Vorbeireden*, which means "looking past the point," or "talking beside the point."

The term was defined by Moeli (1888), as "The answer is wrong, it is true, but it bears, nevertheless, some relationship to the sense of the questions and shows that the sphere of approximate concepts has been touched upon." Anderson and Mallinson (1941) said in describing it that "where the answer is wrong, it is never far wrong, and bears a definite and obvious relationship to the question, indicating that the question has been grasped. The use of the term for any random answer having little or no bearing on the question is considered incorrect."

Other authors, however, question the specificity of the symptom of approximate answers. Nissl (1902), for example, felt strongly that the symptom is identical to that seen in catatonics, and that the Ganser syndrome is schizophrenic and not hysterical.

Whitlock (1967) stressed the fact that patients described as giving approximate answers also gave a significant number of absurd answers, and that these were often the more striking responses. Thus, not all answers have an understandable relationship to the correct answer. He felt that it is difficult to distinguish the speech pattern seen in the Ganser syndrome from other derangements of speech, such as that seen in dysphasia or schizophrenia. Indeed, he considered it a diagnostic dilemma that often can be decided only by observing the course of the illness.

Arieti and Bemporad (1974) pointed out the apparent similarity between answers given in the Ganser syndrome and in schizophrenia. However, they made the point that even the most severely ill schizophrenic does not lose the capacity to perform simple tasks or make obvious identifications: "The Ganserian seems almost to make an effort to give a silly answer. A catatonic would not say that a horse has six legs."

Anderson *et al.* (1959) noted the general agreement that the symptom of approximate answers commonly occurs in the simulation of psychiatric illness. They found that many, but not all, of a group of volunteers who were asked to simulate psychiatric illness gave approximate answers, and indeed more truly approximate than patients in another group diagnosed as having dementia. In a retrospective inquiry, the subjects stated that their answers could not be too wide off the mark if the impression of obvious intent to answer incorrectly was to be avoided.

Several authors (Scott, 1965; Weiner and Braiman, 1955; Anderson *et al.*, 1959) pointed out that the symptom of approximate answers appears in a wide range of conditions, from normal persons simulating mental illness to severe psychotics. Thus, it is clear that the symptom of approximate answers, even when narrowly defined, is itself nonspecific and is found in a wide variety of conditions. It should be noted that Ganser never used the term *Vorbeireden*, and it does not really describe what he meant (Goldin and MacDonald, 1955; Scott, 1965). He did, however, use the word *Vorbeigehen* in a second paper, which translates as "to pass by" (Ganser, 1904).

WHAT IS THE TRUE SYNDROME? A REVIEW OF CASES IN THE LITERATURE

A review of the psychiatric literature indicates a variable definition of what many feel actually constitutes Ganser's syndrome—i.e., its essential symptoms, specificity, and etiology. It is interesting that such differences of opinion exist. (Ganser, as a careful appraisal of his original work shows, was quite clear in his opinion as to what constituted the syndrome.)

Most of the case reports published in English fall into three categories. The first contains 16 cases where care is taken to define the symptom of approximate answers correctly, and not to make the diagnosis of the syndrome unless a substantial number of the other symptoms are present. The second category has 13 case reports where the symptom of approximate answers is correctly defined, and either its presence alone is considered synonymous with that of the syndrome or insufficient data are given to verify the presence of other symptoms. The third category includes 47 case reports where the symptom of approximate answers is said to be present but is incorrectly or inadequately defined, and the examples given are not truly approximate. For some of the cases reported it is difficult to state with conviction whether they do or do not represent the syndrome.

Category I: Clear-Cut Cases

Anderson and Mallinson (1941) reported three cases they felt demonstrated the Ganser syndrome as a circumscribed "psychogenic episode" during the course of a major psychosis. Of these, two were diagnosed as endogenous depression and one as schizophrenia. All were said to demonstrate approximate answers, but specific examples were given in only one case. All demonstrated "hysterical episodes," characterized by histrionic outbursts, hallucinations, catatonic symptoms, echolalia, echopraxia, and loss of continence. The authors noted that depersonalization was present in all three cases, and wondered if this "remarkable disturbance of consciousness forms a suitable soil for the development of Ganser's syndrome." None of the three was charged with any crime or imprisoned, but all were in military service. In the two cases diagnosed as endogenous depression, the patients displayed an obvious wish to be out of their present assignment. In all three there was a history of a recent sexual indiscretion (at least so perceived by the patient) about which there was much self-reproach and guilt, but in none was there a history of severe illness or injury. One of the patients with endogenous depression recovered after ECT. The patient said to be "schizophrenic" recovered spontaneously. There is no mention for any of the cases whether, as part of the recovery, there was amnesia for the Ganser episode. Anderson and Mallison took care to define the symptom narrowly and their examples are correct. Based upon the data given, the diagnosis of endogenous depression is clearly valid. It is questionable, however, whether the third case represented schizophrenia.

Lieberman (1945) described a 39-year-old man with a 17-year history of alcohol abuse and repeated incarcerations for disorderly conduct. Upon examination, he was disoriented, apathetic, and indifferent to his surroundings, and he demonstrated memory loss. He gave clear-cut and typical approximate answers. He identified a matchbox placed in his hand as "dynamite" and "paper." He could not name the months in proper sequence or correctly recite the alphabet. When given simple commands, he always did the opposite. When he was given two-part commands, one response was correct, the other reversed. He identified colors incorrectly and mislabeled coins, and his calculations were truly approximate. No mention was made of hysterical symptoms or hallucinations. The question of clouding of consciousness was not specifically addressed, but the detailed description of the patient's initial presentation suggested cognitive impairment. There was no history of illness or injury prior to the episode, but his EEG was abnormal, showing a pattern similar to petit mal epilepsy. His course was progressively downhill, with no sudden recovery from the episode. Interestingly, the patient was given an amytal interview, during which he became more animated, admitted to his alcoholism, and was oriented to place, time, person, and purpose. He still gave incorrect answers to calculations but answered other questions quickly and accurately. During that interview, he described auditory hallucinations that were very real to him. After a brief period, however, all previous symptoms returned.

This case is a diagnostic dilemma, pointing to the difficulties of evaluating a group of symptoms occurring as part of a long-standing illness. It is reasonable to include this case as an example of the syndrome because the symptom of approximate answers was clearly present, in conjunction with a clouding of consciousness that was not permanent, as evidenced by the dramatic clearing during narcosynthesis.

In a later paper, Lieberman (1954), reported five additional cases. Three were described as typical of Ganser's syndrome and two as malingering. None of the five was a prisoner. In the Ganser group, the syndrome was felt to occur as an interval illness during the longer course of a primary illness. One case was diagnosed as severe depression and two as schizophrenia. The symptom of approximate answers was taken to be present, along with many of the other symptoms Ganser described. For example, patient 2 had disorientation, amnesia for events leading up to admission, anxiety, fearfulness, restlessness, bewilderment, suggestion of olfactory hallucinations, catatonic stupor, analgesia, transitory paralysis, and deafness. In this paper as well, Lieberman clearly used a narrow and specific definition of approximate answers, and many of the other necessary symptoms were described.

Weiner and Braiman (1955) reported six cases demonstrating that the syndrome occurs commonly during the course of other psychiatric disorders, and that the characteristics are unchanged from Ganser's original descriptions. They based their diagnosis upon the presence of the symptom of approximate answers and at least one other symptom described by Ganser. However, in addition to the symptom of approximate answers, they considered the symptom of amnesia with loss of personal identity as essential to the syndrome. They believed that many of the other symptoms, such as anxiety and excitement, are nonspecific.

Of the six, three cases were not described in detail because they were considered so typical of the syndrome. Of these three, one was a prisoner and two were not. All three were said to have symptoms consistent with a severe, long-standing hysterical character disorder. The two nonprisoners specifically demonstrated hysterical conversions prior to and following the episode of Ganser's syndrome. In these same two cases, there was a definite precipitating event. One patient was being pursued by her creditors, and the other was under surveillance for illegally obtaining drugs. In all three, there was an acute onset of the syndrome, and it lasted 48 hours in two and 10 days in one.

Of the three cases described in detail, none was a prisoner or charged with a crime. Case 1 was a 21-year-old man in whom the Ganser syndrome was precipitated after an episode of sexual stimulation. His answers were approximate and absurd. He showed clouding of consciousness, a fugue state, loss of sensation over one-half of his body, and auditory and visual hallucinations. When first seen, he showed amnesia with loss of personal identity. After 24 hours, all Ganser symptoms subsided completely and did not recur. He had total amnesia for all events since his admission. He was given a diagnosis of paranoid character. Cases 2 and 3, one a 30-year-old schizophrenic woman and the other a 40-year-old woman with neurosyphilis, were equally well described and clearly are examples of the syndrome.

Goldin and MacDonald (1955) reviewed both the English and the foreign-language literature and reported an additional case of the syndrome in a 62-year-old man with no previous history of physical or mental illness. The apparent precipitating stress was a requirement by a new shop steward at his place of employment that all the men pay their union dues. The patient was significantly in arrears. He developed a severe agitated depression with derealization, olfactory, visual, and auditory hallucinations, and the delusion that he was to be hanged for killing his wife. He developed a fugue state a few days prior to hospitalization. His answers were clearly approximate, but he was not disoriented and showed no significant memory loss. After three ECT treatments, he made a complete recovery. He had no recollection of the Ganser episode. This case is included as an example of the syndrome, even though a severe disturbance of consciousness was not present. On the basis of the clinical description, the patient had a mild clouding of consciousness, true approximate answers, hysterical symptoms, and recovery with amnesia for the episode.

May *et al.* (1960) reported three cases in which symptoms developed as the patients approached release from a restrictive environment. However, only case 1 fulfilled the criteria for the syndrome. This patient was a 25-year-old man who was brought to the hospital in a daze, disoriented and giving approximate answers, the day after leaving prison. For example, he could not give his age. When he was asked to add 6 and 6, his answer was 25, which was the correct response to the previous question. With patience and coaxing he could correctly answer what had been previously asked, but when he was confronted with this fact, his answers again became more irrelevant. Over a 5-day course, he also demonstrated delusions, hallucinations, hysterical convulsions, and swings in motor activity from agitation to immobility. All symptoms then subsided, and he was amnesic for an episode.

Enoch and Irving (1962) described a case that they called a Ganser syndrome "in pure form," that is, not occurring as part of another psychiatric illness. The patient was a 55-year-old railway worker who 3 years before admission had injured his back. Six months before admission, he was hospitalized for a month with a recurrence of low-back symptoms. A few days before admission, during a routine clinic visit, he was noted by the orthopedist to be mentally disturbed. Later the same day, he went out for cigarettes and did not return for 3 days. When he came back, he showed no ill effects but could not account for his time. Upon admission, he complained of back pain, was anxious and confused, and appeared mildly depressed. He was disoriented to time and place, he complained of memory loss, and his attention and capacity to concentrate were impaired. A few days after admission, while taking the WAIS, he gave typical approximate answers to simple calculations. When asked to count fingers, he always gave the answer as one more or one less than was correct. When asked how many legs a dog has, he thought about it seriously, counted slowly on his fingers, and gave the correct answer. He evidenced no surprise or resentment at being asked such simple questions. Further inquiry revealed that he was disturbed over his wife's attitude toward his illness. He had lived with this woman and her son by another man for 30 years, marrying her after the recurrence of his back symptoms 2 months before admission. He felt that his wife was unsympathetic and favored her son. After his hospitalization, she was more attentive. When retested a month after admission, he gave accurate answers, expressed surprise at being asked such simple questions, and could not believe that he had answered them incorrectly before. He was amnesic for the entire episode.

Category II: Approximate Answers Only

The second category contains 13 additional cases where the symptom of approximate answers is clearly present but where there are insufficient data to confirm the presence of the syndrome.

May *et al.* (1960) reported an additional case of a 15-year-old boy who developed symptoms while discharge plans from a juvenile treatment center were under way. The patient made it clear that he did not wish to leave. He fell to the floor, became catatoniclike, and would not move, but never lost consciousness. However, when firmly questioned, he would answer with irrelevant and incorrect answers. The next morning he stated that he did not know who he was or where he was. He disregarded or answered easy questions approximately but answered more difficult questions both accurately and extensively. In a few days his symptoms cleared, and he claimed amnesia for the episode. Some of his answers were truly approximate and silly; however, his ability to answer difficult questions correctly and extensively ruled out the presence of even mild clouding of consciousness.

Ingraham and Moriaty (1967) described a 20-year-old man with a history, since his early teens, of frequent trouble with the law. He was transferred to the hospital from prison, where he was serving a sentence for assault with a deadly weapon. On admission, he appeared perplexed and zombielike. There was no reference made to the presence or absence of hallucinations, delusions, hysterical symptoms, or amnesia. A lengthy transcript of an interview with the patient showed clear approximate answers. No data were given, however, as to whether other parts of the syndrome were present.

Tsoi (1973) reported 10 cases, but his inclusion criteria are confusing. He acknowledged that his series does not demonstrate all of the "essential clinical features of the Ganser Syndrome." He stated that the "syndrome" varies from those patients who gave an occasional approximate answer to the "full-blown picture." Tsoi did not agree that a disturbance of consciousness is a significant symptom or helpful in a differential diagnosis because he believed it to be too subjective and ill-defined. He arbitrarily excluded from his study 11 patients who presented the same clinical features as the 10 he reported, apparently because of other concurrent medical or psychiatric illness, such as severe head injury, general paresis, and schizophrenia. He stated that, on the one hand, in his 10 cases the "symptom of approximate answers made these patients stand out as a separate clinical entity." On the other hand, he stated earlier in his paper that the symptom of approximate answers is nonspecific and can occur in schizophrenia or chronic brain syndrome, the very diagnoses that he excluded from his series. This obvious contradiction relates to the author's view of the Ganser syndrome and the symptom of approximate answers. It is clear that he considered his 10 cases to be essentially malingerers. Thus, patients with other obvious diagnoses who presented with the same symptoms were excluded because the author could not justify a conclusion of malingering.

Tsoi suggested "probable motivation" for his patients: Three were to be tried for murder, two were dissatisfied with army life, two wished compensation for a head injury, two desired early retirement on medical grounds, and one wished to escape from domestic problems. He described five cases in detail, and all demonstrated the symptom of approximate answers. His summary stated that, in addition, all ten had amnesia, but this was for events prior to the described episode, not for the episode itself. Seven of the patients had fuguelike states, six had hallucinations, and one had a hysterical conversion.

Tsoi's opinion that clouding of consciousness is not a relevant symptom is at variance with Ganser's original description as well as that of most other investigators. His cases clearly demonstrated approximate answers, but not enough data were presented to confirm the presence of other symptoms.

Bustamante and Ford (1977) described a 43-year-old man brought to the hospital dazed, confused, and disoriented as to place and person. His answers were classically approximate. He stated that the color of snow was green and that 9 times 6 was 20. When an informant was found, his real name was discovered and an old hospital record located. It was determined that he was a local resident with a long history of alcohol abuse, suicide attempts, and lengthy jail time. When confronted with these facts, he became very agitated, threatened suicide, and accused the staff of treating him like a dog. The patient subsequently calmed down, continued to give approximate answers, but was more cooperative. Later, even though he professed a memory impairment, he was found to be stealing other patients' belongings and pawning them. He was discharged after refusing treatment at an alcohol rehabilitation program. A few weeks later he reappeared with the same presenting symptoms.

The authors noted that there was much disagreement about this patient's diagnosis. I do not include it in the group demonstrating the true syndrome because his reaction on being confronted with his incorrect answers was not at all consistent with Ganser's original description. In addition, the capacity to steal and pawn other patients' belongings made the presence of significant clouding of consciousness unlikely. The case is more consistent with a diagnosis of pseudodementia or simulation of mental illness by one who was in fact quite psychiatrically disturbed.

Mather et al. (1976) described a case of an 8-year-old who developed symptoms 5 days after his mother gave birth to a second child. He intermittently "fainted," but never lost consciousness. He was responsive and communicative, yet appeared disoriented. Answers to simple calculations were clearly approximate. He counted two windows in a room as four, identified a ring as a watch, and vice versa. He recovered in a week. No mention was made of the presence or absence of amnesia. This case is interesting because it is the only one in the literature of a child presenting with the symptom of approximate answers. However, not enough data were given to confirm the presence of other symptoms.

Category III: Inadequately Described Cases

The third category contains those cases where the symptom of approximate answers is said to be present, but either it clearly is not or insufficient documentation is given. There are 46 examples, the largest number among three categories.

Bender (1934) reported six cases of child murder by a parent, characterized by stupor, a catatonic reaction, or frank depression. This condition was "often initiated with a Ganser twilight state which expresses bewilderment, ideas of punishment and death, and denial of the identity of the individual and also of the deed." She further stated that the patients, who were women with a diagnosis of schizophrenia, claimed amnesia for the act. However, in no case did she give an example of the symptom of approximate answers or explicitly state that the symptom was present. Rather, she gave examples of confusion, disorientation, and probable looseness of associations.

Stern and Whiles (1941) reported three cases. They stated that approximate answers were present, but the few examples given were more consistent with random answers. In one case, they attributed the symptoms to a wish for compensation following an accident by a woman who probably had manic-depressive illness. The second case was a man awaiting trial who was said to have dementia praecox, with no data given to substantiate this diagnosis. The third case was a man who wished to be out of the military, and whose answers were clearly random and not approximate.

Tyndel (1956) noted 25 cases. All were between the ages of 50 and 54 years and were seen as part of the application procedure for pension claims pertaining to work-related psychiatric disability. All were said to heve a history of neurotic disorders, including anxiety and neurasthenia. During the initial part of the interview, the patients behaved in a very helpless manner. (They could, however, give up their helpless behavior and in some instances even stop answering approximately, especially if the overbearing relative who often accompanied them was asked to leave. *Vorbeireden* was said to be typical, but no examples were given.) Clouding of consciousness, hallucinations, and delusions were absent. The patients were oriented. The predominant symptoms were depression, anxiety, and irritability. Since no examples of approximate answers were given and no other symptoms of the syndrome were present, there is no basis for considering these cases as examples of the symptom of approximate answers, much less the Ganser syndrome.

Whitlock's (1967) discussion of the Ganser syndrome is one of the most lucid and comprehensive in the literature. He stated that the symptom of approximate answers is not sufficient to make the diagnosis; clouding of consciousness and the sudden or "brisk" termination of symptoms with amnesia for the episode are also necessary. He presented six cases, none of which, he acknowledged, meet the criteria for the Ganser syndrome. Indeed, they were presented to demonstrate that the symptom can be confused with abnormal speech, such as dysphasia following head injury or stroke.

Doongaji *et al.* (1975) described a 25-year-old man ultimately found to have a Grade IV astrocytoma in the left parietooccipital region. His spontaneous speech was normal, but he mislabeled objects, such as calling keys "tube" and a watch "pen." His calculations were narrowly wrong. There was no mention of any other symptoms.

Latcham *et al.* (1978) described a 20-year-old woman with a hysterical personality and hysterical neurosis who developed what was said to be the symptom of approximate answers following a closed head injury. The descriptions were not detailed enough, however, to distinguish between approximate answers and incorrect answers secondary to transient memory impairment and inability to concentrate.

Reiger and Billings (1978) described a 38-year-old man with sarcoidosis who was involved in three lawsuits, all of which he had brought against his employers, claiming that his illness and other injuries were work-related. Just prior to his psychiatric hospitalization, he suffered a cardiac arrest during heart catheterization. He was oriented in all spheres and denied hallucinations or delusions. He had had an apparent recent dissociative episode and intermittent somatic symptoms, such as blurred vision, dizziness, and fainting. His answers were said to be approximate, yet the main example given was one of incorrect answers to serial sevens. One example is given of a narrowly wrong answer to a calculation. He was said to give ludicrous answers, but no examples are given. The author specifically noted that clouding of consciousness, memory loss, and amnesia were absent. During an amytal interview, he acknowledged sadness, self-pity, and worry about his illness. He recovered with a marked improvement when he received retroactive compensation for his sarcoidosis.

Two brief reports, one claiming the occurrence of approximate answers following carbon monoxide poisoning (McEvoy and Campbell, 1977) and the second describing approximate answers in a 15-year-old

Hispanic girl (Nardi and DiScipio, 1977), did not present sufficient data to confirm the presence of the symptom. A third case by May *et al.* (1960) did not represent an example of true approximate answers.

COMMENT

The Ganser literature contains only 16 cases, in addition to Ganser's 20, where care was taken to give appropriate significance to symptoms other than approximate answers and which thus can be considered true examples of the Ganser syndrome. Of the 60 additional case reports, 13 demonstrate only the symptom of approximate answers, and 47 cases represent neither. Of the 16 full-fledged cases of the syndrome, only 3 were prisoners. This finding is similar to that of Goldin and MacDonald (1955), who reviewed the German literature and cited Flatau (1913), who noted that of the approximately 60 cases reported up to that time, one-third were not prisoners. Thus, the designation of the Ganser syndrome as a "prison psychosis" or as specific to prisoners (Sim, 1968; Meyer-Gross *et al.*, 1960) is obviously inaccurate. In fact, in virtually all cases reported since the early German literature, the syndrome occurred as an interval episode during the course of a major psychiatric illness. Only cases described by Goldin and MacDonald (1955), May *et al.* (1960), and Enoch and Irving (1962) appeared to be an acute illness in an individual with no previous history of psychiatric illness. This nonspecificity of the syndrome was, in fact, commented upon very soon after Ganser's original description. Henneberg (1904) stated that both the symptom of approximate answers and the syndrome appear in various disorders. In fact, virtually all cases reported since the early German literature occurred in the presence of major psychiatric illness (Goldin and MacDonald, 1955).

ETIOLOGY AND CLASSIFICATION

The controversy over etiology began soon after Ganser's publication (Anderson *et al.*, 1959) and generally focused on whether the syndrome was a hysterical illness, a psychosis, or malingering.

Hysteria

When considering the etiology of the Ganser syndrome, it is once again necessary to return to Ganser's original paper. He stated that the nature of his patients' approximate answers appeared to be a "crude malingering," but he felt that they were not deliberately trying to deceive him. He concluded that the syndrome, and specifically the symptom of approximate answers, was a true illness. He believed that his conclusion was supported by the amnesia for the episode and the sudden recovery: "The fluctuating level of consciousness with defects in memory is characteristic for acute hysterical mental illness. In my cases this accompanied the undoubtedly genuine symptoms of hysteria. This combination I consider to be extraordinarily significant and fundamental, at the same time it characterized the syndrome as an hysterical twilight state."

After remarking that hysterical disturbances had once been regarded as malingering, he stated: "So too we are to be misled by our first impression when we are confronted with the symptoms of patients which initially give the appearance of typical deception. Appearance alone in no case suffices to justify the diagnosis of malingering."

Thus, Ganser concluded that the symptom of approximate answers is genuine and part of a true illness because it occurs in the context of a clouded state of consciousness, memory defects, and sudden recovery, with amnesia for the event. He then observed that this clinical state is accompanied by hysterical symptoms. Taken as a whole, this forms the diagnosis of a hysterical twilight state. However, it is important to note that Ganser recognized that the characterization of the syndrome as having clear hysterical symptoms does not totally solve the etiological question.

Anderson and Mallinson (1941) concluded that the syndrome was a hysterical one. They based this conclusion on the presence of "ungenuineness," seen by them as a "hallmark of the hysteric," even though one of their patients was diagnosed by them as schizophrenic. They felt that the Ganser syndrome in their three cases "occurred on the basis of a hysterical disposition, perhaps activated and unmasked by the presence of another psychosis. . . ." That their patients manifested hysterical symptoms during the Ganser episode is clear, but little evidence is given of hysteria in the premorbid history.

Several other authors concurred, concluding that the syndrome is basically a hysterical one and basing this conclusion almost entirely on their assumption that, if the wish for secondary gain can be proven, that is enough to make a diagnosis of hysteria. Goldin and MacDonald (1955), Tyndel (1956), Enoch and Irving (1962), and Latcham et al. (1978) all quoted Skottowe (1964), who postulated four general features likely to be seen in hysteria: "(1) The symptoms are an imperfect representation of the condition that they resemble. (2) The symptoms correspond to the mental image that the patient might be expected to have of the illness or emotional state or the role in life which it resembled. (3) The immediate syndrome or the long-term general attitude and behavior of the patient can be seen to serve some gainful purpose for him. (4) Careful history will generally show a previous clearly hysterical attack, though not necessarily in the same form, and hysterical traits or personality." These authors then stated that the Ganser syndrome fits this definition, i.e., that the symptoms are an imperfect representation of a confusional psychosis, corresponding to the patient's notion of insanity. The purposes served are an abrogation of responsibility and a gaining of attention.

It is clear that numbers 1 through 3 of Skottowe's points refer to secondary gain. Point 4 requires a longitudinal history of hysterical traits or personality. This group of authors totally ignored this feature and focused only on those aspects that fit their notion that the presence of secondary gain is sufficient to make a diagnosis of hysteria. Indeed, among these authors, only Latcham *et al.* presented enough data to verify that their case is one of hysterical personality; however, their case, upon review, is not Ganser syndrome.

Psychosis

Weiner and Braiman (1955) proposed a different hypothesis. In their view, the Ganser syndrome is a psychotic process in reaction to overwhelming stress and helplessness. (It is interesting to note that they came to this conclusion even though three of their patients were described as having typical and long-standing hysterical personalities.)

> This sense of helplessness in some of the cases is imposed by external reality; in others it is secondary to inner impulses which are overwhelming to the individual and have resulted in behavior they cannot understand, or in psychological difficulties leading to accusation on another's part. In this setting the Ganser Syndrome develops. Many of the symptoms such as anxiety and excitement are nonspecific. The two symptoms that are uniformly present and characteristic of the Ganser Syndrome in our series are, (1) amnesia with loss of personal identity, and (2) *Vorbeireden*. It is our proposition that both of the symptoms represent unconscious desperate attempts by the individual to deceive himself and others by casting off or concealing his intellect and personal identity.

Lieberman (1945) reached similar conclusions. The syndrome is a "specific psychological modality available to the patient for use (in the psycho-physiological sense) in an attempt at homeostasis." Bustamante and Ford (1977) concluded that it is "a fairly nonspecific defensive response to threats of interpersonal integrity. They are utilized in order to achieve a sense of mastery by fooling others and simultaneously to obtain secondary gain."

It is the opinion of this author that, when case reports of the Ganser syndrome are critically reviewed with specific attention to the precipitating stress, symptoms, concurrent illness, and course, the definition of the syndrome as a psychotic episode in response to overwhelming stress is the most valid etiologic conclusion. Specifically, as Weiner and Braiman (1955) pointed out, it is a psychosis in which clouding of consciousness is an essential symptom. Indeed, this symptom is the one that distinguishes the full syndrome from the symptom of approximate answers alone.

Clouding of consciousness can be defined as a "potentially reversible global impairment of cognitive processes" (Lipowski, 1967). Even though impaired consciousness is the cardinal symptom of organic delirium, Lipowski pointed out that genuine impairment of cognitive functioning, affecting an individual's capacity to perceive, remember, and think, can occur in susceptible individuals in response to certain types of psychological stress without a specific organic illness or state influencing brain function. The secondary symptoms are strongly influenced by the patient's personality, life experiences, and environmental stimuli. In clouding of consciousness, moreover, psychological symptoms are nonspecific, so that an individual with cognitive impairment may show dysphoric affect, anxiety, or any other symptom of psychiatric illness, such as projection, paranoia, and hysterical or schizophrenic symptoms. Finally, Lipowski pointed out that certain symptoms have consistent diagnostic importance: disorientation, illusions, hallucinations, memory loss, amnesia for the episode, and attention and perceptual deficits. This definition of clouding of consciousness is quite consistent with Ganser's original description.

Malingering

Malingering as an etiologic factor is mentioned by many author's and textbooks. Malingering is itself an indication of serious psychiatric illness and the failure of more adaptive coping mechanisms in response to stress (Karpman, 1926). Braverman (1978) stated that "malingering is the struggle to perserve the self as intact in the fact of knowledge that the self has been damaged." Some consider the Ganser syndrome as an example of conscious simulation (Wertham, 1949; Szasz, 1961). However, it is generally agreed that conscious feigning of psychiatric illness is rare. It is also extremely difficult to convincingly sustain before it becomes obvious to an alert examiner (Anderson et al., 1959; Braverman, 1978).

Organic Brain Syndrome

In terms of clinical relevance and patient care, Ganser syndrome must be distinguished from delirium and dementia. The presence of what was believed to be the Ganser syndrome was reported in patients with brain tumors, strokes, head injury, and carbon monoxide poisoning, as well as various dementias. Thus, there is danger that a diagnosis of

Ganser syndrome may delay a necessary medical evaluation in a patient presenting with approximate answers.

CONCLUSION

A review of the literature confirms that the constellation of symptoms that Ganser believed represented a true illness does occur. It is an extremely rare syndrome, which is itself nonspecific and usually occurs as an interval episode in the course of another major psychiatric illness. Less often, it occurs as an acute or presenting episode in susceptible individuals in response to overwhelming stress.

The *sine qua non* of the syndrome is the symptom of approximate answers occurring in the context of true clouding of consciousness. The presence of hysterical symptoms, hallucinations, delusions, and other psychiatric symptoms, such as catalepsy, are variable. The clinical course is also variable, on a continuum from complete resolution to further psychological deterioration.

The symptom of approximate answers is itself uncommon. Nonetheless, it is nonspecific and occurs in a wide variety of conditions, from conscious simulation to severe psychosis.

The etiology of the Ganser syndrome is, most likely, a psychosis in response to overwhelming stress.

REFERENCES

Anderson, E. W., and Mallinson, W. P., 1941, Psychogenic episodes in the course of major psychosis, *J. Ment. Sci.* 87:383.

Anderson, E. W., Trethowan, W. H., and Kenna, J. C., 1959, An experimental investigation of simulation and pseudo-dementia, *Acta Psychiatr. Neurol. Scand. Suppl.* 132:5.

Arieti, S., and Bemporad, J. R., 1974, Rare unclassifiable and collective psychiatric syndromes, *in* "American Handbook of Psychiatry" (S. Arieti and E. B. Brody, eds.), pp. 710–722, Basic Books, New York.

Bender, L., 1934, Psychiatric mechanisms in child murderers, *J. Nerv. Ment. Dis.* 80:32.

Braverman, M., 1978, Post-injury malingering is seldom a calculated ploy, *Occup. Health Safety* 47:36.

Bustamante, M. D., and Ford, C. U., 1977, Ganser's syndrome, *Psychiatr. Opinion* 14:39.

Curran, D., and Partridge, M., 1963, "Psychological Medicine an Introduction to Psychiatry," E. Livingston, Edinburgh and London.

Doongaji, D. R., Apte, V. S., and Bhat, R., 1975, Ganser state (syndrome) an unusual presentation of a space occupying lesion of the dominant hemisphere, *Neurol. India* 23:143.

Enoch, M. D., and Irving, G., 1962, The Ganser syndrome, *Acta Psychiatr. Scand.* 48:213.

Flatau, G., 1913, Ueber den Ganserschen Symptom Complex, *Z. Gesamte Neurol. Psychiatr.* 15:122. (Cited in H. Weiner and A. Braiman, 1955.)

Ganser, S.J., 1898, Ueber einen eigenartigen hysterischen daemmerzustand, *Arch. Psychiatr. Nervenkr.* 30:633. (Translated by C. E. Shorer, 1965, *Br. J. Criminol.* 5:120.)

Ganser, S. J., 1904, *Arch. Psychiatr. Nervenk.* 38:34 (Cited in S. Goldin and J. E. MacDonald, 1955.)

Goldin, S., and MacDonald, J. E., 1955, The Ganser state, *J. Ment. Sci.* 101:267.

Henneberg, R., 1904, *Charate Ann.* 28:593. (Cited in E. W. Anderson, W. H. Trethowan, and J. C. Kenna, 1959.)

Ingraham, M. R., and Moriaty, D. M., 1967, A contribution for the understanding of the Ganser syndrome, *Compr. Psychiatry* 8:35.

Karpman, B., 1926, Psychosis in criminals: Clinical studies in the psychopathology of crime, *J. Nerv. Ment. Dis.* 64:331, 482.

Kolb, L. C., 1977, "Modern Clinical Psychiatry," W. B. Saunders, Philadelphia.

Latcham, R., White, A., and Sims, A., 1978, Ganser syndrome: The aetiological argument, *J. Neurol. Neurosurg. Psychiatry* 44:851.

Lehmann, H. E., 1975, Unusual psychiatric disorders and atypical psychoses, *in* "Comprehensive Textbook of Psychiatry" II (A. M. Freedman, H. I. Kaplan, and B. J. Sadock, eds.), Williams and Wilkins, Baltimore.

Lieberman, A. A., 1945, The Ganser syndrome, *Ill. Med. J.* 88:302.

Lieberman, A. A., 1954, The Ganser syndrome in psychosis, *J. Nerv. Ment. Dis.* 120:10.

Lipowski, Z. J., 1967, Delirium clouding of consciousness and confusion, *J. Nerv. Ment. Dis.* 145:227.

Mathur, S., Rostogi, C. K., Singh, Y. D., Singh, R. N., and Mathur, G. P., 1976, Ganser's syndrome: A rare psychiatric disorder, *Indian Pediatr.* 13:947.

May, R. H., Volgele, G. E., and Paolmo, A. F., 1960, The Ganser syndrome: A report of three cases, *J. Nerv. Ment. Dis.* 130:331.

McEvoy, J., and Campbell, T., 1977, Ganser-like signs in carbon monoxide encephalopathy (Letter), *Am. J. Psychiatry* 134:1448.

Meyer-Gross, W., Slater, E., and Roth, M., 1960, "Clinical Psychiatry," Williams and Wilkins, Baltimore.

Moeli, C., 1888, "Ueber Ire Verbrecher," Fischer, Berlin. (Cited in H. Weiner and A. Braiman, 1955.)

Nardi, T. J., and DiScipio, W. J., 1977, The Ganser syndrome in an adolescent Hispanic-black female, *Am. J. Psychiatry* 134:453.

Nissl, F., 1902, Hysterische Symptome bei einfachen Seelenstoerimgen, *Zentralbl. Nervenbeilkr. Psychiatr.* 25:2. (Cited in H. Weiner and A. Braiman, 1955.)

Reiger, W., and Billings, C. K., 1978, Ganser's syndrome associated with litigation, *Compr. Psychiatry* 19:371.

Scott, P. D., 1965, The Ganser syndrome, *Br. J. Criminol.* 5:127.

Sim, M., 1968, "Guide to Psychiatry," E. and S. Livingstone, Edinburgh and London.

Skottowe, I., 1964, "Clinical Psychiatry," Eyre and Spotteswoode, London.

Stern, E. E., and Whiles, W. H., 1941, Three Ganser states and Hamlet, *J. Ment. Sci.* 88:134.

Szasz, T. S., 1961, "The Myth of Mental Illness," Hoeber-Harper, New York.

Tsoi, W. F., 1973, The Ganser Syndrome in Singapore: a report of ten cases, *Br. J. Psychiatry* 123:507.

Tyndel, M., 1956, Some aspects of the Ganser state, *J. Ment. Sci.* 102:324.

Weiner, H., and Braiman, A., 1955, The Ganser syndrome, *Am. J. Psychiatry* 111:767.

Wertham, F., 1949, "The Show of Violence," Doubleday, Garden City, New York.

Whitlock, F. A., 1967, The Ganser syndrome, *Br. J. Psychiatry* 113:19.

4

Psychiatric Syndromes in Prisoner of War and Concentration Camp Survivors

RANSOM J. ARTHUR

One of the most tragic of the extraordinary syndromes of psychiatry is one brought about by prolonged exposure to extreme stress in captivity. The extraordinary feature of the syndrome lies in the horrifying levels of stress that produce it rather than its rarity. In fact, millions of humans in our century exhibit features characteristic of this entity. The syndrome has various names: concentration camp syndrome, repatriation neurosis, concentration camp survivor syndrome, or KZ syndrome, whcih is abbreviated from the German word *Konzentrationslager* (Arthur, 1974; Bloch, 1946–47; Chodoff, 1959, 1963; Dor-Shav, 1978; Eitinger, 1964, 1975; Hoppe, 1971b; Krystal, 1968; Strom, 1968). The existence of this sickness stands as evidence of massive brutality on an unprecedented scale. That there are lasting effects of such cruelty upon virtually all who were incarcerated in concentration camps or certain prisoner-of-war camps for a period longer than a few weeks is now incontrovertible. In past centuries, humans who suffered as prisoners of the Inquisition or as galley slaves in situations with a high incidence of torture and death doubtlessly had adverse somatic and psychological consequences, but their later suffering was not recorded. However, in the 20th century there have been captivity experiences on a scale without precedent, as well as systematic refinements of cruelty. The permanent injury suffered by the

RANSOM J. ARTHUR • The Oregon Health Sciences University, Portland, Oregon.

survivors of our time have been amply recorded and documented (Eitinger, 1964, 1975; Mattussek et al., 1975).

After the initial euphoria incident to the ending of World War II had
dissipated, it became clear that individuals who had survived the concentration camps of Nazi Germany or the prisoner of war camps of the
Japanese were continuing to suffer from many residual pathological
manifestations (Anderson et al., 1954; Arntzen, 1948; Brill, 1946; Segal et
al., 1976; Wolf and Ripley, 1947).

At the time of release from imprisonment and for a number of years
thereafter, the former prisoners exhibited a plethora of overt signs of
physical disease. This was to be expected in view of the physical hardships, such as starvation, beatings, excessive work, and exposure to the
elements, that were a part of the concentration camp and certain prisoner
of war camp environments. Medical problems included premature aging,
visual difficulties, extreme loss of weight, wasting, abnormal liver function, peripheral neuritis, bronchitis, emphysema, and tuberculosis, as
well as evidence of traumata such as fractures, hemorrhages, and contu-
sions. Suppression of normal menstrual function in many of the females
was seen.

In addition to physical sequelae, the former inmates manifested psychopathological features resulting from the experiences of captivity. All
authorities who have studied the concentration camp survivors report a
very high prevalence of chronic depression among them. Anxiety, sleep
disturbances, easy fatigability, recurring nightmares, anhedonia, isolation, restlessness, rumination, preoccupation, irritability, and startle reactions are almost universal. In addition, brain functioning seems
impaired. The released inmates displayed difficulties in concentration,
memory, and calculation. Additionally, there are psychosomatic manifestations such as anorexia, digestive problems, hypochondriacal preoccupation, vague pains in various parts of the body, difficulties in breathing, and cardiovascular manifestations of anxiety such as dyspnoea,
tachycardia, and palpitations.

Many former prisoners of war who were imprisoned by the Japanese
or by the Koreans developed a similar set of symptoms to those of the
concentration camp survivors. However, there is one psychological phenomenon, survivor's guilt, which is most marked in the concentration
camp survivors as compared to former prisoners of war (Carmelly, 1975;
Hoppe, 1966). Because so many former inmates suffered the loss of family
and friends, some of whom may also have been imprisoned under similar circumstances, it is entirely understandable that an individual might
feel that he or she was wrongfully spared while better people died. Survivors may believe that some act committed in camp had been wrong,
even though it might have ensured the individual's survival. Whatever

the reasons, guilt is a manifestation commonly seen in survivors of concentration camps and one that persists decades after their release. In addition to the necessity of understanding survivor guilt, Hoppe has stressed the importance of understanding the underlying and often hidden aggressive feelings of the survivors. The examiners in the early follow-up studies saw the survivors as individuals with little aggression; that observation, however, was not accurate. More careful examination naturally showed that there were many survivors with large amounts of unexamined rage.

Studies of mortality have shown that prisoners of war who were interned by the Japanese in the Second World War experienced a much higher mortality rate than other veterans of comparable age and service who were not prisoners (Beebe, 1975; Nefzger, 1970). The principal causes of death among the returned prisoners of war were tuberculosis and accidents. Former prisoners of war from the Pacific died of cardiovascular disease, cancer, and suicide at a higher rate than did the comparison subjects. Interestingly enough, American prisoners of the Germans suffered no increased mortality after their release from captivity as compared to controls. This is because the Germans, however vile they were in their treatment of Russian and Polish prisoners of war, as well as in their treatment of Gypsies, Jews, and other minority groups, attempted, by and large, to adhere to the Geneva Convention in their treatment of American and English prisoners of war. Conditions in those particular POW camps were not as appalling as those in the concentration camps or the POW stockades run by the Japanese or the Koreans. The American prisoners of the Koreans also showed a strikingly increased death rate compared to controls. Accidents, tuberculosis, trauma, suicide, and cirrhosis of the liver were the principal causes of death. Violent accidents, suicide, and murder accounted for more than 50% of the total mortality.

The high incidence of psychiatric disorders among concentration camp and prisoner-of-war survivors was soon noted. For example, by 1960 Bensheim reported that over half of the patients in his clinic in Israel were under treatment for psychiatric problems resulting from their persecution (Bensheim, 1960). It was already apparent that a characteristic syndrome resulting from the concentration camp experience existed. Hocking (1970) indicated that the appearance of the ex-concentration camp inmates was sufficiently obvious that they could be identified while sitting in the waiting room prior to the examination.

It was not only the concentration camp survivors from Europe and American prisoners of war of the Japanese and Koreans who had a strikingly high incidence of psychiatric hospital admissions and psychological impairment after World War II and the Korean War. Indeed, the Navy

crew of the U.S.S. *Pueblo* showed many untoward physical and psychological aftereffects from their brutal captivity experience in North Korea
(Spaulding, 1977). The same problem was noted in a 20-year follow-up
study (Kral *et al.*, 1967) of a group of Canadian former prisoners of war.
They, too, showed the same manifestations of irritability, poor memory,
slow thinking, depression, social isolation, and anxiety that is so well
documented in the other groups. Former prisoners of war from New Zealand (Mason, 1954) had similar residual manifestations.

It is apparent that evidence from over the globe documents the existence of a clear-cut syndrome that follows a certain kind of experience
in a very large number of individuals who have undergone brutal captivity. The syndrome consists of psychological manifestations such as
problems in mentation, memory, and concentration, as well as anxiety,
depression, guilt, startle reactions, insomnia, anhedonia, recurrent nightmares, social isolation, and psychosomatic manifestations such as pain,
exhaustion, and digestive difficulties. The psychiatric problems may be
accompanied by evidence of residual physical defects, such as decreased
vision or hearing, premature aging, liver damage, poorly healed fractures, joint problems, and pulmonary diseases. If KZ syndrome occurs in
the vast majority of individuals who underwent the concentration camp
and similar experiences, then, if one wishes to understand its genesis,
one must necessarily concentrate first on the nature of the stressors.

EXAMINATION OF STRESSORS

Let us now turn to an examination of the stressors that appear to
produce this tragic, monotonic, and chronic syndrome. We will first
describe the stresses associated with the concentration camp experience
(Adler, 1958; Foreman, 1959; Matussek *et al.*, 1975). The three major stressors mentioned by the inmates were a constant and pervasive fear for
one's life; physical depletion brought on by hunger, work, and frequent
beatings; and a poisoning of interpersonal contacts and relations.

The camps themselves were not uniform in their policies and procedures. Some were used almost exclusively as venues for the mass extermination of inmates. Very few individuals indeed survived. There were
other camps where more than half of the inmates were murdered and
yet others in which 30 to 50% were killed and at least one other where
the death rate was about 20%. In any case, death was ubiquitous. Work
was in many ways a fundamentally purposeless activity used by the
authorities to further harass and degrade the prisoners as part of the general persecution. Hunger and starvation were routine, and very severe
beatings were given at the whim of the guards or of prisoners who acted
as assistant guards. Infectious diseases were common, and climatic inju-

ries such as frostbite occurred. Menstrual function ceased in virtually all female inmates. Certain authors who were themselves prisoners report that sexual thoughts and activity were largely suppressed by cold, hunger, exhaustion, fear, and lacerating work. The atmosphere of the camp was such that the prisoners were constantly indoctrinated with the idea that they were inferior beings and deserved to suffer and even die. Selection for death was often carried out in an enigmatic way that increased the sense of nightmare, uncertainty, and doom.

Prisoner of war camps run by the Japanese and by the North Koreans had many similar stressors to those found in the Nazi camps (Beebe, 1975; Nardini, 1952). Death rates were very high, up to 50% in some compounds in Southeast Asia. Beatings were common, humiliation of prisoners was routine, hard work was often required, as, for example, on the railroad line that the Japanese built in Siam. Starvation was also routine. The prisoners were spared the concentration camp victims' agony of seeing their relatives and family friends murdered and their very dwellings destroyed. However, the POWs did witness the deaths of their military comrades. The Japanese made no attempt to indoctrinate the American, English, and Caucasian British Empire prisoners, but they did convey to them their contempt for anyone taken prisoner. The Japanese military code at that time required that a soldier die in action and never be captured under any circumstances. If he were captured, he was to be considered dead and as having dishonored his oath to the emperor. The arrogant and contemptuous treatment of the prisoners by the Japanese sprang, at least in part, from that particular code of beliefs.

During the Korean War, those imprisoned by the North Koreans experienced the hardships mentioned above, plus the intense cold of the Korean winter. Along with their Chinese allies, the Koreans attempted a systematic indoctrination of the prisoners (Chodoff, 1959). Popularly called "brainwashing," it was in fact simply a method of forceful persuasion using coercion, sleep deprivation, torture, starvation, and repetitive propaganda. The Chinese and Koreans attempted to convince American and British prisoners that they should become Communist sympathizers and help to bring about an end to the war. This indoctrination attempt was a lamentable failure in the permanent sense because only a handful of men remained behind at the time of repatriation and, of the 21 who stayed, only 1 did so for years.

The descriptions we have of the camps of the Gulag Archipelago in the Soviet Union, the reeducation camps of China and Vietnam, not to mention similar institutions elsewhere in the world, confirm that the same set of stressors are present in many other nations, but there is no medical and psychiatric follow-up of former inmates of those camps. The horrendous conditions of camp life provide implacable stress for all the inmates. However, the question arises as to whether there are individual factors that predisposed certain individuals to the development of the KZ syndrome. The issue of predisposition and premorbid emotional liabilities arose particularly in connection with reparations for the victims. Compensation was initially refused to some individuals because of alleged preexisting psychiatric disorder. However, the similarity and chronicity of manifestations in the victims gradually convinced most authorities that the intensity of the victim's camp experience was the primary factor in the genesis of the disorder, rather than preexisting individual problems. No one doubts that there are indeed individual differences in susceptibility. However, these seem to pale in comparison to the duration and magnitude of the stressors. Almost everyone who spent a year or more in a concentration camp or several years as a prisoner of the Japanese or North Koreans had residual and chronic symptoms following release. Even so, one can find exceptional individuals who appear to have survived such experiences without much in the way of sequelae. The author knows of one such individual but such humans are indeed the exception. The universality of the syndrome, its relatively stereotypic character, the fact that its variants occur in many different populations—Norwegians, Jews from Eastern Europe, Black and white Americans, Canadians—all argue strongly that the bulk of the variance must be accounted for by the magnitude and duration of the stress situation rather than by underlying neurotic susceptibility, which undoubtedly existed in some prisoners, but certainly not in all.

Among all the stressors, the pervasive, constant, unyielding terror posed by the ubiquity of death in the camps seems to be the most potent. The imminent and constant threat of death is a stressor that the combat fatigue syndrome and the KZ syndrome have in common. Soldiers with combat fatigue have insomnia, startle reactions, overwhelming anxiety, shaking, dissociative phenomena, exhaustion, guilt, and depression. This kind of behavior is regularly seen in infantry soldiers who spend months in constant battle (Southard, 1919/1973). The ability to tolerate active service on the front line varied greatly among individuals, but the experience of both world wars confirmed that even the most stable and hardened of men began developing adverse psychological and psychophysiological manifestations after several months of constant combat. A detailed discussion of persistent symptoms in individuals who developed traumatic neuroses of combat is beyond the scope of this chapter. However, many military men who had extensive combat experience, particularly those who finally broke down under the weight of repetitive stress, have often manifested chronicity of symptoms (Bourne, 1969, 1970; Van Putten, 1973). They may continue for years to show some of the features of the concentration camp syndrome: nightmares, startle reactions, irritability, and psychophysiological problems. Such individuals may have an increased incidence of alcoholism and of psychoticlike attacks with flashbacks, paranoid manifestations, and persecutory hallucinations. However, the pure combat-produced neurosis syndrome, in its later stages, generally does not have the pervasive depression and sense of guilt that characterizes the KZ syndrome patients. Of course, there are times when the combat fatigue patient relives his combat experiences just as the KZ patients relive their camp experiences. The combat neurosis patient also may have deep anger toward authority figures. But if one interviews a half dozen concentration camp survivors and then a half dozen veterans with combat-related neuroses who were not prisoners of war, one will note profound differences of life approach and configuration of symptoms between the two groups. In both the front line trench and the concentration camp, death was a constant neighbor, and a direct threat to one's very being was inescapable. Although denial was a common defense, it is hard to sustain against this kind of overwhelming reality. The other stressors such as sleep deprivation, cold, infectious disease, beatings, and starvation are corrosive in themselves. However, these hardships primarily enhance the traumatic nature of the threat to survival by weakening the individual. These other stresses made him even more conscious of his vulnerability and of the thin thread on which his life hung.

METHODS OF COPING

During their time in the camps, the inmates used various defensive maneuvers as a means of coping with intolerable situations (Dimsdale, 1974; Chodoff, 1959). The initial stage was one of shock, terror, stupor, and depersonalization. This initial period of turmoil and fear might be followed by a time of apathy, depression, guilt, and mourning. Some inmates became so apathetic that they seemed to give up the struggle to live, and quickly died. This was true of both concentration camp inmates and prisoners of war. This "giving up" syndrome seems to occur regularly in situations like concentration camps or the Bataan "Death March." Among those who did not initially die, behavior often became selfish and regressive, marked by envy, concentration on food, lack of compassion, and seeking of preferential treatment. Chodoff indicates that this regression might be adaptive. The prisoner immersed in fantasies was likely to behave with appropriate deference and submission toward the SS. In fact, many prisoners not only did not manifest overt anger toward the SS, but some actually identified with the aggressor and aped the attitudes and behavior of their captors. Other defenses used for survival included denial, reduction of emotionality, and, in some incidences, sublimation. New psychiatric disorders were not seen and psychosomatic or psychoneurotic problems already existing were ameliorated to some degree. It would not, of course, have been possible to survive with a mental illness because the Nazis immediately exterminated anyone with such a condition.

SUBSEQUENT COURSE OF ILLNESS

The clinical course of individuals released from different prisoner-of-war camps or concentration camps naturally shows some variability. It is not possible to clearly delineate when the symptoms characteristic of the KZ syndrome began, although, certainly, anxiety, restlessness, apprehension, and irritability were all present during the camp experience. Similarly, the fatalism, helplessness, apathy, suspicion, hostility, bitterness, and distrust originated during the time of the experience. Other features, such as psychosomatic problems or the obsessive ruminative state with preoccupation about the camp experience, doubtless appeared later. In any case, even by a year or two after the end of the war, many of the symptoms were already in place. While prisoners of war were generally youthful males, there were some female nurses among them, and some older noncommissioned and commissioned officers in their 40s. On the other hand, the concentration camps imprisoned individuals of all ages, including young children. Those who were children during the time of incarceration often developed later character difficulties and a sense of bitterness and pervasive dissatisfaction in addition to the usual anxiety and depressive features of the KZ syndrome. Those who were young adults during the war have developed the full-blown syndrome, with anxiety as the predominant manifestation. In those who were imprisoned at an older age, depression seemed to be the chief impairment. For some individuals there was a latent period after the war before major symptoms appeared.

The war's end did not bring to a close the stress on the former inmates (Zwingmann and Pfister-Ammende, 1973). The concentration camp victims reentered the world only to find, in many instances, that their previous dwellings had been destroyed and their communities liquidated, and that their families were dead. Many had to enter displaced-persons camps, which did not have the survival stress of the concentration camps but did pose another set of problems for the released prisoners. The displaced-persons camps were not really supportive at a time when the emotional needs of the victims were immense. Many of the former prisoners saw that they had suffered a loss of status. Many were without money or other material possessions. Large numbers of individuals subsequently emigrated, particularly to Israel and to the United States. This meant, in many instances, moving to a wholly different environment with strange languages, customs, and ways of doing business. It was also soon apparent that the vision of a perfect world, which had helped sustain many of the individuals during their camp experience, had been an illusion, and that the postwar world would be, in its own way, grim. Inmates were moving out into a world that could never completely understand all they had undergone and in which they would necessarily be alien. Above all, the extent and nature of their suffering could not be totally comprehended by others, and the response of the outside world was seen as inadequate in the face of the magnitude of the crimes against them.

Similarly, reentry into society was difficult for returning prisoners of war. The released prisoners of the Japanese were initially described as showing the same features of apathy, remoteness, and detachment that were seen in the concentration camp survivors. In addition to the increased mortality and morbidity described earlier, released prisoners of war had an unfavorable occupational experience. Canadian POWs and American POWs from World War II and Korea had high rates of unemployment and inability to adapt to a work environment. Concentration camp survivors in the United States also have had difficulties in vocational and social adjustment. Released prisoners from both types of camps felt a profound difference between themselves and those who had not undergone similar experiences. For example, New Zealand prisoners of war saw civilians as self-centered and society as unduly materialistic. In all instances, the former prisoners felt as if they had been left behind by profound societal changes that occurred during their absence. Naturally, some prisoners made apparently good adjustments to the postwar world and have done well. Others have only apparently done well. For instance, a group of former concentration camp survivors have been described as suffering from a "synecdoche of success" (Ostwald and Bittner, 1969). These are individuals who have done extremely well economically but who carry a heavy burden of symptoms, poor interpersonal relationships, and a feeling of emptiness and futility.

It is understandable that the children of former inmates might be expected to have an increased incidence of emotional trouble (Barocas, 1975; Hendrix, 1978a, 1978b; Hochman, 1978; Sigal and Rakoff, 1971; Sigal et al., 1973). Either one or both parents may suffer the KZ syndrome, with excessive rumination about the past, depression, fatigue, and anxiety. Such parents may find the demands of children in the areas of nurturance and aggressive independence unduly burdensome. Sigal et al. have stated that children of parents who are survivors of Nazi persecution appear in child psychiatric clinics at a greater rate than does the general population, with symptoms of depression, inability to handle aggression, and impairment in coping ability. Similarly, studies of American POW families from World War II and Korea have shown that the father traditionally had difficulty disciplining the child. The irritability, fatigue, and emotional instability of the father were reflected in adverse consequences in the children. The intense preoccupation with past experiences on the part of so many ex-prisoners provided a very considerable barrier to full intimacy in the parent–child relationship. The parents might be physically present but emotionally absent because of constant rumination. Thus, psychiatric troubles seem to extend into the next generation even while the syndrome persists in the aging survivors.

THE VIETNAM WAR

During the course of the Vietnam War, many hundreds of American military men were captured by the Communist forces (Anderson, 1975; Berg and Richlin, 1977a, 1977b, 1977c, 1977d). A small number (77) of youthful Army men (28 officers and 49 enlisted men) survived capture by the Vietcong. However, the majority of the American prisoners were air crews. These were commissioned officers of the Navy and Air Force who were shot down over the North. Some of these men were in captivity for 7 to 9 years.

The morbidity rate among those captured in the south was quite high. The Vietcong were in constant motion and living in the midst of guerilla warfare. Disease and hardship were common to both captor and captive, and the situation was highly lethal.

In the North, the prisoners were concentrated in a few stockades. They were eventually seen by their captors as being highly valuable for propaganda and bargaining purposes. Nevertheless, during the era between 1964 and 1973, treatment of the prisoners was harsh, particularly in regard to restricted diet, physical abuse, lack of medical care, and extensive use of solitary confinement. Some of the captives withstood 4 years of solitary confinement. However, death rates were not high by the standards of concentration camps and Japanese or Korean prison camps. In fact, they were less than 5%.

In the planning for the repatriation of the prisoners, those charged with developing medical and psychosocial rehabilitation plans naturally had to assume a "worst case" approach. The authorities had to be prepared to treat individuals who might be suffering from the initial features of the concentration camp syndrome. In many ways, the stressors appeared to be comparable and, in terms of duration of incarceration and time spent in solitary confinement, perhaps greater than elsewhere.

After release of the American prisoners, it was found that the prisoners who had been held primarily in the south were suffering from very severe physical and psychological disabilities quite comparable to those described in the captives of the past. They showed evidence of parasitic disease, malnutrition, skin disease, pulmonary disease, visual difficulties, and injuries, as well as residual psychiatric manifestations.

Released prisoners from North Vietnam, however, appeared remarkably healthy and fit, considering the duration and intensity of their ordeal. Regardless of how healthy their initial appearance, it was necessary to have a complete medical and psychosocial evaluation of each returnee. A large measure of supportive services was provided. The approach was highly successful. Systematic data of medical importance were gathered and recorded in a way that will prove to be of great utility to each individual returnee in the future. Many of the prisoners of war from Japan and Korea had been penalized later in life because of the grossly inadequate medical records that had been constructed at the time of their release. A number of disabilities had been overlooked at the time of the initial examinations in 1945 or 1953, respectively. For the released Vietnam prisoners, these mistakes and omissions were corrected. Additionally, the planners considered evidence that suggested that concentration camp victims who had been given supportive services might have made a better adjustment than those who did not receive such services (Eitinger, 1975). Accordingly, the released Vietnam prisoners were given a full measure of support of all kinds and have been followed periodically as they have reintegrated themselves into society with a considerable measure of success. Subsequent follow-up studies of the released naval aviator prisoners confirm that they are not developing the KZ syndrome. They have also had considerable occupational success, whether or not they remained in the Navy. The released Army prisoners of war held in South Vietnam, on the other hand, continued to have many residual problems.

Many of the repatriated prisoners of war from North Vietnam fulfilled the precepts of Nardini (1952), who was himself a POW of the Japanese during World War II, as to the qualities that most favorably influenced the survival of a prisoner. These included a strong motivation to live, good general intelligence, emotional insensitivity or well-controlled and balanced sensitivity, sense of humor, controlled fantasy life, successful active or passive resistance to the captors, and several years of prior military experience. The aviators were men who were characterized in other studies as being aggressive, assertive, energetic, and action-oriented individuals whose coping style was to make attempts to control, change, or master the environment, rather than resorting to fantasy or other kinds of passivity (Deaton et al., 1977).

They used various methods to defeat the sensory isolation of solitary confinement. Among the popular modes were attempts at communication with other captives, physical activity, concentration on maintaining one's health, mental exercises, the construction of mental diaries, and the planning of escapes. These men, indeed, were individuals who were well suited to cope with the stressors of the North Vietnamese prison camps. It must be reemphasized that because the North Vietnamese found the prisoners to be of value to them, they did not engage in the systematic extermination or lethal torture that characterized the Nazi concentration camps. In fact, the captors proved unable to break up the invisible disciplinary networks that bound the prisoners of war together in a military formation, even in captivity, and that provided enormous emotional support for the men. On the other hand, no matter how tough, mature and experienced the human, the policies of the Nazi concentration camps prevented use of coping strategies that were successful in other situations of incarceration.

Additionally, the imprisoned group consisted of men of mature years, the bulk of whom were over 30. They were regular military officers with a firm set of values and a definite sense of patriotic commitment. Among those most resistant to the pressures of prison camps are individuals with strong social convictions. Dedicated communists, for example, proved to be very difficult people to crush in prison camps. On the other hand, during the Korean War, the youths who appeared to defect to the communists were generally highly immature individuals from deprived backgrounds and with poorly formed values. This was also the kind of individual who was most likely to die during the prisoner of war experience. Individuals with a high degree of inner strength and discipline or, in some instances, a high degree of defiance and an inner rebelliousness were maximally resistive to either the torture or the propaganda attempts of the enemy. In this instance, aviators formed very strong military groups in the camp and maintained a considerable degree of order and covert resistance to their captors. This military cohesiveness carried over into the postrelease phase. Many of the individuals were able to resume their flight duties and their careers with normal prospects of promotion.

The only sector in which there appeared to be difficulties for the released prisoners was the family area (Dahl et al., 1976; Hall and Simmons, 1973). Some of the family problems were the kind that appear when the father is absent for a number of years. Other problems arose because of the rapid transmogrification of American society and its values that occurred entirely during the years of captivity. In any case, there was some degree of family turmoil after release, and a certain number of divorces ensued. It is not precisely clear, however, whether there was any more trouble and divorce in the families of the released prisoners than might be found elsewhere in America during the same period.

GENESIS OF SYNDROME

It would now be appropriate to examine evidence about the genesis of the KZ syndrome. This particular syndrome is obviously similar to combat neurosis and to posttraumatic states seen in victims of severe natural disasters. However, it does have certain unusual features: virtual universality and chronicity. It is seen in almost all survivors of concentration camps and prisoner-of-war camps in which there is a very high death rate. It can appear in individuals who were not actually in concentration camps but who fled from the Nazis and hid throughout Europe with the constant danger of exposure and consequent death. The condition cannot be merely a result of captivity *per se*, because the syndrome is not seen in its full-blown form in former prisoners of war who were treated with some degree of humanity in prison camps in which the death rate was below 5%. It is also not seen in individuals imprisoned in civilian jails in which there is a low death rate. Additionally, this syndrome has not yet been seen in the officers who were former prisoners of the Vietnamese, some of whom spent as many as 9 years in captivity. The weight of evidence certainly argues against the simplistic notion of incarceration itself being the major causative factor in the disorder. Similarly, solitary confinement does not seem to produce the syndrome. The constellation of symptoms begins in a situation in which the individual's life is under constant threat, the stress of which is reinforced by seeing others constantly dying. The person must be further depleted by the lack of normal environmental and social supports and by adverse conditions such as humiliation, physical torture, malnutrition, sleep deprivation, and vicious work requirements. The early theory that the KZ syndrome could be explained as a residual of brain trauma resulting from frequent beatings does not appear to be a believable explanation of so variegated a group of symptoms. On the other hand, some of the former prisoners' problems with memory, concentration, calculation, and abstract thought might represent an organic brain syndrome secondary to trauma and malnutrition. This syndrome would appear to be close in character to a traumatic neurosis. Brain patterns or engrams seem to be encoded through constant repetition until they acquire autonomy, activation, and persistence through time. It is probable that the symptoms are exacerbated by postcaptivity events: further incarceration, emigration, social isolation, and failure of social supports. The full-blown picture appears only over the course of the years, with further elaboration of defense maneuvers to ward off the terror, guilt, dysphoria, and low self-esteem.

If appropriate psychotherapeutic intervention and strong social supports had been available at the time of release, some of the victims would not have developed the full measure of impairment, even though they doubtless would have had some depression, anxiety, and rumination. It would be hard to imagine escaping absolutely unscathed from years in hell.

TREATMENT OF SYNDROME

Various approaches to the psychiatric treatment of patients with concentration camp syndrome have been described (Berger, 1977; Hoppe, 1966, 1971a; Koenig, 1964; Krystal, 1968). The patients show a lack of basic trust and often a submissive and fearful attitude. They are often terrified of authority. It is also common to see distortions of body imagery. Depersonalization and derealization are frequently encountered along with the feeling that the present life is dreamlike compared to the life in the camps. The therapist must understand the sociocultural backgrounds of the victims and be aware of the distortions of the superego, particularly in relationship to the loss of the ego ideal and the masochistic attitude toward authority figures. The therapist must, of course, listen to sometimes repetitious material about persecution and death and be able to work through his own guilt feelings about the events of the war. There should be a sense of permanent attachment to the patient and a careful examination of the mental associations between the concentration camp experience and childhood problems. The necessity of dealing with the underlying suspicion, regression, guilt, and covert aggressive feelings, including identification with the aggressor, is stressed. Similarly, the patients' massive dependency needs and unremitting preoccupation with the past must be recognized. The author has not been impressed with the efficacy of psychotropic medication in dealing with the long-term characterological and neurotic phenomena in such patients, although, to be sure, the patients may develop a new depression on top of the old chronic depressive feelings. Constancy, patience, and kindness, and an attempt to understand the inner horror posed by the reminiscences of the patient are all necessary attributes of the therapist. Startling results are not to be looked for, but considerable help can be given by steady, individualized, and long-term therapy.

Even the youngest of those who were imprisoned during the Second World War are now approaching middle age. Those who were young adults at the time of incarceration are now at the edge of old age. Many who were middle-aged are now dead. Each year more prisoners of the Second World War will be dying. Nonetheless, the memory of what was suffered and the pain that accompanied it has not diminished at all. The world must still remember what happened between 1939 and 1945 so as not to repeat the same crimes. There could be a time when there would be no more new KZ syndrome patients. The disease is, after all, preventable.

REFERENCES

Adler, H. G., 1958, Ideas toward a sociology of the concentration camp, *Am. J. Soc.* 63:513.

Anderson, C. L., Boysen, A. M., Esensten, S., Lam, G. N., and Shadish, W. R., 1954, Medical experiences in Communist POW camps in Korea, *J. Am. Med. Assoc.* 156:120.

Anderson, R. S., 1975, Operation homecoming: Psychological observations of repatriated Vietnam prisoners of war, *Psychiatry* 38:65.

Arntzen, F. I., 1948, Psychological observations of prisoners of war, *Am. J. Psychiatry* 104(7):446.

Arthur, R. J., 1974, Extreme stress in adult life and its psychic and psychophysiological consequences, *in* "Life Stress and Illness" (E. K. E. Gunderson and R. H. Rahe, eds.), pp. 195–207, Charles C Thomas, Springfield, Illinois.

Barocas, H. A., 1975, Children of purgatory: Reflections on the concentration camp survival syndrome, *Soc. Psychiatry* 21(2):87.

Beebe, G. W., 1975, Original contributions: Follow-up studies of World War II and Korean war prisoners, *Am. J. Epidemiol.* 101:400.

Bensheim, V. H., 1960, Die KZ-Neurose rassisch Verfolgter, *Nervenarzt* 31:10.

Berg, S. W., and Richlin, M., 1977a, Injuries and illnesses of Vietnam War POW's I: Navy POW's, *Mil. Med.* 141:514.

Berg, S. W., and Richlin, M., 1977b, Injuries and illnesses of Vietnam War POW's II:Army POW's, *Mil. Med.* 141:598.

Berg, S. W., and Richlin, M., 1977c, Injuries and illnesses of Vietnam War POW's III:Marine Corps POW's, *Mil. Med.* 141(9):678.

Berg. S. W., and Richlin, M., 1977d, Injuries and illnesses of Vietnam War POW's IV:Comparison of captivity effects in North and South Vietnam, *Mil. Med.* 141(10):757.

Berger, D. M., 1977, The survivor syndrome:A problem of nosology and treatment, *Am. J. Psychother.* 31:238.

Bloch, H. A., 1946–47, The personality of inmates of concentration camps, *Am. J. Soc.* 52:335.

Bourne, P. G. (ed.), 1969, "The Psychology and Physiology of Stress: With reference to special studies of the Vietnam War," Academic Press, New York.

Bourne, P. G., 1970, "Men, Stress, and Vietnam," Little, Brown, Boston.

Brill, N. Q., 1946, Neuropsychiatric examination of military personnel recovered from Japanese prison camps, *Bull. U.S. Army Med. Dept.* 5(4):429.

Carmelly, F., 1975, Guilt feelings in concentration camp survivors:Comments of a "survivor," *J. Jewish Comm. Serv.* 52(2):139.

Chodoff, P., 1959, Effects of extreme coercive and oppressive forces:Brainwashing and concentration camps, *Am. Handbook Psychiatry* 3:385.

Chodoff, P., 1963, Late effects of the concentration camp syndrome, *Arch. Gen. Psychiatry* 8:323.

Dahl, B. B., McCubbin, H. I., and Lester, G. R., 1976, War-induced father absence:Comparing the adjustment of children in reunited, non-reunited and reconstituted families, *Int. J. Soc. Family* 6(1):99.

Deaton, J. E., Berg, S. W., and Richlin, M., 1977, Coping activities in solitary confinement of U.S. Navy POW's in Vietnam, *J. Appl. Soc. Psychol.* 7(3):239.

Dimsdale, J. E., 1974, The coping behavior of Nazi concentration camp survivors, *Am. J. Psychiatry* 131(7):792.

Dor-Shav, N. K., 1978, On the long-range effects of concentration camp internment of Nazi victims:25 years later, *J. Consult. Clin. Psychol.* 46(1):1.

Eitinger, L., 1964, "Concentration Camp Survivors in Norway and Israel," Oslo Universitetsforlaget, Oslo.

Eitinger, L., 1975, Jewish concentration camp survivors in Norway, *Isr. Ann. Psychiatry Relat. Discip.* 13(4):321.

Foreman, P. B., 1959, Buchenwald and modern prisoner-of-war detention policy, *Soc. Forces* 37(4):289.

Hall, R. C. W., and Simmons, W. C., 1973, The POW wife: A psychiatric appraisal, *Arch. Gen. Psychiatry* 29:690.

Hendrix, K., 1978a, Children of holocaust survivors:Making peace with the past, *Los Angeles Times*, November 30, pp. 1, 18–21.

Hendrix, K. 1978b, Holocaust aftermath:The 2nd generation speaks out, *Los Angeles Times*, December 1, pp. 1, 8–15.

Hochman, J., 1978, On the analysis of a child of holocaust survivors with some notes on countertransference problems, *Bull. South. Calif. Psychoanal. Inst. Soc.* 53:7.

Hocking, F., 1970, Psychiatric aspects of extreme environmental stress, *Dept. Psychiatry, Alfred Hospital, Melbourne, Australia*, 542–545.

Hoppe, K. D., 1966, The psychodynamics of concentration camp victims, *Psychiatr. Forum* 1(1):76.

Hoppe, K. D., 1971a, Chronic reactive aggression in survivors of severe persecution, *Compr. Psychiatry* 12(3):230.

Hoppe, K. D., 1971b, The aftermath of Nazi persecution reflected in recent psychiatric literature, *Internat. Psychiatr. Clin.* 8:169.

Koenig, W., 1964, Chronic or persisting identity diffusion, *Am. Psychiatr. Assoc.* 120(11):1081.

Kral, V. A., Pazder, L. H., and Wigdor, B. T., 1967, Long-term effects of a prolonged stress experience, *Can. Psychiatr. Assoc. J.* 12:175.

Krystal, H. (ed.), 1968, "Massive Psychic Trauma," International Universities Press, New York.

Mason, W. W., 1954, "Prisoners of War: Official history of New Zealand in the Second World War 1939–45," War History Branch, Department of International Affairs, R. E. Owen, Government Printer, Wellington, New Zealand.

Matussek, P., Grigat, R., Haiböck, H., Halbach, G., Kemmler, R., Mantell, D., Triebel, A., Vardy, M., and Wedel, G., 1975, "Internment in Concentration Camps and Its Consequences," Springer-Verlag, New York.

Nardini, J. E., 1952, Survival factors in American prisoners of war of the Japanese, *Am. J. Psychiatry* 109(4):241.

Nefzger, M. D., 1970, Follow-up studies of World War II and Korean war prisoners: I. study plan and mortality findings, *Am. J. Epidemiol.* 21:123.

Ostwald, P., and Bittner, E., 1969, Life adjustment after severe persecution, *Am. J. Psychiatry* 124:1393.

Segal, J., Hunter, E. J., and Segal, Z., 1976, Universal consequences of captivity:Stress reactions among divergent populations of prisoners of war and their families, *Int. Soc. Sci. J.* 28(3):593.

Sigal, J. J., and Rakoff, V., 1971, Concentration camp survival:A pilot study of effects on the second generation, *Can. Psychiatr. Assoc. J.* 16:393.

Sigal, J. J., Silver, D., Rakoff, V., and Ellin, B., 1973, Some second-generation effects of survival of the Nazi persecution, *Am. J. Orthopsychiatry* 43:320.

Southard, E. E., 1919, "Shell-Shock and Other Neuropsychiatric Problems: Presented in five hundred and eighty-nine case histories from the war literature, 1914–1918," W. M. Leonard, Boston. (Reprinted, 1973, "Mental Illness and Social Policy: The American experience," Arno Press, New York.)

Spaulding, R. C., 1977, The Pueblo incident:Medical problems reported during captivity and physical findings at the time of the crew's release, *Mil. Med.* 141:681.

Strom, A., 1968, "Norwegian Concentration Camp Survivors," Universitetsforlaget, Oslo/Humanities Press, New York.

Van Putten, T., and Emory, W. H., 1973, Traumatic neuroses in Vietnam returnees: A forgotten diagnosis?, *Arch. Gen. Psychiatry* 29:695.

Wolf, S., and Ripley, H. A., 1947, Reactions among allied prisoners of war subjected to three years of imprisonment and torture by the Japanese, *Am. J. Psychiatry* 104:180.

Zwingmann, C., and Pfister-Ammende, M., 1973, "Uprooting and After . . . ," Springer-Verlag, New York.

5

Autoscopic Phenomena

JAMES S. GROTSTEIN

Autoscopy, or heautoscopy, is one of the most fascinating and uncanny of the rare syndromes of the mind. One may call it the idosyncratic quintessence of self-consciousness. It has intrigued and perplexed writers and philosophers across the centuries, as evidenced by Lhermitte's (1951) review of world literature. His review of the literature on the "double" cited Aristotle, who told the story of a man who could not go for a walk without seeing his own image coming toward him (Todd and Dewhurst have indentified this man as Antipheron); Hoffmann (the story of the lost reflection); Chamisso (the story of Peter Schlemyl, who was haunted by having sold his shadow to the devil); Gabriele d'Annunzio *(Notturno)*; Wilde *(The Picture of Dorian Gray)*; Poe (especially the tale of William Wilson); Steinbeck *(Great Valley)*; Dostoyevsky *(The Double, The Idiot,* and *The Brothers Karamazov)*; Kafka *(The Trial)*; de Maupassant *(La Horla)*; Balzac *(Peau de Chagrin)*; Goethe *(Der Erlkoenig)*; and de Musset *(La Nuit de Décembre)*. In an interesting aside, Lhermitte pointed out that many of the authors noted above were, in fact, victims of mental illnesses secondary to epilepsy or syphilis.

Autoscopic phenomena consist of the observation of one's own phantom self by hallucination, illusion, or fantasy. In most instances the person who experiences autoscopy reports that he perceives his double, in part or in whole, as in a mirror. Lhermitte (1951) informed us that the subject of an autoscopic phenomenon not only believes that he can see his own image as if it were reflected in a mirror but also has a special sense that in this image there is a part of himself: he feels connected to this image by "spiritual and material" links (p. 432). Lhermitte stated that this is never found in any other sensory hallucination and that it is an essential characteristic of the autoscopic hallucination.

JAMES S. GROTSTEIN • Department of Psychiatry, University of California at Los Angeles, Los Angeles, California.

The phenomenon usually occurs at dusk or against a twilight-hyp-nagogic-hypnopompic background. The hallucinations are generally translucent, mainly emphasize the bust and torso, and most commonly occupy the visual sphere, although the auditory and kinesthetic senses may be involved as well. The latter is demonstrated by the fact that the patient may be able to predict his twin's motion. When the auditory sense is involved, the patient may have the curious and eerie experience of hearing his own voice within himself, but without his ears being affected (pseudoauditory perception).

Lukianowicz (1958) wrote perhaps the most definitive account of autoscopy to date. He defined autoscopy as a complex psychosensorial hallucinatory perception of one's own body image projected into the external visual space. He reported seven cases of autoscopic phenomena. In his comments on these and other cases, he pointed out that the double usually appears suddenly and without any warning, although it may at times appear with a sensory aura in migraine patients or may in fact be a migraine equivalent. He pointed out that the person sees mainly the head and the bust of the figure and less commonly the whole figure of his double. He described the color of the double as being gray or misty. The texture of the double may be either transparent, semitransparent, "jelly-like," or solid, so that it eclipses everything behind it. Yet, he points out, no matter how dense the texture of the double, it does not seem to cast a shadow. This latter phenomenon is an important differential feature between an autoscopic double and an "apparition."

Lukianowicz pointed out that the autoscopic double faithfully repeats the movements and facial expressions of the subject, not unlike echopraxia, and the movements are copied in a "mirror-writing" fashion. His own patients perceived the double multisensorily—that is, through visual, auditory, and kinesthetic modes. The person has many different reactions to seeing the double. Often it is one of sadness, and other times, amazement. On other occasions there may be indifference or even narcissistic satisfaction. Persons perceiving the double attribute sensory feeling of coldness and/or weariness to the double, almost like the experience of the presence of a ghost. At these times the person himself may also feel cold and lifeless. There may also be the attribution of qualities of mind to the double; one of Lukianowicz's patients believed that the double contained her mind.

Lukianowicz stated:

> The subject remains aware of his psycho-physical identity and of his actual, "real" body, as well as of its position in space, throughout the whole experience, and seems to be conscious "at the back of his mind" of the unreality of his experience. This peculiar detached "insight" in autoscopy is entirely different from the attitude shown by a hallucinating psychotic patient, who has an unshakable belief in the reality of his experience. It is also unlike the

critical insight of a hallucinating organic patient, who is mostly aware of the unreal character of his vision. Thus, the insight in autoscopy lies somewhere between a complete acceptance and a complete rejection of the reality of the hallucinated phenomena. It resembles the "very private" notion on the part of some children of the make-believe nature of their "imaginary companions."

The phantom generally appears in the visual space directly in front of the person and usually about a yard away. In other cases there may be no spatial correlation or localization. The double phenomenon generally lasts only a few seconds, but this is debatable, according to Lukianowicz, because of the possible impairment of the appreciation of time in patients in the emotionally stressful situations that precipitate autoscopic phenomena.

He quoted Leaning in stating that the frequency of these phenomena may vary all the way from once in a lifetime to a habitual presence, by day whenever the eyes are closed and by night with the eyes open or shut. Generally, however, twilight or dawn favors the appearance of a double.

Autoscopic phenomena are sometimes associated with the Capgras syndrome, the illusion that an object is a double of a real object. Although the phenomena are similar and parallel, they only rarely occur together.

EPIDEMIOLOGY

Autoscopic phenomena are rare and are often benign. They can, however, be associated with migraine headaches, various forms of epilepsy (particularly temporal lobe types), brain tumors, and degenerative states of the brain (particularly of the parieto-temporo-occipital area). Autoscopy may also occur in psychosis in association with other hallucinations, depersonalization, and other aspects of ego-boundary loss, but it is not necessarily indicative of a psychotic state in itself. It has often been associated with the phantasmagoria of imaginary twins or companions, eidetic imagery, hypnagogic and hypnopompic imagery, "phantom limbs," and "astral projections." Persons who use so-called consciousness-expanding drugs such as mescaline and lysergic acid diethylamide also frequently report autoscopic phenomena.

REVIEW OF THE LITERATURE ON CAUSATION

Organic

Wigan (1844) was probably the first physician to explore autoscopy. He related it to the splitting of functions of the two cerebral hemispheres. Lhermitte (1951) and Hecaen and de Ajuriaguerra (1952) high-lighted the importance of labryinthitis, anxiety, fatigue, and infectious-toxic states in the development of isolated episodes of autoscopy in otherwise normal subjects. At the same time they called attention to the relatively high incidence of recurrent autoscopy in patients with epi-lepsy, syphilis, dementia paralytica, encephalitis lethargica, chronic alco-holism, drug addiction, and schizophrenia. Menninger-Lerchenthal (1935) claimed that autoscopic phenomena occur in cerebral lesions, whether infective, traumatic, vascular, or neoplastic, especially in the right parieto-occipital area.

Dewhurst and Pearson (1955), in reviewing the organic contribu-tions to autoscopy, reported three patients, one of whom had a small vas-cular lesion in the brain that produced the phenomenon, a second of whom had a tumor in the left temporal area, and a third of whom had experienced an injury to the cortex by shrapnel and experienced autos-copic phenomena 13 years afterward. In their commentary on these cases, and on the autoscopic phenomenon in general, Dewhurst and Pearson noted, "These strictly neurological hypotheses fail to explain fully individual variations and the degree of complexity of hallucina-tions in general, and the recurrence of autoscopy in particular. It has long been known that, together with cerebral irritation, such individual vari-ances, visual memory, and the degree of visual imagery constitute a pecu-liarly subjective undertone to hallucinosis." Galton (1908) was the pioneer in investigating the degree to which people can recall past sen-sations and see images in the mind's eye. He observed that visual mem-ory varied greatly. To some people it had no meaning, whereas others were able to revive an early visual experience with hallucinatory clarity. The latter he called "visualizers"; at the other extreme are the congeni-tally blind, who never experience visual hallucinations (p. 56). Dewhurst and Pearson further stated, "It would seem probable that amongst the visualizers are some who possess this faculty of seeing a spatially local-ized mirror image of themselves, and we believe that it is amongst these subjects that the phenomenon of autoscopy is to be found."

Thus, Dewhurst and Pearson, like Todd and Dewhurst (1955), believe that autoscopy, whatever the precipitating organic focal factor, can occur only in a group of subjects with a highly developed visual memory sense of their corporal being.

Todd and Dewhurst (1955) cited the role of disturbances in the brain's somatognostic areas. Lesions in various areas of the brain, partic-ularly in the temporo-parieto-occipital zones, may affect the integration of the body schema or body image. In this regard, they stated, "This inte-gration of sensory impulses from the various parts of the body into a body image is accompanied by the development of a complementary psychical component which imbues it with *personal* significance. As a result, the individual is not merely aware of the external appearance, position, and 'feeling' of his body, but also bears toward it a sentiment of ownership with all the emotional and ideational accompaniments" (p. 53). Thus, they seem to believe that a somatognostic disturbance can contribute to the experience of autoscopy by creating a defective sensory construction of the body image.

Schilder (1933, 1935) has contributed to our knowledge about autoscopic phenomena through his pioneering work on the development of the concept of the body scheme or body image. The body image is a mental representation that, when projected outward, becomes the autoscopic phenomenon. The body image is formed, according to Schilder, by a consensual validation of all the senses, and it is subject to constant revision during the person's growth and development. Schilder's most poetic insight into autoscopic phenomena lies in his statement about imagination and hallucination in general. "They are, so to say, varied expressions of the 'unconscious' parts of sensual perception; they are the 'dream' of the senses" (1933, p. 609).

Narcissism

Todd and Dewhurst (1955) paralleled the findings of Lhermitte but also cited narcissism as an important condition in autoscopy. They stated:

> It should be stressed that in some of the illustrative cases quoted there is an interplay of factors ... narcissism, fear, anxiety, wish-fulfillment, or the super-normal power of visual imagery ... in projecting the autoscopic double. Whilst super-normal power of visual imagery may be regarded as a factor likely to facilitate the appearance of visual hallucinations *in general* ..., narcissism should be regarded as a *specific* factor facilitating the appearance of visual hallucinations *of the self*. In view of this, the high incidence of autoscopia amongst creative writers is not surprising, as they frequently possess both these factors as traits of their personality and occupation. (p. 50)

Todd and Dewhurst also implicated the role of archetypic thinking in autoscopy. They stated:

> In the process of dissolution, the central nervous system exhibits a hierarchical devolution, as phylogenetically older mechanisms are progressively released from the control of higher centers ... similarly, archaic modes of thinking are released in the process of the accompanying dissolution of the personality, As a result, bizarre hallucinatory-delusional themes invade consciousness. Visual hallucinations originating in this way may assume any form, but man's ancient preoccupation with his reflection and shadow particularly favors the appearance of the autoscopic double. (p. 51)

They supported this thesis by their review of the myths and religious beliefs of primitive tribes, which shed light on the origins and importance of the "double" motif.

Psychoanalytic Theory

The first psychoanalytic study of the double was written by Rank (1914), who believed that the double, as manifested in shadows, mirror reflections, and guardian spirits, was the origin of the idea of the immortal soul and, therefore, constituted a denial of one's mortality.

Freud (1919) connected the phenomenon of the double with the termination of primary narcissism and the inchoation of secondary narcissism with the development of the ego ideal. He stated:

> A special agency is slowly formed there, which is able to stand over against the rest of the ego, which has the function of observing and criticizing the self and of exercising a censorship within the mind, and which we become aware of as our "conscience." . . . the fact that an agency of this kind exists, which is able to treat the rest of the ego like an object—the fact, that is, that man is capable of self-observation—renders it possible to invest the old idea of a "double" with a new meaning and to ascribe a number of things to it— above all, those things which seem to self-criticism to belong to the old surmounted narcissism of earliest times. . . .
>
> I believe that when poets complain that two souls dwell in the human breast, and when popular psychologists talk of the splitting of a person's ego, what they are thinking of is this division between the critical agency and the rest of the ego, and not the antithesis discovered by psycho-analysis between the ego and what is unconscious and repressed. It is true that the distinction between these two antitheses is to some extent effaced by the circumstance that is foremost among the things that are rejected by the criticism of the ego derivatives of the repressed. (p. 235–236)

Freud (1919) called attention to the "extraordinarily strong feeling of something uncanny that pervades the conception" of the double, but believed that this very quality of its uncanniness must be due to the fact that the "double" is a creation in the primitive stage of development of the ego and is a result of the deterioration following the collapse of primary narcissism. Doubling, therefore, according to Freud, is both a manifestation of primary narcissism and a denotation of its dissolution.

Ostow (1960) revived psychoanalytic interest in autoscopy. He pointed out that rebirth as well as death are the aims of the autoscopic experience. He believed that autoscopic phenomena occur in patients who are depressed and/or who use extreme splitting mechanisms. He stated, "We have, then, in melancholia an ego suffering great pain, eager to act to destroy something or someone in order to eliminate the pain, but 'knowing' only itself as the source and the seat of the pain." Thus, according to Ostow, in the absence of any external object cathexis, the ego must reproject into its own reconstituted double.

Winnicott's (1967) work also has bearing on the subject of autoscopy. He has written in depth about the mirroring phase as a state in which the infant discovers himself in his first mirror, the mother's face. Winnicott stated:

> In the early stage of the emotional development of the human infant, a vital part is played by the environment which is in fact not yet separated off from the infant by the infant. Gradually the separating-off of the not-me takes place, and the pace varies according to the infant and according to the environment. The major change takes place in the separating-out of the mother as an objectively perceived environmental feature. . . . What does the baby see when he or she looks at the mother's face? I am suggesting that, ordinarily, what the baby sees is himself or herself. In other words, the mother is looking at the baby and *what she looks like is related to what she sees there.* (p. 111–112)

Thus, according to Winnicott, the mirroring phase is not merely a matter of looking into a physical mirror. Rather, it is the mirroring of mother's response to the infant in terms of her being a holding, handling, and object-presenting person who represents to the infant her impressions of him.

Thus, autoscopic phenomena can be seen to derive from the mirroring phase of ego development and may constitute a regression back to that time. They may also reflect an incompleteness of integration of the mirroring phase when an identification with the mirror image of the object reflection may not have been totally acceptable to the subjective "I." In short, autoscopy can be thought of as the hallucinatory epiphany of the breakdown between the "I" and "self."

CASE EXAMPLES

R.J. A 21-year-old single woman consulted me in regard to her conflicts about her forthcoming marriage. In the course of treatment, she revealed that she had taken considerable amounts of lysergic acid diethylamide (LSD) in the preceding years in order to relieve depression. During our second visit, she told me the following story: "As I was leaving your office yesterday, I went into the exit hall, looked in the mirror to adjust my hair, and then opened the door. In the outer hallway I saw an apparition or ghost—but it was me! It seemed to be waiting for me to fuse with it so that we could go on our way together!"

As her analysis progressed, I deduced that this autoscopic event represented a drug-induced projective identification of her more primitive self, which she had put into "safekeeping" while she remained identified with her corrupt, depressed, worthless self. Having decided to enter analysis, she felt it was safe for her to rejoin her positive self.

L.Y. A 45-year-old television director consulted me for anxieties relative to his work situation. During the consultation, he revealed a good deal about his early family life, and I was able to make interpretations about his avoidance of painful depressive feelings as a child by imaginative flights of fantasy in which he would "jump into his imaginary heroes and fly away from his depressed self." The next day he informed me that, after the hour, while walking down the hallway toward the elevator, he had a "visitation of a scene from my earliest childhood. I recognized myself in my bedroom. I seemed to open the door—and there stood my child-self! It was very moving! I really felt I had found myself!"

This patient, too, had probably rid himself of a portion of his personality because of a lifelong depression and, like R. J., was able to feel safe enough to rejoin that self upon deciding to undertake analysis.

R.N. A young screenwriter came into analysis because of a success neurosis involving his burgeoning career. It gradually emerged in the analysis that, although he was seemingly well-adjusted and outgoing on the surface, there seemed to be another split-off, hidden self that was experienced by him as introverted, introspective, and "grand." He called this portion of his personality "the prince." There then emerged another personality split, "the pauper." The patient had been deeply ashamed of his father for having been a lackey for his mother's family's business. This shame caused the patient to correct his identification with a devalued father by flight into a grand inner world in which he was the young prince, the monarch-to-be. The pauper represented his attempt to correct his father's image omnipotently, by absorbing the poor, shameful features of his father, thereby appropriating them for himself in order to spare his father these traits. One day, after several analytic hours that had clarified these separate selves, the patient reported that he was given the name of an airline stewardess to call for a date, and he thereupon heard the vivid voices of his two split-off selves. He himself listened in as an amazed, but separated-off, audience to the following conversation: "What are you doing wasting your time calling an airline stewardess? Don't you know they're common? And besides, they often are hooked up with gangsters and do a lot of sex trips. She'll be out of your league." (This apparently was the voice of the "prince.") The "pauper" answered: "She's just a person like any other person. There is no magic to people. Stop looking for the special one. You're calling her because you're lonely. Why do you have such high standards? What are your criteria?"

P.D. A bright, highly confident attorney consulted me for depression. His depression quickly lifted in the analysis when I was able to interpret to him his fear of death, which was precipitated by his father's illness. As the analysis progressed, he informed me of how gifted an attorney he was, especially in court. He reported an incident in which he was cross-examining an adversary and became aware that he was also a detached spectator observing his own brillance. He frequently observed himself say, "Great job!" and he noted that these episodes were often visual as well. The shift in perspective from the observer to the observed is interesting in this case. The patient experienced himself as the brilliant lawyer *and* as the observer at the same time. While relating this to me, he stated, "My mind is now moving to the left, and I see myself lying on the couch and yet I can feel myself to be on the couch at the same time. I guess the maniac is watching the real me—or is the maniac the real me?"

This observation of self corresponds to his assuming the role of an idealized object admiring a grandiose self. All his object relations seem to be superficial, expedient, and self-serving. He never had trusted anyone but himself and so had developed the notion that he had to be a parent to his own child-self, so to speak.

DISCUSSION

Autoscopy emerges, perhaps, as a curiously less rare phenomenon than has hitherto been thought. When we stop to consider it more carefully, we can readily find daily evidence for its occurrences in dreams, where the observing self gazes disinterestedly upon an acting or participating self. If we were to expand the definition of autoscopy to include such ultrasensual phenomena as fantasies (intrapsychic experiences), we might say then that autoscopic phenomena include the whole spectrum of self-consciousness, "normal" through "abnormal." The "sensual band" (visual, kinesthetic, and auditory) of autoscopy proper would then be located on one position of this spectrum. We could then state that autoscopy seems to be a manifestation of a difficulty in the *tone* of narcissistic well-being and reveals a state of *alienation*. The autoscopic phenomenon ultimately expresses the "self" as the "ghost" of the subjective "I." In this regard, much of the romantic literature of the 19th century, as stated earlier, has chosen to explore the phenomenon of autoscopy, especially as seen in *Doctor Jekyll and Mr. Hyde, The Vampire, The Double,* etc., all of which seemed to have anticipated the great "autoscopic discovery," "the unconscious."

As outlined in the introduction, autoscopy seems to follow from migraine, epilepsy, and CNS affections of the temporo-occipito-parietal lobes of either hemisphere; may occur in dissociated states such as in hysteria, borderline and psychotic states, and drug-induced states; and is also a variant in normal personalities that are easily prone to imaginative visualization and audition. Faguet (1979) suggested that autoscopic hallucinations represent a "unique retention of critical insight and judgment" by the subjects who experience them, and that autoscopy therefore lies "somewhere between perception and representation, akin to hypnagogic hallucinations." In that regard, they "recapture an important object relation . . . the image of the self as it once was believed to be or still possibly could be." He concluded that autoscopic phenomena represent a transitional position between sensation and thought.

Autoscopy involves primarily a splitting of consciousness and a *projective identification* (externalization) of one's body image. Secondarily, we can see the derivative defense mechanisms of detachment, alienation, isolation, displacement, and reversal. One of the patients, P.D., demonstrated the unusual phenomenon of shifting perspective in which he identified with the observer and the participant at the same time. This represents, I believe, an extreme degree of ambivalence of consciousness. The other patients in this series did not experience that phenomenon, nor is it reported in the literature. Psychodynamically, autoscopy demonstrates the sensory epitome of self-consciousness and, as such, reveals affective attitudes toward the observed self. Generally, these attitudes are critical and unfavorable, but, in rare instances, they are highly complimentary.

At other times the phantom seems to be a benign ghost by daytime, corresponding to the apparition of a loved one who is either absent or dead, but who is now returning in a silent, but comforting, visitation. This aspect of autoscopy represents Freud's conception of the infant's capacity to hallucinate the presence of mother in her absence and constitutes the beginning of symbolization and the capacity to represent objects in their absence.

It is my impression that the split-brain phenomenon may also play a role in its causation. We know that the corpus callosum and the deep cerebral commissures do not myelinate until about 4 to 5 months of age and do not complete their myelination until adolescence (see LeCours, 1975). The significance of this fact is that the infant seemingly has two separate minds, a left-hemispheric organization *and* a right-hemispheric organization, which only slowly begin to come together. (In another contribution, Grotstein, 1979, I have cited this phenomenon as corresponding to a natural neuronal precursor for the mental phenomenon of splitting.) The long delay in myelination in interhemispheric associational fibers may be an important factor in the phenomenon of the imaginary twin of childhood, and consequently, the completion of myelination in adolescence may explain why this phenomenon seemingly dissolves in most cases at that time.

I postulate that the phenomenon of the double, as evinced in autoscopy, may be a manifestation of the breakdown of the function of this interhemispheric coordination and integration. It can be thought of as "interhemispheric diplopia" and is therefore more apparent in fugue states and in dreams when the interhemisphere connections seemingly dissolve temporarily. This interhemispheric disconnection can be brought about by drugs, seizures, organic lesions, congenital absence, surgery, and by states of mind in themselves. The latter may function in the form of a "conversion paralysis" of function of the interhemispheric connection. What then emerges is a release phenomenon, an externalization of one's self-image representation. This latter notion is in keeping with Schilder's (1933, 1935) important statement that autoscopic phenomena represent a breakdown in the body image that itself is the dream of the senses. For a similar view from the standpoint of schizophrenia, see Green (1978).

Autoscopic phenomena probably represent more than just an interhemispheric split. Katan (1954) and Bion (1957) have talked about the dissociation between the psychotic and the nonpsychotic portions of the personality. The autoscopic phenomena of schizophrenics and manics, as well as of borderline patients, may easily reflect this duality. Elsewhere, I have posited that split personalities or dissociated states emerge from a sense of a defective Background Object of Primary Identification, which is believed by the patient to be no longer able to protect him or "back him up" in his life situation (Grotstein, 1977a, 1977b, 1979). At the same time, I have postulated a dual track of mental existence from birth onward in which, on one track, there is immediate postnatal separateness and, on another track, there is the continuation of primary identification.

Autoscopic phenomena may reveal a breach or a discrepancy between these two tracks secondary to a nonharmonious or defective background object. The experience of a defective Background Object of Primary Identification can seemingly emerge when there is a premature abruption of the sense of primary oneness with mother, as when the infant is overwhelmed by stimuli from both within and without. This abruption of primary oneness precipitates a precocious two-ness. The dissociated state that results may precipitate autoscopic phenomena, as well as other types of similar states. By virtue of its being a phenomenon of dissociation, autoscopy therefore characterizes a special form of *depersonalization*.

SUMMARY

Autoscopy is thought to be a rare phenomenon in which a person visualizes a veritable hallucinatory image of his double. It may be more common than hitherto has been thought, however. It has no pathological significance, generally, as compared with its counterpart, and Capgras' syndrome, but it can occur in psychotic and borderline states and affections of the CNS. Autoscopy has been known since ancient times but has come into prominence in the last century, both in the romantic literature of the double and in neuropsychiatric investigation.

It is the contention of the author that the phenomenon is far more common as an intrapsychic (nonhallucinatory) experience and that it is especially common in dreams. Autoscopy can ultimately be considered the quintessence of Cartesian artifice in which one mind-body ("I") is caught in the act of regarding its compatriot self as another mind-body. A theory is offered that autoscopy is a special form of depersonalization which may be related to the "split-brain" phenomenon neurophysiologically and to splitting and projective identification psychically.

REFERENCES

Bion, W. R., 1957, Differentiation of the psychotic from the non-psychotic personalities, in "Second Thoughts," pp. 43–64, William Heinemann, London.

Dewhurst, K., and Pearson, J., 1955, Visual hallucinations of self in organic disease, J. Neurol. Neurosurg. Psychiatry 18:53.

Faguet, R. A., 1979, With the eyes of the mind: Autoscopic phenomena in the hospital setting, Gen. Hosp. Psychiatry 1(4):311–314.

Freud, S., 1919, "The uncanny," S.E. 17:217.

Galton, F., 1980, "Inquiries into Human Faculty and Its Development," E. P. Dutton, New York.

Green, P., 1978, Defective inter-hemispheric transfer in schizophrenia, J. Abnorm. Psychol. 87:472.

Grotstein, J., 1977a, The psychoanalytic concept of schizophrenia: I. The dilemma, Int. J. Psycho-Anal. 58:403.

Grotstein, J., 1977b, The psychoanalytic concept of schizophrenia. II. Reconciliation, Int. J. Psycho-Anal. 58:427.

Grotstein, J., 1979, "Splitting and Projective Identification," Jason Aronson, New York.

Hecaen, H., and de Ajuriaguerra, J., 1952, "Meconnaissances et Hallucinations Corporelles," Masson, Paris.

Katan, M., 1954, The importance of the non-psychotic part of the personality in schizophrenia, Int. J. Psycho-Anal. 35:119.

LeCours, A., 1975, Myelogenetic correlates of the development of speech and language, in "Foundations of Language Development: A Multi-Disciplinary Approach," Vol. 1, Academic Press, New York.

Lhermitte, J., 1951, Visual hallucinations of the self, Br. Med. J. 1:431.

Lukianowicz, N., 1958, Autoscopic phenomena, AMA Arch. Neurol. Psychiatry 80:199.

Menninger-Lerchenthal, E., 1935, "Das Truggebilde der eigenen Gestalt (Heautoskopie, Doppelgänger)," S. Karger, Berlin.

Ostow, M., 1960, The metapsychology of autoscopic phenomena, Int. J. Psycho-Anal. 41:619.

Rank, O., 1914, Der Doppelgaenger, Imago 3(97):234.

Schilder, P., 1933, Experiments on imagination, after-images, and hallucinations, Am. J. Psychiatry 13:597.

Schilder, P., 1935, "The Image and Appearance of the Human Body," George Routledge, London.

Todd, J., and Dewhurst, K., 1955, The double: Its psychopathology and psychophysiology, *J. Nerv. Ment. Dis.* 122:47.

Wigan, A., 1844, "The Duality of the Mind: A New View of Insanity," Longman, Brown, Green & Longman, London.

Winnicott, D., 1967, Mirror-role of mother and family and child development, *in* "The Predicament of the Family: A Psycho-Analytical Symposium" (P. Lomas, ed.), Hogarth Press and The Institute of Psycho-Analysis, London.

6

Gilles de la Tourette Syndrome or Multiple Tic Disorder*

F. S. ABUZZAHAB, SR.

Gilles de la Tourette syndrome is the eponymous designation for multiple tic disorder, after Georges Gilles de la Tourette, a French neurologist. Although this disorder had been described previously by Itard in 1825, Dr. Georges Gilles de la Tourette (1885), under the tutelage of Jean-Martin Charcot at the Salpétrière, Paris, France, published the classical treatise that to this day gives an accurate description of this disorder.

DEFINITION

The criteria for the diagnosis of Gilles de la Tourette syndrome, or multiple tic disorder, have been clearly spelled out by Shapiro et al. (1978). The criteria have been slightly modified but follow three sets of requirements.

The Essential Requirements

1. The usual onset is between the ages of 2 and 15. There have been rare cases of onset after adolescence.
2. The patient has multiple, rapid, stereotypic, involuntary tics, which tend to follow a cephalocaudal distribution, appearing first in the

*Supported in part by Pharmacopsychiatry Fund, University of Minnesota Medical Foundation; and Psychopharmacology Fund, Minneapolis, Minnesota 55455.

F. S. ABUZZAHAB, SR. • Departments of Psychiatry, Pharmacology, and Family Practice and Community Health, University of Minnesota Hospitals, Minneapolis, Minnesota.

head muscles and then spreading to the neck and upper extremities. At times they occur in startling, explosive fashion. Ninety-three percent of patients reported worsening of tics during emotional stress (Brunn *et al.*, 1976).

3. There are usually verbal tics that take the form of grunting, sniffing, and clearing the throat. Occasionally, flagrant symptoms appear that sound like animal noises, e.g., barking. These involuntary vocalizations are produced at the level of the glottis during expiratory air flow (Okamura *et al.*, 1976), a fact confirmed by fluoroscopic, aerodynamic, and sonographic examinations.

4. Voluntary effort can completely control or reduce symptoms for brief periods, and occasionally for prolonged periods, but this results in subsequent tension and ultimate increase in discharged symptomatology.

5. Nonanxious concentration or preoccupation is associated with a decrease in symptoms, and a variety of psychosocial factors may be associated with an increase or decrease in symptoms.

6. Symptoms always disappear during sleep and orgasm.

7. The illness is usually lifelong and chronic, although some lifelong remissions have been reported. Carney (1977) reported a remission of 18 years.

8. The tics tend to be aggravated by dopamine enhancers such as methylphenidate (Golden, 1974, 1977a; Fras and Karlavage, 1977; Pollack *et al.*, 1977) and amphetamine (Woodrow, 1974).

9. The tics tend to be suppressed, and at times completely controlled, by dopamine blockers, such as haloperidol, as well as other neuroleptics, e.g., pimozide (Ross and Moldofsky, 1978).

10. There is an increase in dopamine metabolites in the cerebrospinal fluid of afflicted patients.

Confirmatory, but Not Essential for a Diagnosis

1. The coprophenomena: (a) coprolalia and coprophrasia—the uttering of obscene words—or, at times, an unexpressed urge to utter such words; (b) copropraxia—obscene gestures; (c) coprographia—writing obscene words.

2. The echopathy or echophenomena: (a) echolalia and echophrasia—mimicking words; (b) echopraxia, echokinesis, echomatism, echomimia—mimicking gestures; (c) echopalilalia—the morbid repetition of words spoken by another person.

3. Other obsessive-compulsive symptoms: (a) palilalia—rapid repetition of a word or phrase; (b) haphemania—compulsion to touch; (c)

arithromania—obsession with numbers and counting; (d) autopero-mania—self-mutilation (Shapiro and Shapiro, 1977b).

Frequent Concomitants of the Disorder, but Not Essential for a Diagnosis

1. History of hyperactivity or behavioral problem in childhood or organic stigmata in adulthood (Shapiro et al., 1973b).
2. Abnormal, nonspecific EEG changes (Sweet et al., 1973).
3. Soft signs of neurologic abnormality (Golden, 1977).
4. Subtle signs of organic dysfunction on psychological testing (Logue et al., 1973; Shapiro et al., 1974).
5. Familial history of tics.

CASE HISTORY

The case presented here is rather typical of the syndrome and will present points to be discussed in the remainder of the chapter.

In 1966, at the age of 6, this white male patient (J. S.) began to walk with a double-step type of skipping. Shortly thereafter, he began to demonstrate eye blinking, facial and neck tics, sniffling, and vocalizations. IQ tests done at the time were in the "low-average" range. A few months later he developed coprolalia, expressed in the form of "goddamn." The patient was started on haloperidol, 2 to 3 milligrams daily, in the fall of 1967, with a 90 to 95% reduction in symptoms after 4 to 6 weeks. His symptoms remained under good control until late in 1968, when they began to increase in frequency, especially when he was fatigued or stressed. His dosage of haloperidol was subsequently increased to 24 milligrams per day, but the symptoms came only partially under control. Nonetheless, the patient made adequate progress in school and was able to progressively lower the dosage of the drug. At present, he is on 6 milligrams of haloperidol per day. He has graduated from high school and plans to enter the University of Minnesota in the fall of 1979.

The parents were both dependent and tended to be overly protective. The father expressed some hostility toward the patient and his behavior, while the mother tended to be more passive in her attitude. The parents separated in the fall of 1973.

HISTORY

The clinical features of Gilles de la Tourette syndrome were baffling to the observers and physicians alike. The etiology of this disorder tended to be colored by the prevailing theories of the specific historical era. For simplicity's sake, the disorder can be seen as having passed through four main stages.

Mysticoreligious Stage

The earliest written record of a possible case of Gilles de la Tourette syndrome appeared in Sprenger (1489/1948) in the *Malleus Maleficarum*. A priest was afflicted with uncontrollable thrusting of his tongue. This was attributed to the devil making his tongue thrust; he apparently was cured by exorcism. More recent interest in this disorder appeared in the popular movie, *The Exorcist*, which is based on an exaggerated description of a patient with Gilles de la Tourette syndrome.

Religious dogma played a very important role in the daily lives of the people of the Middle Ages, and religious convictions permeated their intellectual formulations. Therefore, an explanation of this disorder on the basis of possession by demons or the devil, and hence amenable to exorcism, was an accepted explanation of the times. The mysticoreligious phase should be viewed as an essential incubation phase of human knowledge, which paved the way for the Renaissance or Age of Reason.

Clinical-Descriptive Stage

Early 19th-century France was fertile soil for the development of this clinical-descriptive era. The postrevolutionary atmosphere perhaps incited the medical establishment to reject past dogmatic beliefs and pay more attention to what they could detect themselves through accurate clinical observations.

Bouteille (1810) published the book *Treatise on Chorea*, in which he described involuntary movements. He borrowed the word *chorea* from the Greek, which means "dance."

J. M. G. Itard (1825), director of the Royal Institute for Deaf Mutes, Paris, France, described the Marquise de Dampierre, a noblewoman who had involuntary movements and obscene utterances. It is interesting that this lady survived to be studied by Charcot and eventually by Gilles de la Tourette himself.

It appears that Georges Gilles de la Tourette was sidetracked in his article of 1884, when he included the Jumping Frenchmen of Maine, myriachit of Siberia, and latah of Malaysia as similar to multiple tic disorder (see chapter 13). His second paper in 1885 seemed to overemphasize the uncoordinated nature of this movement, a point that was attacked by his contemporary Guinon (1886, 1887). Finally, in his last paper of 1899, he tended to agree with Guinon that the movements were coordinated and systematized. Catrou (1890) consolidated the existing knowledge about this disorder in a thesis submitted to the Faculty of Medicine of Paris.

Psychoanalytic-Psychosocial Stage

The third stage in the history of this disorder is the psychoanalytic-psychosocial stage. Since the group of French neurologists did not have any definitive explanation for multiple tic disorder other than the tics being viewed as possibly a symptom of degeneration, it fell on the psychoanalysts to seek a psychological basis for disorders of unknown etiology. In 1893 Freud wrote that the multiple tic disorder was neurotic in nature. He felt that the cause of this illness could be found by delving into the unconscious. Ferenczi (1921) believed that tiqueurs were narcissistic and that tics were "stereotyped masturbatory equivalents." The initial symptom of eye tic was viewed as an attempt at unconscious repression by the patient, who, as a child, had witnessed his parents having sexual intercourse. The spread of the tics to other muscles of the body and their explosive clinical appearance were viewed by some psychoanalysts as implying an orgasmic equivalent. Ascher (1948) felt that the symptoms of echolalia and coprolalia appeared when the patients developed unacceptable attitudes or feelings toward one or both parents and attempted to suppress them.

Since psychotherapy produces improvement in only 45% of the cases (Abuzzahab and Anderson, 1976), it is rarely used at present as the only modality of treatment. However, it has tremendous value as a form of supportive treatment for patients when used in conjunction with pharmacotherapy (Clements, 1972; Goforth, 1974).

The salient contribution of psychoanalytic theory was to help us accept these patients as human beings and delve into their unconscious to interpret the symptoms of their disease. Prior to the psychoanalytic approach, these patients were shunned by the medical establishment and even imprisoned or chained. Therefore, the psychoanalytic movement should be viewed as the pinnacle of the humanistic treatment of patients with symptoms that were difficult to explain. In this regard, it was a definite advancement over the mysticoreligious approaches. Psychoanalytic theory should be viewed not as harming patients (Shapiro et al., 1978) but as an essential stage in the history of this disorder without which we could not have approached the current genetic and neurochemical theories.

Genetic and Neurochemical Stage

This era was heralded by Seignot's report (1961) of a case of Gilles de la Tourette syndrome cured with R-1625, which was the code for haloperidol. His observation was replicated throughout the world, starting with Caprini and Melotti (1961). Overall success from the application of haloperidol is in the range of 89% (Abuzzahab and Anderson, 1976).

Since one of the principles of pharmacology is that a drug does not act in a vacuum but alters preexisting neurochemical pathways, the success of haloperidol in controlling tics in a clinical setting was used by the neurochemist as a key to unlock the secrets of the brain. Abuzzahab speculated in an abstract submitted to the American Psychiatric Association in 1968 that haloperidol blocked dopamine receptors in the brains of Gilles de la Tourette syndrome victims, and that the underlying disorder might therefore be an excess of CNS dopamine. The speculation was later confirmed by the work of Messiha et al. (1971) and Snyder et al. (1970).

Since genes cannot transmit any trait unless it is chemical in nature, the neurochemical theory led to the birth of a new field known as behavior genetics. A parallel phenomenon has occurred in schizophrenia, manic depressive disorders, sleep disorders, and presenile and senile dementias. In other words, the introduction of a pharmacologic agent to control these diseases led to speculation about a neurochemical substrate upon which these drugs are working. This, in turn, kindled interest in tracing genetics of Gilles de la Tourette syndrome. Friel (1973) reported three cases with familial incidence, Sanders (1973) reported two cases in father and son, Frost et al. (1976) had one case of familial incidence, and Merskey (1974) reported on Gilles de la Tourette syndrome with XYY karyotype. Eldridge et al. (1977) studied 21 families in the New York area. In 12 of 13 Jewish families, there were multiple members with motor and vocal tics. Wassman et al. (1978) replicated this study in Minneapolis and found 13 out of 14 families affected.

EPIDEMIOLOGY

The mean age of onset is 7.2 years. Thirty percent of patients develop Tourette syndrome before age 6, 58% by age 7, 80% by age 9, and 90% by age 11. These figures of Shapiro et al. (1978) agree with the figures of Abuzzahab and Anderson (1976). Less than 4% of all cases have symptom onset beyond the age of 20. Araneta et al. (1975) described a case with symptom onset at age 35.

The Tourette Syndrome Association, Inc., estimates that there are 10,000 cases in the United States of America. This is probably a conservative estimate. Estimates of its incidence worldwide range from 0.005 to 0.8 per 1,000 population (Shapiro et al., 1978).

Seventy-one percent of 439 cases reported in the literature were male (Abuzzahab and Anderson, 1976). This is similar to the ratio of males to females of 3:1 reported by Shapiro et al. (1978).

When 426 cases in the literature were divided by country of origin, 137 came from the United States, 105 from France, 57 from Germany, 52 from the United Kingdom, 46 from Italy, 13 from Eastern Europe, 9 from Scandinavia, 5 from India, and 2 from Japan (Abuzzahab and Anderson, 1974). This indicates that the disorder is not limited to the Caucasians in the Western world, as was originally thought. Carroll (1974) reported a case in a 12-year-old black male. Interest in publishing might reflect a higher incidence in the literature from the Western world, although there are several reports in the literature from non-Western countries (Verma and Magotra, 1976; Yamane et al., 1977).

In spite of minor variations, there was a high correlation between samples from different cultures. For example, the male–female ratio showed an excellent fit. Cases from the United States had earlier age of onset than European cases, which was statistically significant. The Italian sample showed a significantly higher incidence of eye tics, while the French showed significantly fewer. There were more neck tics observed in the United States sample than in the French sample. The British sample displayed less echophenomena, while the other vocal phenomena fit closely. The French showed more echokinesis. Coprolalia was found to occur in the United States sample to a significantly higher frequency than elsewhere.

The lack of major variation of symptoms in this cross-cultural analysis points to the fact that neurochemical factors are more important than cultural factors in the evolution of the disease.

SYMPTOMS

The initial symptom is a head tic in 20% of the cases, a facial grimace in 11%, and other types of tic in 42% of the cases (Shapiro et al., 1978). Nineteen percent of the cases begin with sounds. Coprolalia as an initial symptom occurs in only 6.2%.

It usually takes several years for a full clinical picture to evolve. Coprolalia develops in 55.3% of the cases, according to Shapiro et al. (1978), with average year of onset at 13.5 years. Thus, not all patients develop these symptoms (Abuzzahab and Anderson, 1976), underscoring the error in calling this illness the "cursing disease," as some have done. The expletives tend to be monosyllabic and repetitive, as well as stereotyped. In other words, children expressing coprolalia do not tend to vary the expletive. This is in marked contrast to the use of expletives in certain segments of our society where the use of obscene utterances varies with the occasion.

Therefore, while the occurrence of a monosyllabic, stereotyped expletive—coprolalia and coprophrasia—with multiple tics might lead to the diagnosis of Gilles de la Tourette syndrome with a neurochemical disturbance, the reverse is not true. Use of obscene language—coprophemia—without motor tics does not indicate a neurochemical disorder but rather points to an acquired habit depending upon the subculture of the individual.

EXPERIMENTAL AND LABORATORY INFORMATION

The Wechsler Intelligence Scale (WISC) for children, with 45 full-scale scores reported, indicates an almost normal distribution. In 66 cases, intelligence was described as "average," in 26 "above average," and in 14 "below average" (Abuzzahab and Anderson, 1976). Shapiro *et al.* (1978) reported a significant deficit in performance ability in the adult patients on the Wechsler Adult Intelligence Scale (WAIS).

Organic impairment based on the Bender Gestalt, WAIS, and WISC scales was reported as high as 68% in patients with Gilles de la Tourette syndrome versus 28% in a control group (Shapiro *et al.*, 1978). In addition, psychological testing to reveal schizophrenia, underlying psychosis, obsessive-compulsive traits, inhibition of aggression, or hysteria did not characterize subjects who had Gilles de la Tourette syndrome (Shapiro *et al.*, 1978).

Martindale (1976) suggested that tics vary in form independent of lexical environment, based on his analysis of 2 hours of speech by a patient who was not being treated with any medication. Further analysis (Martindale, 1977) showed tics occurring in longer sentences. This led Martindale to hypothesize that, normally, the need for coordination of material in long sentences activates a subcortical center, causing momentary cortical inhibition to prevent cognition from outracing phonation. In Gilles de la Tourette syndrome, the subcortical area, he speculated, malfunctions and tics are injected into speech. Frank (1978) speculated that Gilles de la Tourette syndrome represented a malfunctioning of the extrapyramidal tracts resulting in exaggeration and distortions of normal phenomena within all functions of speech.

Of 102 patients with electroencephalograms (EEG), 45% were reported as "abnormal" (Abuzzahab and Anderson, 1976). This percentage compared with 57.1% of abnormal EEG, reported by Shapiro *et al.* (1978). Abnormalities included bilateral sharp waves, diffuse background, disorganization, slowing, and frequent unilateral temporal-occipital slowing and sharp waves.

It should be noted that Gilles de la Tourette syndrome is *not* a convulsive disorder. These tics are usually absent during sleep and there are no focal abnormalities. Furthermore, anticonvulsive treatment does not control the symptoms.

Left-handedness and ambidexterity were reported in 22.8% (Shapiro *et al.*, 1978) of these patients. The authors felt the incidence high enough to warrant speculation about early brain injury and Gilles de la Tourette syndrome. The finding of minor asymmetries in 57.1% of carefully examined patients may also indicate such a relationship.

Neuropathological findings in Gilles de la Tourette syndrome are rare. The first autopsy was reported by Bing (1925), who found specific meningitic thickening upon gross examination of the brain. No microscopic examination was performed.

The second autopsy was by DeWulf and van Bogaert (1940), who found no extrapyramidal lesion. Balthasar (1956–57) described generalized encephalitic changes in the corpus striatum. Borak (1969) demonstrated congenital vasculopathy in all areas of the cortex and in subcortical structures. There are two unpublished reports of autopsies in the international registry that were negative, and, overall, there has been no conclusive evidence found on autopsy. What is really needed is neurochemical study of brain tissue, rather than histologic and gross anatomic findings.

DIFFERENTIAL DIAGNOSIS

The differential diagnosis of Gilles de la Tourette syndrome can be subdivided into intoxications, "common" disorders, and "rare" disorders.

Common Disorders

The three common disorders with which Gilles de la Tourette syndrome is confused are the simple transient tic of childhood, the hyperkinetic syndrome, and Sydenham's chorea.

Simple Transient Tic of Childhood. The simple tic is usually transient (Bachman, 1977). It is generally not multiple or vocal. Although there is some feeling that there is a spectrum of tic disorders, starting with the simple transient tic at one extreme to Gilles de la Tourette syndrome at the other end of the spectrum (Golden, 1978), consensus is that this is a separate entity.

The Hyperkinetic Syndrome. The hyperkinetic syndrome, or minimal brain dysfunction syndrome, is a very popular diagnosis these days. Consequently, many mild cases of Gilles de la Tourette syndrome initially are labeled "hyperkinesis." A differential point is that patients with

Gilles de la Tourette syndrome will get worse when they are treated with methylphenidate. This is sometimes the clue that leads parents to seek other opinions. In addition, hyperkinetic children do not usually have multiple muscular and vocal tics.

Sydenham's Chorea. Sydenham's chorea, previously known as "chorea minor," is more predominant in females than in males. Manifestations include streptococcal septicemia and eosinophilia. Seventy-five percent are associated with rheumatic fever. Its course is generally self-limiting.

Rare Disorders

Shapiro *et al.* (1978) have listed some rare disorders with which Gilles de la Tourette syndrome can be confused.

Athetoid Type of Cerebral Palsy. The athetoid type of cerebral palsy (Boshes, 1976) occurs between birth and age 3 and usually is static after age 3. It includes features of mental retardation, and movements tend to be athetoid.

Dystonia Musculorum Deformans. DMD occurs between the ages of 5 and 15, with a characteristic torsion dystonia, usually progressive until death. It seems to have familial occurrence, with a high incidence in Russian Jews.

Encephalitis Lethargica. Encephalitis lethargica, or Von Economo's encephalitis, can affect any age. There usually are Parkinsonian symptoms. There have been no recent occurrences of this encephalitis.

Hallervorden-Spatz Disease. This disease usually occurs around the age of 10 and is associated with choreic and athetoid myoclonic movements, optic atrophy, clubbed feet, retinitis pigmentosa, dysarthria, dementia, and emotional lability. It is usually progressive.

Huntington's Chorea. Huntington's chorea is extremely rare in childhood. The usual age of onset is between 30 and 50, with familial and choreiform movements being prominent. It is estimated that about 1% of cases occur in childhood.

Pelizaeus-Merzbacher's Disease. This illness occurs in infancy, is familial, and occurs predominantly in males. Choreoathetoid movements are prominent and progressive to ages 5 and 6, at which point the disease becomes static.

Spastic Torticollis. Spastic torticollis affects any age and manifests itself as a torsion or dystonia of the neck. Usually there are no vocal tics associated with it.

Status Dismyelinatus. Status dismyelinatus occurs in the first year, with abnormal movements that are gradually replaced by rigidity, leading to death in the second decade.

Wilson's Disease. Wilson's disease, or hepatolenticular degeneration, occurs between the ages of 10 and 25 and has a pathognomonic Kayser-Fleischer ring in the eye, with liver cirrhosis and a low blood ceruloplasmin. The disease is due to deposition of toxic amounts of copper in various tissues.

Leysch-Nyhan's Disease. This syndrome occurs in the second year. Its cause is a hypoxanthine phosphoribosyl transferase enzyme defect. It is a recessive disease, sex-linked in males, and includes mental retardation, self-mutilation, biting, screaming, spasticity, and coprolalia. It is usually progressive to death. Some recent authors have suspected that Gilles de la Tourette syndrome might be related to this disorder (Van Woert *et al.*, 1977), but the finding is not confirmed by others (Moldofsky *et al.*, 1974; Johnson *et al.*, 1977; Singer *et al.*, 1979).

Intoxications. Of all toxic disorders, manganese poisoning most closely resembles Gilles de la Tourette syndrome, as it often causes choreiform movements. Usually there is an extrapyramidal rigidity.

TREATMENT

There is no cure for multiple tic disorder. Several methods, however, have been developed for the diminution of its frequency and intensity. Three of these approaches will be discussed here: psychosurgery, behavior modification, and pharmacology.

Psychosurgery

Beckers (1973) reported three patients with Gilles de la Tourette syndrome who improved after stereotactic surgery. De Divitiis, *et al.* (1977) reported on three patients who underwent surgery on the right thalamus. One case had a small reduction in symptomatology. The other two had a complete remission that lasted 2 years, after which the tics gradually returned.

In view of the national concern regarding psychosurgery, as well as the above literature, it is felt that psychosurgery should be used only as a last resort and only in the most severe cases when all other modalities have been exhausted.

Behavior Modification

Several reports of behavior modification in individual patients have been made. Reinforcement contingency management, self-recording, and mass practice were used in controlling tics in a 9-year-old boy. Mass practice seemed to have a greater effect on tic frequency and topography than did the other behavior therapy (Sand and Carlson, 1973). Fernando (1976) advocated the use of mass practice as an alternative to medication.

Another approach (Rosen and Wesner, 1973) employed a patient's peers as a reinforcer for the control of coprolalic behavior. Doleys and Kurtz (1974) reported success with one patient in significantly reducing gutteral sounds and in increasing acceptable social behaviors, eye contact, and personal hygiene by using reinforcement contingencies over a 5-month treatment period.

In still another case, Cohen and Marks (1977) reported on the use of operant conditioning employed by the parents of the patient in the home. A system of stars and money for a tic-free period was employed. In still another patient, participation in high-probability activities like playing pocket billiards when tics were low was made contingent upon low-probability activities like bowling when tics were worse (Jansma, 1978).

Although the data are slim, behavior modification seems to offer an ingenious and elegant approach to the reduction of tics. In clinical practice, however, it is rarely possible to utilize such a modality unless one is dealing with a highly motivated child and parents. Massed practice, which includes asking the tiqueur to indulge to his heart's content in deliberately inducing the tic, is usually followed by a tic-free period. In children with vocal tics, the use of a tape-recording device during massed practice might increase compliance.

Pharmacologic Control of Tics

There is much evidence that central nervous system monoamines play a role in the pathophysiology of Gilles de la Tourette syndrome. Drugs that block dopamine in the brain, such as neuroleptics, or drugs that inhibit synthesis of dopamine e.g., alphamethylparatyrosine (Sweet et al., 1974) or inhibit storage, e.g., tetrabenazine (Sweet et al. 1974) and reserpine, decrease the tics (Gonge and Barbeau, 1977a). Thus, dopamine hyperactivity may well be the underlying basis of the illness. Indeed, dopamine metabolite excretion is related to treatment response in Gilles de la Tourette syndrome (Messiha and Knopp. 1976). Van Woert *et al.* (1976) found elevated HVA, the major metabolite of dopamine, in the cerebrospinal fluid of Gilles de la Tourette patients.

Haloperidol, as well as all neuroleptics, produces its effect by blockage of dopamine receptors. For example, flupenthixol 6 mg for 2 weeks was used in controlling tics (Cookson, 1975). Lithium treatment in Gilles de la Tourette syndrome was suggested by Dalen (1973). Messiha *et al.* (1976) showed that when lithium blood levels stabilized at 0.8–1.0 mEq/ 1, the major tics and involuntary sounds cleared dramatically in two patients. Erickson *et al.* (1977) reported similar results in three patients.

GABA-mimetic drugs can indirectly decrease dopamine hyperactivity. Benzodiazepines seem to increase the efficiency of GABAergic transmission when these synapses are activated. The benzodiazepines increase the affinity of GABA receptors for GABA and therefore act with precision, providing a fine tuning at the level of synapses where small amounts of the neurotransmitter are released (Costa and Guidotti, 1979). Gonge and Barbeau (1977b) reported that seven patients received partial relief with clonazepam.

Since dopamine receptor blockade by haloperidol tends to increase dopamine receptor sensitivity, Friedhoff (1977) advanced the possibility of giving levodopa to increase the supply of ligand dopamine. After initial worsening of symptoms, there was improvement in Gilles de la Tourette syndrome.

Kondo and Kabasawa (1978) reported improvement in Gilles de la Tourette syndrome with corticosteroid therapy.

Other medications that have been reported are carbamazepine (Lutz, 1977) and chlorimipramine (Yaryura-Tobias, 1975).

Initiation of Pharmacologic Treatment

Patients whose tics are interfering with their general functioning— school, job, or social interaction—should be started on medication. Haloperidol has been the most widely used dopamine blocker for the control of tics. Patients with mild forms of the disorder should not be given neuroleptics.

The initial dose is 0.25 to 0.5 mg (Shapiro and Shapiro, 1977a) at bedtime. This can gradually be increased to reach a therapeutic level (Lawall and Pietzcker, 1973; Alliez and Audon, 1975; Asam and Trager, 1975; Perera, 1975; Erenberg and Rothner, 1978; Murray, 1978). The end point is control of tics or the emergence of disabling side effects, such as Parkinsonian symptoms or sedation. The akathisia that sometimes occurs from haloperidol can be controlled with diphenhydramine, and the akinesia and dystonia can be controlled with anticholinergic agents such as benztropine mesylate. It is wise not to give anticholinergic agents on a routine basis, however, since they tend to increase dopamine hypersensitivity and thus lead to tardive dyskinesia.

Concomitant administration of lithium carbonate with neuroleptics has been postulated to reduce the incidence of tardive dyskinesia. It is, however, too early to state with certainty that this is a useful combination, since the incidence of tardive dyskinesia in patients treated for Gilles de la Tourette syndrome remains very low (Caine et al., 1978). In advising parents and patients about treatment, one should bear in mind that the benefit of tic control with haloperidol on the general functioning of the patient with severe tics far outweighs the possible risk of tardive dyskinesia.

Long-Term Pharmacology

Since there are no tests or factors that help the clinician determine whether the multiple tic disorder is going to progress throughout life or disappear, it becomes essential that haloperidol, when used in the control of the tics, be gradually reduced to the minimum effective dose. Since haloperidol has a long half-life, it can also be omitted on weekends, provided tics do not recur. During long school holidays, the patients could be taken off haloperidol to see if they still needed it. If tics recur, the medication can be reinstated (Jeste, et al., 1973). In this manner, the least amount of neuroleptic is given over a long period of time, thus minimizing the chances of side effects from the haloperidol (Gittelman-Klein, 1978). The tendency of haloperidol to produce overcontrol and impairment in temporal processing will also be minimized (Goldstone and Lhamon, 1976).

Monitoring patients on haloperidol for possible emergence of depression is also indicated in adults (Penna and Lion, 1975). Shapiro et al. (1973a) followed 21 patients with Gilles de la Tourette syndrome treated with 6–180 mg haloperidol in the acute phase of their illness for between 2 months and 5 years. Depression occurred in all who took more than 8 mg haloperidol per day.

PROGNOSIS

The international registry for Gilles de la Tourette syndrome was founded at the University of Minnesota in an attempt to collect cases of this rare disorder and establish the natural history of the syndrome (Abuzzahab and Ehlen, 1971; Abuzzahab and Anderson, 1973).

To date, we have 110 unpublished cases of Gilles de la Tourette syndrome that have come to our attention. It seems that prognosis is significantly better for girls than for boys (Shapiro et al., 1978; Zausmer, 1954). The prognosis is also better for those whose tics began at between 6 and

8 years of age (Shapiro et al., 1978; Corbett, et al., 1969). Adolescent onset had poor outcome (Milman, 1975). Recent publicity in the lay press about this disorder has led to earlier recognition and treatment of the disease (Shapiro and Shapiro, 1974). We hope that this will result in better outcomes. If tics are controlled early in life and not permitted to become ingrained in the personality of the child, the outcome is usually favorable.

TOURETTE SYNDROME ASSOCIATION, INC.

In 1971 parents of patients suffering from Gilles de la Tourette syndrome organized a meeting in New York. The association was incorporated March 21, 1972, and now has several local chapters. Through articles in the lay press (Martin, 1977), they have been able to educate the public and physicians. The association was able to call for a national conference in May 1979 for all chapters. Their efforts to secure research funds for Tourette's syndrome have to be complimented. Furthermore, the local chapters have provided social support for the children, instead of hiding them in seclusion for fear that they might be shunned (Abuzzahab et al., 1975).

Aside from the introduction of haloperidol for tic control, the Tourette Syndrome Association, Inc., should be viewed as the most important development in the history of Gilles de la Tourette syndrome.

CONCLUSION

Gilles de la Tourette syndrome is a rare disorder manifested by multiple tics, including vocalizations and, at times, coprolalia. Its usual onset is in childhood and early adolescence, with a preponderance of 3:1 in male versus females. Symptoms of this disorder have a variable course and can be controlled with dopamine blocking agents such as haloperidol. The most accepted hypothesis is that there are genetic neurochemical disturbances leading to dopamine hyperactivity in the brain. It has not been determined whether psychological and social stresses by themselves could induce such neurochemical disturbances in the brain. A combination of psychosocial support and haloperidol seems most efficacious in controlling severe cases.

REFERENCES

Abuzzahab, F. S., Sr., and Anderson, F. O., 1973, Gilles de la Tourette's syndrome, Minn. Med. 56:492.
Abuzzahab, F. S., Sr., and Anderson, F. O., 1974, Gilles de la Tourette's syndrome: Cross-cultural analysis and treatment outcome, Clin. Neurol. Neurosurg. 1:66.

94   F. S. ABUZZAHAB, SR.

cultural analysis and treatment outcome, *Clin. Neurol. Neurosurg.* 1:66.

Abuzzahab, F. S., Sr., and Ehlen, K. J., 1971, The clinical picture and management of Gilles de la Tourette's syndrome, *Child Psychiatry Hum. Dev.* 5:224.

Abuzzahab, F. S., Sr., and Anderson, F. O., 1976, "Gilles de la Tourette's Syndrome," Vol. 1, Mason, St. Paul.

Abuzzahab, F. S., Sr., and Anderson, F. O., and Sekhon, S. M., 1975, Multiple tic disorder: Gilles de la Tourette's syndrome, *Pract. Psychol. Phys.* 2:58.

Alliez, J., and Audon, S., 1975, Gilles de la Tourette's disease, *Ann. Med. Psychol. (Paris)* 2:489.

Araneta, E., Magen, J., Musci, M. N., Jr., Singer, P., and Vann, C. R., 1975, Gilles de la Tourette's syndrome symptom onset at age 35, *Child Psychiatry Hum. Dev.* 5:224.

Asam, U., and Trager, S.-E., 1975, Therapeutische Aspekte der Gilles de la Touretteschen Erkrankung, Nervenarzt 46:361.

Ascher, E., 1948, Psychodynamic considerations in Gilles de la Tourette's disease (maladie des tics), *Am. J. Psychiatry* 105:267.

Bachman, D. S., 1977, Gilles de la Tourette's syndrome, *Ohio State Med. J.* 74:429.

Balthasar, J., 1956–57, Ueber das anatomische Substrat der generalisierten Tic-Krankheit, *Arch. Psychiatr. Nervenkr.* 195:531.

Beckers, W., 1973, Zur Gilles de la Touretteschen Erkrankung anhand von fünf eigenen Beobachtungen, *Arch. Psychiatr. Nervenkr.* 217:169.

Bing, R., 1925, Ueber lokale Muskelspasmen und Tics, *Schweiz. Med. Wochenschr.* 55:993.

Borak, W., 1969, Przypadek encefalopatii z tikami Tourette'a zespolem anankastycznym i impulsywymi tendencjami do samouszkodzen, *Psychiatr. Pol.* 3:111.

Boshes, L. D., 1976, Gilles de la Tourette's syndrome, *Am. J. Nurs.* 76:1637.

Bouteille, E. M., 1810, *"Traite de Chorée,"* Vicard Press, Paris.

Brunn, R. D., Shapiro, A. K., Shapiro, E., Sweet, R. D., Wayne, H, and Solomon, G. E., 1976, A follow-up of 78 patients with Gilles de la Tourette's syndrome, *Am. J. Psychiatry* 133:944.

Caine, E. D., Margolin, D. I., Brown, G. L., and Ebert, M. H., 1978, Gilles de la Tourette's syndrome, tardive dyskinesia, and psychosis in an adolescent, *Am. J. Psychiatry* 135:241.

Caprini, G., and Melotti, V., 1961, Un grave sindrome ticcosa guarita con haloperidol, *Riv. Sper. Freniatr.* 85:191.

Carney, P. A., 1977, Recurrence of Gilles de la Tourette syndrome, *Br. Med. J.* 1:884.

Carroll, W. J., 1974, Gilles de la Tourette syndrome, *Va. Med. Mon.* 101:672.

Catrou, J., 1890, *Etude sur la maladie des tics convulsifs (jumping, latah, myriachit),* Thèse, Henri Jouve Press, Paris.

Clements, R. O., 1972, Gilles de la Tourette's syndrome—An overview of development and treatment of a case, using hypnotherapy, haloperidol, and psychotherapy, *Am. J. Clin. Hypn.* 14:167.

Cohen, D., and Marks, F. M., 1977, Gilles de la Tourette's syndrome treated by operant conditioning (Letter), *Br. J. Psychiatry* 130:315.

Cookson, I. B., 1975, Speech disorder, partial syndrome of Gilles de la Tourette, and drug therapy (Letter), *Br. J. Psychiatry* 126:395.

Corbett, J. A., Mathews, A. M., Connell, P. H., and Shapiro, D. A., 1969, Tics and Gilles de la Tourette's syndrome: A follow-up study and critical review, *Br. J. Psychiatry* 115:1229.

Costa, E., and Guidotti, A., 1979, Molecular mechanisms in the receptor action of benzodiazephines, *Annu. Rev. Pharmacol. Toxicol.* 19:531.

Dalen, 1973, Gilles de la Tourette's disease, *Br. J. Psychiatry* 123:378.

de Divitiis, E., D'Errico, A., and Cerillo, A., 1977, Stereotactic surgery in Gilles de la Tourette syndrome, *Acta Neurochir.* (Suppl. 24):73.

DeWulf, A., and van Bogaert, L., 1940, Etudes anatomo-cliniques de syndromes hyper-cinetiques complexes, *Mschr. Psychiatr. Neurol.* 103:53.

Doleys, D. M., and Kurtz, P. S., 1974, A behavioral treatment program for the Gilles de la Tourette syndrome, *Psychol. Rep.* 35:74.

Eldridge, R., Sweet, R., Lake, C. R., Ziegler, M., and Shapiro, A. K., 1977, Gilles de la Tourette's syndrome: Clinical, genetic, psychologic, and biochemical aspects in 21 selected families, *Neurology (Minn.)* 27:115.

Erenberg, G., and Rothner, A. D., 1978, Tourette syndrome: A childhood disorder, *Cleveland Clin. Q.* 45:207.

Erickson, H. M., Jr., Goggin, J. E., and Messiha, F. S., 1977, Comparison of lithium and haloperidol therapy in Gilles de la Tourette syndrome, *Adv. Exp. Med. Biol.* 90:197.

Ferenczi, S., 1921, Psycho-analytical observations on tic, *Int. J. Psychol.* 2:1

Fernando, S. J. M., 1976, Six cases of Gilles de la Tourette's syndrome, *Br. J. Psychiatry* 128:436.

Frank, S. M., 1978, Psycholinguistic findings in Gilles de la Tourette syndrome, *J. Commun. Disord.* 11:349.

Fras, I., and Karlavage, J., 1977, The use of methylphenidate and imipramine in Gilles de la Tourette's disease in children, *Am. J. Psychiatry* 134:195.

Friedhoff, A. J., 1977, The psychiatric clinical syndrome and essential corresponding qualities of an animal model of receptor sensitivity modification, *in* "Animal Models in Psychiatry and Neurology" (I. Hanin and E. Usdin, eds.), pp. 51–59, Pergamon Press, Oxford.

Friel, P. B., 1973, Familial incidence of Gilles de la Tourette's disease, with observations on aetiology and treatment, *Br. J. Psychiatry* 122:655.

Frost, N., Feighner, J., and Schuckit, M. A., 1976, A family study of Gilles de la Tourette syndrome, *Dis. Nerv. Syst.* 37:537.

Gilles de la Tourette, G., 1884, Jumping, latah, myriachit, *Arch. Neurol. (Paris)* 8:68.

Gilles de la Tourette, G., 1885, Etude sur une affection nerveuse, caracterisée par de l'incoordination motrice, accompagnée d'echolalie et de coprolalie, *Arch. Neurol. (Paris)* 9:19, 158–200.

Gilles de la Tourette, G., 1899, La maladie des tics convulsifs, *Sem. Med. (Paris)* 12:153.

Gittelman-Klein, R., 1978, Psychopharmacological treatment of anxiety disorders, mood disorders, and Tourette's disorder in children, *in* "Psychopharmacology: A Generation of Progress," (M. Lipton, A. DiMascio, and K. F. Killam, eds.), pp. 1471–1480, Raven Press, New York.

Goforth, E. G., 1974, A single case study: Gilles de la Tourette's syndrome, *J. Nerv. Ment. Dis.,* 158:306.

Golden, G. S., 1974, Gilles de la Tourette's syndrome following methylphenidate administration, *Dev. Med. Child Neurol.* 16:76.

Golden, G. S., 1977a, The effect of central nervous system stimulants on Tourette syndrome, *Ann. Neurol.* 2:69.

Golden, G. S., 1978, Tics and Tourette's: A continuum of symptoms? *Ann. Neurol.* 4:145.

Goldstone, S., and Lhamon, W. T., 1976, The effects of haloperidol upon temporal information processing by patients with Tourette's syndrome, *Psychopharmacologia* 50:7.

Gonge, M., and Barbeau, A., 1977a, La maladie de Gilles de la Tourette, *Union Med. Can.* 106:559.

Gonge, M., and Barbeau, A., 1977b, Seven cases of Gilles de la Tourette's syndrome: Partial relief with clonazepam: A pilot study, *Can. J. Neurol. Sci.* 4:279.

Guinon, G., 1886, Sur la maladie des tics convulsifs, *Rev. Med. (Paris)* 1:50.

Guinon, G., 1887, Tics convulsifs et hysterie, *Rev. Med. (Paris)* 7:509.

Itard, J. M. G., 1825, Memoire sur quelques fonctions involuntaires des appareils de la locomotion, de la prehension, et de la voie. *Arch. Gen. Med.* 8:387.

Jansma, P., 1978, Operant conditioning principles applied to disturbed male adolescents by a physical educator, *Am. Correct. Ther. J.* 32:7178.

Jeste, D. V., Sule, S. M., Apte, J. S., and Vahia, M. S., 1973, Gilles de la Tourette's disease. Multiple vocal and motor tics, *Indian J. Pediatr.* 40:435.

Johnson, G. G., Pepple, J. M., Singer, H. S., and Littlefield, J. W., 1977, HGPRT in the Gilles de la Tourette syndrome (Letter), *N. Engl. J. Med.* 297:339.

Kondo, K., and Kabasawa, T., 1978, Improvement in Gilles de la Tourette syndrome after corticosteroid therapy, *Ann. Neurol.* 4:387.

Lawall, P. Ch., and Pietzcker, A., 1973, Das Gilles de la Tourettesche Syndrom, *Fortschr. Neurol. Psychiatr.* 41:282.

Logue, P. E., Platzek, D., Hutzell, R., and Robinson, B., 1973; Neurological, neuropsychological and behavioral aspects of Gilles de la Tourette's syndrome: A case, *Percept. Mot. Skills* 37:855.

Lutz, E. G., 1977, Alternative drug treatments in Gilles de la Tourette's syndrome (Letters), *Am. J. Psychiatry* 134:98.

Martin, A., 1977, Tourette's syndrome, *Child. Today* 6:26.

Martindale, C., 1976, The grammar of the tic in Gilles de la Tourette's syndrome, *Lang. Speech* 19:266.

Martindale, C., 1977, Syntactic and semantic correlates of verbal tics in Gilles de la Tourette's syndrome: A quantitative case study, *Brain Lang.* 4:231.

Merskey, H., 1974, A case of multiple tics with vocalisation (Partial syndrome of Gilles de la Tourette) and XYY karyotype, *Br. J. Psychiatry* 125:593.

Messiha, F. S., and Knopp. W., 1976, A study of endogenous dopamine metabolism in Gilles de la Tourette's disease, *Dis. Nerv. Syst.* 37:470.

Messiha, F. S., Knopp, W., Vanecko, S., O'Brien, V., and Corson, S. A., 1971, Haloperidol therapy in Tourette's syndrome: Neurophysiological, biochemical and behavioral correlates, *Life Sci.* 10:449.

Messiha, F. S., Erickson, H. M., Jr., and Goggin, J. E., 1976, Lithium carbonate in Gilles de la Tourette's disease, *Res. Commun. Chem. Pathol. Pharmacol.* 15:609.

Milman, D. H., 1975, Gilles de la Tourette syndrome, *N.Y. State J. Med.* 75:892.

Moldofsky, H., Tullis, C., and Lamon, R., 1974, Multiple tic syndrome (Gilles de la Tourette's syndrome), *J. Nerv. Ment. Dis.* 159:282.

Murray, T. J., 1978, Tourette's syndrome: A treatable tic, *Can. Med. Assoc. J.* 118:1407.

Okamura, H., Kitazima, K., and Isshiki, N., 1976, Involuntary vocalization: Two cases of Gilles de la Tourette's disease, *Folia Phoniatr.* 28:182.

Penna, M. W., and Lion, J. R., 1975, Gilles de la Tourette's syndrome and depression: A case report, *Dis. Nerv. Syst.* 36:41.

Perera, H. V., 1975, Two cases of Gilles de la Tourette's syndrome treated with haloperidol, *Br. J. Psychiatry* 127:324.

Pollack, M. A., Cohen, N. L., and Friedhoff, A. J., 1977, Gilles de la Tourette's syndrome. Familial occurrence and precipitation by methylphenidate therapy. *Arch. Neurol.* 34:630.

Rosen, M., and Wesner, C., 1973, Case report. A behavioral approach to Tourette's syndrome, *J. Consult. Clin. Psychol.* 41:308.

Ross, M. S., and Moldofsky, H., 1978, A comparison of pimozide and haloperidol in the treatment of Gilles de la Tourette's syndrome, *Am. J. Psychiatry* 135:585.

Sand, P. L., and Carlson, C., 1973, Failure to establish control over tics in the Gilles de la Tourette syndrome with behaviour therapy techniques, *Br. J. Psychiatry* 122:665.

Sanders, D. G., 1973, Familial occurrence of Gilles de la Tourette syndrome. Report of the syndrome occuring in a father and son, *Arch. Gen. Psychiatry* 28:326.

Seignot, N. J., 1961, Un cas de maladie des tics de Gilles de la Tourette gueri par le R-1625, *Ann. Med.-Psychol.* 119:578.
Shapiro, A. K., and Shapiro, E., 1974, Gilles de la Tourette's syndrome, *Am. Fam. Physician* 9:94.
Shapiro, A. K., and Shapiro, E., 1977a, Treatment of Gilles de la Tourette syndrome (Letter), *J. Am. Med. Assoc.* 238:29.
Shapiro, A. K., and Shapiro, E., 1977b, Subcategorizing Gilles de la Tourette's syndrome, *Am. J. Psychiatry* 134:818.
Shapiro, A. K., Shapiro, E., and Wayne, H., 1973a, Treatment of Tourette's syndrome with haloperidol: Review of 34 cases, *Arch. Gen. Psychiatry* 28:92.
Shapiro, A. K., Shapiro, E., Wayne, H., and Clarkin, J., 1973b, Organic factors in Gilles de la Tourette's syndrome, *Br. J. Psychiatry* 122:659.
Shapiro, E., Shapiro, A. K., and Clarkin, J., 1974, Clinical psychological testing in Tourette's syndrome, *J. Pers. Assess.* 38:464.
Shapiro, A. K., Shapiro, E. S., Bruun, R. D., and Sweet, R. D., 1978, "Gilles de la Tourette Syndrome," Raven Press, New York.
Singer, H. S., Pepple, J. M., Ramage, A. L., and Butler, I. J., 1978, Gilles de la Tourette syndrome: Further studies and thoughts, *Ann. Neurol.* 4:21.
Snyder, S. H., Taylor, K. H., Coyle, J. T., and Meyerhoff, J. L., 1970, The role of brain dopamine in behavioral regulation and the actions of psychotropic drugs, *Am. J. Psychiatry* 127:199.
Sprenger, J., 1489, "Malleus Maleficarum" (Trans. by M. Summers, 1948), Pushkin Press, London.
Sweet, R. D., Solomon, G. E., Wayne, H., Shapiro, E., and Shapiro, A. K., 1973, Neurological features of Gilles de la Tourette's syndrome, *J. Neurol. Neurosurg. Psychiatry* 36:1.
Sweet, R. D., Bruun, R., Shapiro, E., and Shapiro, A. K., 1974, Presynaptic catecholamine antagonists as treatment for Tourette syndrome, *Arch. Gen. Psychiatry* 31:857.
Van Woert, M. H., Jutkowitz, R., Rosenbaum, D., and Bowers, M. P., Jr., 1976, Gilles de la Tourette's syndrome: Biochemical approaches, *in* "The Basal Ganglia" (M. D. Yahr, ed), pp. 459–465, Raven Press, New York.
Van Woert, M. H., Yip, L. C., and Balis, M. E., 1977, Purine phosphoribosyltransferase in Gilles de la Tourette syndrome, *N. Engl. J. Med.* 296:210.
Verma, K. C., and Magotra, M. L., 1976, Gilles de la Tourette's syndrome with review of literature, *Indian Pediatr.* 13:871.
Wassman, E. R., Eldridge, R., Abuzzahab, F. S., Sr., and Nee, L., 1978, Gilles de la Tourette syndrome: Clinical and genetic studies in a midwestern city, *Neurology (Minn.)* 28:304.
Woodrow, K. M., 1974, Gilles de la Tourette's disease—A review, *Am. J. Psychiatry* 131:1000.
Yamane, H., Katoh, N., Tani, N., Iwase, N., Takahashi, S., Haga, H., and Abe, T., 1977, A case of Gilles de la Tourette's syndrome accompanied with alcoholism, *Folia Psychiatr. Neurol. Jpn.* 31:167.
Yaryura-Tobias, J. A., 1975, Chlorimipramine in Gilles de la Tourette's disease (Letter), *Am. J. Psychiatry* 132:1221.
Zausmer, D. M., 1954, Treatment of tics in childhood. *Arch. Dis. Childr.* 29:537–542.

7

The Paranoid-Erotic Syndromes

F. DAVID RUDNICK

The paranoid-erotic syndromes are examples of psychiatric entities that defy precise classification. While all present with a dominant paranoid flavor and are primarily delusional in nature, the erotic overtones are variably manifest. Furthermore, each of the syndromes excites legitimate controversy as to its ability to stand alone diagnostically. The syndromes are generally considered rare, and the literature, especially in recent years, is correspondingly sparse. The Capgras syndrome is an exception and will be discussed in detail. Other syndromes described are the Fregoli syndrome, the intermetamorphosis syndrome, the syndrome of Cotard, and de Clerambault's syndrome.

THE CAPGRAS SYNDROME

In 1923 the French psychiatrists Capgras and Reboul-Lachaux published the first case report of a syndrome they referred to as an "illusion des sosies" or the illusion of doubles. Their patient, a woman with a chronic paranoid psychosis, including delusions of persecution and grandeur, became convinced that her daughter had been replaced by a series of as many as 1000 different "doubles." This syndrome, in which the subject holds a delusional belief that a person or persons familiar to him has been replaced by an imposter of identical physical appearance, has come to be known as the Capgras syndrome.

As initial case reports were presented in the European literature, it appeared that several features were universal, thus validating the concept of a self-contained syndrome. These features included the restriction

F. DAVID RUDNICK, • Department of Psychiatry, University of California at Los Angeles-Neuropsychiatric Institute, Los Angeles, California.

of the delusion to objects with whom the subject maintained a close, emotionally charged relationship; the setting of a clear sensorium; the existence of the delusion in women only; and the absence of concomitant organic disease. Since 1936, however, when Murray described the syndrome in a male patient, the literature has become rich with cases that underscore the variability of these features. As a result, considerable controversy exists as to whether Capgras is in fact a separate syndrome or a symptom complex that can arise in a background of several functional and organic illnesses. This issue will be discussed in detail at the end of this section. There is even discussion in the literature as to whether Capgras represents an illusion or a delusion. Since, in fact, the subject does visually perceive the object correctly as a virtually identical double, it seems appropriate, as Christodoulo (1977b) pointed out, to refer to the syndrome as a *delusional* negation of identity.

While it is impossible to review all cases reported in the literature, several cases can be cited as landmarks in the present understanding of the syndrome. In 1924 Capgras and Carette described a second case in which a woman with schizophrenia simultaneously developed intense incestuous desires toward her father and the delusion that her parents had been replaced by impostors. In 1931 Larrive and Jasienski described a woman who believed that her impoverished lover had been replaced by a rich, powerful, and handsome double. These two cases provided typical material for psychodynamic explanations based on ambivalence, splitting, and projection, which will be discussed in more detail later. Murray's 1936 case report of a male with the Capgras delusion overturned early psychoanalytic explanations based on the syndrome occurring only in females.

All adult age groups are represented, including a few cases in childhood and adolescence (Moskovitz, 1972; Nikolovski and Fernandez, 1978; Rosenstock and Vincent, 1978), with the youngest being a 9-year-old boy whose syndrome appeared as a sequel to chickenpox encephalitis. Moskovitz's case is noteworthy in that once the syndrome subsided in the original patient, a 12-year-old boy, it resurfaced in a younger brother (Moskovitz, 1975).

Gluckman (1968) is generally credited with the first report of the syndrome having an organic basis, but Weston and Whitlock (1971) claimed to have studied the first case in the presence of unequivocal brain damage. MacCallum (1973) described five cases with a variety of concomitant organic illnesses; in three of these, he felt that the delusional system could definitely be attributed to the illness. Hay et al. (1974) described an interesting case of a woman with pseudohypoparathyroidism who developed the delusion on two occasions following ECT treatments for depression, each time accompanied by EEG changes that resolved when the syndrome remitted.

When the syndrome appears in the setting of a functional disorder, schizophrenia comprises the majority of diagnoses. In the extensive review by Merrin and Silberfarb (1976), other psychiatric diagnoses cited include schizoaffective disorder, major affective disorders, and paranoid state. They also pointed out that males and females are nearly equally represented in all diagnostic categories (overall, 41% of the 46 patients they described were males). Finally, two cases have been reported in which patients saw themselves (as well as others) as impostors (Fialkov and Robins, 1978; Siomopoulous and Goldsmith, 1975).

No review would be complete without mention of the colorful appearance of the concept of the double in lay writing. Several authors, including Coleman (1934), referred to the work of Dostoyevsky, who is described an in introvert in whom a moral sense conflicted with sexual impulses. In his writings, he created a double who indulged in exhibitionistic outbursts. In *The Possessed*, he had Marya accuse Stavrogin, to whom she was secretly married, of being an impostor: " . . . mine is a bright falcon and a prince, and you're an owl and a shopman." Guy de Maupassant was also described by Coleman as a man who lived in morbid fear of the consequences of his own potential for sexual excesses. He hallucinated his own double in the setting of a mounting paranoid psychosis, probably syphilitic in nature, as "a projection of the sex libido as enemy and destroyer" (Coleman, 1934). (For a more complete review of this literature, see chapter 5.)

CASE REPORT

The following case illustrates several representative features of the syndrome and also raises questions of an etiologic and psychodynamic nature to be discussed later.

Mrs. M., a 37-year-old Egyptian-born married woman with a 17-year-old daughter, was admitted to the UCLA Neuropsychiatric Institute on two occasions between June 1977 and September 1977 for treatment of depression and the delusion that her husband and daughter had been kidnapped and replaced by impostors. Prior psychiatric history included two suicide attempts by analgesic overdose in 1965 and 1969 with no psychiatric follow-up, and psychiatric hospitalizations in 1974 and 1976 for depression accompanied by the delusion that her husband had been kidnapped from an airport in Libya in 1968 and replaced by an impostor. In each of these hospitalizations, both the depression and the delusion responded to ECT and the patient was able to return to her normal level of functioning. In the 6 weeks prior to her first UCLA admission, out-patient treatment had included amitryptiline and thioridazine, but the patient became increasingly more depressed and her delusion returned, this time extended to include her daughter. She believed that five different men had serially replaced her husband and seven different girls had posed as her daughter, all looking alike, with the exception of minor physical differences such as skin markings and color. On admission, she denied suicidal ideation, sleep disturbance, appetite disturbance, or weight loss. Her family reported, however, that she had restlessness at night and a 10-pound weight loss. Family history was negative for psychiatric disorders.

Mental status examination on the first admission revealed a depressed and anxious woman who appeared older than her stated age. She manifested hand wringing and head holding, with occasional tearful outbursts. She was generally withdrawn, but submissive and responsive to questions. She spoke softly, often whispering, but speech was coherent and connected with normal vocabulary and syntax. There was no looseness of associations or thought blocking. Psychotic content consisted only of the delusional system described above. There were no active hallucinations and no other paranoid ideation, but she admitted to having heard voices in the past of her husband and daughter crying out to her in Arabic. She expressed extreme guilt over having slept with her husband's impostors and now insisted on separate bedrooms and abstinence from sexual activity. She admitted that each of the impostors had been kind and generous and had honored her wishes to avoid sexual contact. She also expressed love for all her daughter's impostors and expressed a desire to care for all of them. There was no suicidal ideation present. Her sensorium was clear and intellectual functioning adequate. Physical examination was noncontributory, as was the neurological examination and its supportive lab work.

In-depth interviews with Mrs. M. and her family (including one under sodium amytal with Mrs. M.) during the first admission revealed potentially important dynamic influences. She was born in Egypt and raised in the strict atmosphere of the Coptic Orthodox church. She was especially close to her father, who was her mother's cousin. Mrs. M. noted that her father frequently went alone to movies because her mother was "too tired." In retrospect, Mrs. M. felt that her father may have been having an affair. Mrs. M.'s marriage to Mr. M., who was her first cousin and 15 years her senior, was arranged by her family. Sexual activity was limited in the early years of their marriage, and Mrs. M. often retired to bed just as her husband returned from work. Her daughter was born 2 years into the marriage, and, in the years to follow, Mrs. M. underwent two illegal abortions at her own insistence in order to avoid the financial burden of additional children and also because she felt that the confinement of motherhood was making her uninteresting to her husband: "I stayed home and took care of my daughter, and this was not enough for a husband. Working women dress well, act very well." The second abortion was particularly traumatic, due to severe hemorrhaging. The abortions, along with subsequent use of birth control pills, brought her into conflict with her deep religious convictions.

The course of Mrs. M.'s first UCLA hospitalization was marked by unsuccessful trials of doxepin and low doses of haloperidol. She remained withdrawn, pacing and praying. She would use photographs taken years earlier to point out subtle physical differences between her real family and the present impostors. She also called the police, asking for help. She received seven ECT treatments but refused additional treatment; her depression and delusional system remained intact. She was even willing to deny her priest's ability ot communicate with God in order to rationalize his support of her husband. She asked to be allowed to live alone to carry out the search for her family, but ultimately she agreed to return home if she could avoid any contact with her husband.

Her second UCLA admission was arranged when Mrs. M. apparently agreed to undergo another ECT series. Her mother, who had been instrumental in persuading Mrs. M. to consent to ECT in 1976, was again flown out from Egypt. This time, however, Mrs. M. greeted her mother by incorporating her into the delusional system, claiming that she was a physically larger woman than her real mother. Mrs. M. had also called her brother in North Carolina, and when he was not sympathetic, she concluded that he too had been kidnapped and replaced.

Once on the ward, she steadfastly refused ECT, dwelling instead on nonspecific somatic complaints. Videotape confrontation, with participation in the taping by Mrs. M.'s husband, daughter, and mother, did not shake the delusion.

The patient was discharged to the care of her family and priest, who immediately placed her in a private hospital. The last contact with Mrs. M. was an anxious phone call stating that her doctor and most of the staff were all impostors. A later report from her family indicated, however, that she had ultimately again agreed to ECT, this time with successful resolution of her delusion. The discharge diagnosis was unipolar depression with a circumscribed Capgras delusion.

Theoretical Considerations

Coleman (1933) organized processes of misidentification into three categories: (1) hyperbolic misidentification, the "facetious and flippant" errors seen in manic states; (2) amnesic misidentification, seen in dementia and confusional states; and (3) delusional misidentification, a subjective evaluation made in the setting of normal perception and memory, as seen in psychosis. The Capgras syndrome, he felt, belonged in this last category.

Neurological considerations of misidentification are contained in discussions by Ellinwood (1969) and Gerstmann (1958). Ellinwood described the important phenomenon of *prosopagnosia*, a specific agnosia for familiar faces, first reported by Charcot (1883) and named by Bodamer (1947), who cited evidence that it could be a separate deficit from general object agnosia. In prosopagnosia, lesions are primarily located in the right parietooccipital cortex. That this is *not* the basis of Capgras is supported by Ellinwood's statement that facial agnosia is generally accompanied by a loss of emotional investment in the unrecognized objects. Unlike Capgras, estrangement exists in both prosopagnosia and paranoid psychosis. In prosopagnosia, it is a "bewildered, unknowing estrangement" from a "colorless, emotionally detached world of objects," while in the paranoid psychosis, it is an "evil, unnatural" estrangement associated with a "sense of intense reality and significance." He pointed out that in paranoid schizophrenia there is often a restitutional "hypercathexis" of faces as a means of regaining contact with outside objects.

Other phenomena that may produce distorted perceptions of faces include the epileptic psychoses, temporo-parieto-occipital lesions producing autoscopy, and various toxic psychoses. Of considerable interest in delineation of major and minor hemispheric functions is the finding of Kimura (1963) that major hemispheric lesions tend to affect perceptions of *emotionally neutral* familiar and ordinary objects, as opposed to the emotionally charged faces that are invariably involved in the Capgras delusion.

Gerstmann discussed disorders of body image, pointing out that it is a dynamic process repatterned by afferent impressions and perceptions. Disorders of the body image proper are bilateral and related to lesions in the dominant parietal or parieto-occipital region, while defects in the accurate recording of a bodily alteration occur in nondominant lesions and are unilateral. An interesting case example of the latter type, cited by Gerstmann, has some suggestive features of Capgras: A patient denies his left hemiplegia by insisting the affected limbs were someone else's. "I can feel they are not [mine] and I can't believe my eyes." Here an accurate visual analysis could not perserve the unity of the body image in the tactile-kinesthetic sphere. With Capgras, visual perception is intact but may be overridden by emotional distortions.

Several authors have paid attention to themes in primitive thinking that may become manifest in a delusion of doubles. Todd and Dewhurst

(1955) and Todd (1957) pointed out that in primitive folklore and tribal religions an individual's soul ghost was often believed to be able to act as the double of its host. Ancient mythology offers numerous accounts of gods taking the identical form of a mortal. In the monkish anthology of the *Gesta Romanorium*, the emperor Jovinian is replaced by a double as punishment for excessive pride. Todd (1957) concluded: "In the disintegration of the nervous system, the destruction of higher and more recently acquired neurological mechanisms releases lower and more primitive ones. Similarly, the disintegration of the personality doubtless sets free primitive modes of thoughts, which include the tendency to think in terms of doubles and dualisms."

A final interesting insight was offered by Davidson (1941), who pointed out that, in Egyptian theology, "to die" meant to become one's double, which, as a distinct entity, then wandered away. This suggests that the phenomenon of doubles could, on a primitive level, be a homocidal wish or, in the case of self-replacement, a suicidal wish.

Etiological Considerations

While case reports through the mid-1960s linked the Capgras syndrome exclusively to functional disorders in the setting of a clear sensorium, subsequent literature attested to a range of organic causative factors as well. This development alone supports the notion of Capgras as a symptom complex rather than a self-contained syndrome, for in the latter interpretation it would have to exist simultaneously with a large group of totally unrelated illnesses. That the nosological controversy persists is in part due to the fact that the treatment course of the delusion does not always follow the course of the identified underlying disease. This aspect will be discussed later.

Merrin and Silberfarb (1976) reviewed 46 cases from the English-language literature. Of these, 19 had pure diagnoses of schizophrenia, 5 more were diagnosed as "paraphrenics," 4 carried diagnoses of schizophrenia with organic factors, 4 were diagnosed as schizoaffective, 7 were purely affective disorders, and 7 were purely organic. Interestingly, the mean age for schizophrenic patients manifesting Capgras is 41 years, significantly higher than the average age of hospitalized schizophrenics who do not have the delusion. Indeed, a typical case report may describe a patient with one or more psychotic breaks preceding the onset of the Capgras delusion. Mrs. M., the patient described in this chapter, had two suicide attempts 9 and 5 years before the onset of her delusion, the latter attempt having possibly been prompted by a paranoid psychosis. Christodoulou (1977b) reported on 11 cases (6 schizophrenic, 4 depressed, 1 organic) in which there was an average duration of 5 years between the onset of the basic illness and the onset of the syndrome. Again, the average age for the schizophrenic patients was 43 years in his series.

Christodoulou also emphasized the nearly universal feature of a marked paranoid component in patients with the syndrome. This is borne out by the literature and is independent of etiology. Stern and MacNaughton (1945), in an in-depth study via Rohrschach testing on one patient, reported a large number of "di responses" in which a subject saw structure in a blot area that is usually perceived as unbroken. This response was interpreted as a magical attempt to diffuse the threat of shading. The authors pointed out that to see something "inside" an area that is not discerned by others is a classic paranoid response.

Leonhard (1975) described a group of nonschizophrenic paranoid psychoses that he called the "cycloid psychoses." These were characterized by the presence of easily recognized external etiological factors, often of a somatic nature. Included in this were most puerperal psychoses and a specific subcategory he called "confusion psychosis," marked by stupor and, often, misidentification of persons. A specific example of the Capgras syndrome occurring in the setting of a cycloid psychosis was the case report by Cohn et al. (1977) of a 25-year-old woman who developed the delusion as part of her second postpartum psychosis.

There appears to be no consistent diagnostic pattern to organic illnesses associated with Capgras. MacCallum (1973) reported on five diverse cases. In three of them, a 71-year-old man with chronic lung disease and bacterial pneumonia, a 28-year-old woman with a right hemiplegia secondary to basilar migraine, and a 45-year-old man with alcohol intoxification, treatment of the underlying illness abolished the delusion. Two others had suggestive causes of diabetes mellitus with a buttock abscess, and malnutrition. Complicating somewhat the conclusions of his report was the fact that each patient had some background suggestive of psychiatric problems, including depression, bipolar illness, alcoholism, and paranoid state. This at least raises the possibility of an acute organic insult unleashing psychosis in a premorbidly susceptible individual.

Perhaps more convincing are case reports of Capgras in association with documented brain dysfunction. The case of Weston and Whitlock (1971) has already been mentioned in which a 20-year-old man with no prior psychiatric history sustained diffuse brain damage in an auto accident. Deficits included memory loss, mixed dysphasia, and generalized intellectual impairment. Two months after the accident, apparently as a sequel to an in-hospital hallucinatory experience during a posttraumatic delirium, the patient manifested a delusion that his family had been killed by Chinese Communists and replaced by identical impostors. Hay-

man and Abrams (1977) reported two more cases of Capgras in association with gross right-sided dysfunction and suggested that prosopagnosia formed the basis for delusional formulation. The cases of Hay *et al.*
(1974) previously cited, Hugonena (1969) (associated with postencephalitic Parkinson's disease), and Nikolovski and Fernandez (1978) (following varicella encephalitis) can also be considered to have a neurological
basis.

In an attempt to explain the fact that this rare syndrome is often
coupled with relatively more common disease entities, some authors concluded that both brain dysfunction and a psychotic process are necessary.
In a remarkable study of his 11 patients, Christodoulou (1977b) performed extensive EEG studies, echoencephalograms, pneumoencepha-
lograms, brain scans, and neuropsychological testing. Abnormalities of
one type or another were found in most patients, including EEG abnormalities, enlargement of the third cerebral ventricle, and marked differences between verbal and performance IQ, the latter being lower. As
described earlier, all but one patient had major psychiatric diagnoses as
well. Of striking similarity is the case of Nilsson and Perris (1971) who
reported pneumoencephalogram findings of enlarged ventricles and
slight atrophy of the right temporal lobe in a patient with a history of
recurrent psychotic depressions. Waziri (1978) reported the case of a
schizophrenic woman who evidently developed the Capgras delusion
and an organic brain syndrome as a result of a central anticholinergic
toxicity to thioridazine. He pointed out that patients who have no history
of psychosis and develop localized brain lesions may display prosopagnosia and accuse close relatives of being doubles, without formulating an
elaborate delusional system.

At this point, few definitive conclusions can be drawn about a specific etiological environment in which the Capgras syndrome appears. At
best, the delusional system may represent a final common pathway for a
wide spectrum of disorders. That this specific psychosis develops in some
individuals and not in others with similar underlying illness no doubt
reflects, in part, the psychodynamics of the individual.

Psychodynamic Formulation

Probably the earliest attempt to formulate a dynamic understanding
of the Capgras syndrome was that of Coleman (1933), who proceeded
from a classical analytic standpoint. His work is primarily of historical
interest in that it was based on case reports available at that time that
described only women. Coleman felt that the crucial difference between
men and women that predisposed only the latter to Capgras-like delusions occurred in the Oedipal phase. He felt that, at that time, the female

child undergoes a jolting transfer of libidinous desires from mother to father. Previously a loved object, mother suddenly becomes a hated rival, and the child becomes subject to the development of ambivalence and mistrust of significant objects. Similarly, other objects may not be what they appear. For the male child, on the other hand, mother remains the loved object throughout the Oedipal phase. Hence, in times of stress, the male maintains object constancy and instead turns inward to search for anomalies. Interestingly, Murray (1936), in reporting the first case of a male patient, attempted to maintain Coleman's formulation by pointing out that the patient had poor premorbid heterosexual adjustment. He believed that his patient's infantile psychosexual developmental occurred along the lines of a typical female.

The psychodynamic explanation of Capgras now generally advanced is based on ambivalence, splitting, and projection. Moskovitz (1973) put it succinctly that "in the face of unacceptable sexual or hostile feelings, an ambivalently held object is split into good and bad objects." Vogel (1974) stated that the psychosis is often preceded by the patient's desperate, but unsuccessful, attempt to achieve tighter emotional bonds with a love object, who is entreated to change his rejecting and hurting responses. When this fails, the object is split into the "alter" and the "alias." Into the former are projected all virtues and the patient continues to love this projection, who is actually removed (in Mrs. M.'s case, kidnapped) from the patient's emotional experience. The latter physically remains in the patient's environment and is hated for his cruelty and rejection, but with a characteristic coldness of affect. In the example of Mrs. M., this is consistent with her position vis-à-vis her husband. However, with respect to her daughter, she seems to have maintained the warm and loving feelings for the double and projected out into the alter any hostility. Vogel pointed out that the dividend in this mechanism is that the patient is allowed to retain the love object and yet be spared a persistent intolerable conflict between love and hate. Interestingly, Cavenar et al. (1977) felt that only schizophrenia as an etiology can give rise to such powerful ambivalence. Siomopoulous and Goldsmith (1975) emphasized projective mechanisms. They reported a male patient with paranoid schizophrenia who saw himself as an impostor, and they postulated that his delusion was a defense against a self-image that had been damaged by insight into his mental illness and by frustrated professional ambitions. He embodied the good aspects of himself in the impostor and banished the deficient aspects into his departed real self. The authors felt that, in the more classical Capgras syndrome involving external objects, the patient sees unacceptable changes in himself and projects them outward, probably onto the persons he considers responsible for the change.

Then, through denial and rationalization, he concludes that those persons have been replaced by impostors.

Merrin and Silberfarb (1976) suggested a dynamic theory based on a change in the affective response of the individual to an object whose physical identity has not changed. Here there is a creation of a cognitive dissonance, which is resolved by paranoid projection: The object, rather than the patient's internal milieu, is altered. It follows that only objects that evoke strong subjective experiences are involved. A variation of this theme proceeds from postulating a subtle change in the patient's perception of his own body that then triggers a sequence of depersonalization followed by misidentification. The original disturbance could reflect a basic parietal lobe dysfunction.

Many of the foregoing ideas were restated in the paper by Mikkelsen and Gutheil (1976). In addition, they pointed out the crucial element of family dynamics during the patient's upbringing. That the Capgras delusion is manifest rather than any other psychotic construct may be in fact a valid communication about the patient's early experience of significant objects. The patient may be expressing profound disappointments in his previous expectations of family members or displaying a tendency to impermanent identification of objects due to early loss (through death, abandonment, separation) of family members. It is interesting to speculate on the fact that Mrs. M.'s husband was much older than she was and, like her father, was suspected of being unfaithful. Her delusion could in part represent a psychotic transference of her unresolved conflicts about her father.

Treatment and Prognosis

The literature survey in this area produces no conclusions about definitive treatment or prognosis. This probably reflects the wide variety of underlying illnesses. The mainstays of treatment, when clear organic causes are not identified, include neuroleptic and antidepressant medication and electroconvulsive therapy. Christodoulou's (1977c, 1978) results in a series of 20 patients with Capgras and similar delusions of misidentification (see subsequent sections in this chapter) are representative. Not surprisingly, he concluded that the preferred treatment was dictated by the underlying diagnosis and favored tricyclic antidepressants in depressed patients and neuroleptics in the setting of schizophrenia or organicity. Of the neuroleptics, trifluoperazine seemed most correlated with improved outcome. He also noted the benefical effect on the delusional system of treating any accompanying medical conditions—in 3 cases, remission of both conditions coincided. Two patients with EEG abnormalities were treated with anticonvulsants and were reported to show less impulsive behavior and less pronounced delusions.

Most authors agree that the course and prognosis of the Capgras syndrome generally, but not always, follow the overall clinical status. Merrin and Silberfarb (1976) reviewed 26 cases of nonorganic patients. In 20, the progress of the delusion paralleled the general clinical response. In 17 patients in which the underlying illness was successfully treated, the Capgras syndrome also remitted. In several case reports, usually patients with a clear psychiatric diagnosis, recurrence of the illness was accompanied by recurrence of the Capgras delusion in similar form to previous presentations. This is well illustrated in the case of Mrs. M., who manifested the delusion on three occasions, each time accompanied by clinical depression, and each time responding ultimately to an adequate series of electroconvulsive treatments.

Psychotherapy with Capgras patients probably differs little from therapy with other patients having fixed delusional systems, and there is little in the literature devoted specifically to this aspect of treatment. A key question is whether or not the delusion can be directly challenged. In the early literature, especially Coleman (1933), it was felt that the patient would respond to such a challenge with rationalization and further delusional elaborations. Enoch (1963) emphasized that the misidentification was selective and therefore could be confronted in psychotherapy. An attempt at confrontation was made in the case of Mrs. M. A video tape of her together with her husband, daughter, and mother was made and then played back in a session with only Mrs. M. and two therapists. Her tear-laden affective response was dramatic, and on several occasions she appeared to reembrace her family. However, in the end, she steadfastly clung to her delusion. Further attempts to involve the authority of the church by including her priest in therapy sessions resulted in his being incorporated into the delusion, much as Coleman suggested.

Moskovitz (1972, 1975) used family therapy in addition to pharmacological agents in his successful treatment of a 12-year-old boy. Mikkelsen and Gutheil (1976) emphasized that attention to family history and dynamics may reveal the specific meaning and role of the delusion.

Discussion

In conclusion, the nosological issue of whether Capgras is indeed a separate syndrome or a symptom complex should be readdressed. As previously indicated, the delusion has now been reported in a wide spectrum of both organic and functional disorders, and, in reviewing the English language literature, the clinical symptomatology of all patients described extends beyond the Capgras delusion itself. It would appear then that in the Capgras syndrome a final common pathway is reached from diverse directions, beginning in some cases with a genetic vulnerability followed by acute stress and in others with an organic insult. This weakened state then combines with the individual's intrapsychic and interpersonal dynamics, along with influences of environment, to produce psychosis with a specific delusional content.

It is, in this author's opinion, a mistake to consider the syndrome a self-contained entity. Such an assumption could restrict diagnostic inquiry to the extent that the patient may be deprived of definitive treatment. The more inclusive view outlined above may in fact underlie all fixed delusional systems and, in particular, explain rarer syndromes to be described in the remainder of this chapter.

SYNDROME OF FREGOLI

Closely allied to the Capgras syndrome is the illusion of Fregoli, first described by Courbon and Fail in 1927. They reported the case of a schizoid woman who attended the theater regularly and became convinced that she was being persecuted by the actor, Fregoli, who was a master of rapid facial changes on stage. She felt that Fregoli was appearing to her in the bodies of a succession of persons in her environment.

The syndrome is now classified by Christodoulou (1977a) as an example of delusional hyperidentification. The patient identifies a familiar person, usually seen as a persecutor, in the bodies of various strangers, claiming they are psychologically identical, while recognizing their physical differences.

The rarity of the syndrome is reflected in the paucity of English-language literature. Comprehensive textbooks of psychiatry (Lehmann, 1975; Arieti and Bemporad, 1974) define the symptom without devoting a separate section to it, underscoring the conclusion that, like Capgras, Fregoli is only a symptom complex in a primary disease process. The discussion here is based largely on Christodoulou's (1977a) systematic study of seven patients.

Theoretical and Etiological Considerations

Coleman (1933) felt that the Fregoli syndrome represented a disorder of misidentification advanced beyond that of Capgras. He considered it a case of false recognition, but with accurate physical identification. As with Capgras, a marked paranoid element underlies the delusion, although in Christodoulou's series, three of his seven patients had a *positively* charged emotional attachment to the identified object.

Six of Christodoulou's patients were male, all were single, and they were between the ages of 17 and 33. These demographic data are in marked contrast to those of the typical Capgras patient. Six of the patients were diagnosed as having schizophrenia and one as having an epileptic psychosis. As with his series of Capgras patients, Christodoulou systematically searched for organic factors. A history of potential CNS contributions was elicited from five patients, including head injuries, febrile convulsions, one case of documented major motor seizure disorder, and paroxysmal headaches. Objective findings included "mild and diffuse abnormalities" in the EEGs of five patients, echoencephalogram findings of enlarged third ventricles in four patients, and negative brain scans on all patients. A pneumoencephalogram done on one patient showed enlargement of the suprapineal recess, a finding reported in epilepsy, in spinocerbellar ataxia, and in the aftermath of cranial injury. A consistent finding on psychological testing was a significant increase in verbal over performance IQ. Other, more spotty findings generally implicated functions that required processing visual input. Overall, these results were similar to those of Christodoulou's (1977b) series of Capgras patients and again suggest an interplay of functional and organic factors in patients with delusions of this type.

Treatment and Prognosis

The available data are again from Christodoulou's series and conclusions are identical to those reached in Capgras patients. The success of somatic treatments including neuroleptics, antidepressants, and ECT is linked to the response of the underlying illness.

THE INTERMETAMORPHOSIS SYNDROME

Courbon and Tusques (1932) were the first to describe this syndrome. They reported on the case of a depressed woman with delusions of persecution who was convinced that several objects in her environment had been interchanged. She felt that her two young hens had been replaced by two older ones, that her new coat had been replaced by an old, shabby one, that women had been interchanged with men, young people with old, and that a neighbor had been incarnated into her husband.

Coleman (1933) considered intermetamorphosis the complete loss of coenesthesia, combining both false psychological and physical recognition. He described the case of a 55-year-old married woman who combined both Capgras and intermetamorphosis delusions. She felt that both her husband and sister had been replaced by doubles and that, at various times, a neighbor, whom she considered to be her chief persecutor, had become interchanged with her servant and her doctor. She purported to perceive physical changes in both these persons to support her contention.

While the literature is even more scanty for this syndrome, the same etiological and treatment conclusions apply here as do for Capgras and Fregoli. Christodoulou (1977c) had one case in his series with a diagnosis of schizophrenia who improved on trifluoperazine. Malliaras *et al.* (1978) described the case of a 19-year-old female who manifested diffuse epileptiform EEG activity (most prominent in temporal areas), had a 38-point deficit between verbal IQ (120) and performance IQ (82), and showed a variety of deficits in neuropsychological testing involving visual performance. The authors diagnosed an epileptic psychosis but noted that the patient's delusions responded to neuroleptic medication.

COTARD'S SYNDROME

This syndrome was first described in 1880 at a meeting of the Société Medico Psychologique in Paris. The French psychiatrist Cotard reported on several cases of what he referred to as "délire de négation," or delusional state of negation. Since then, similar delusions have appeared in diverse settings, particularly involutional depression and organic brain syndromes, where they are now usually called nihilistic delusions. Arieti and Bemporad (1974) pointed out that only in France and Italy is the condition still considered to be a separate entity by some psychiatrists.

The essential content of the delusion is that nothing exists—the physical reality of the patient along with the world around him has disappeared into nothingness. He even denies the possibility of death and thus paradoxically in his own view becomes immortal. According to Arieti and Bemporad, the typical patient is a woman in the involutional age who is depressed with usual endogenous features and a paranoid psychosis that may include hallucinations. In a series of 10 patients described in the Spanish literature by Saavedra (1968), 8 were female, and diagnoses included melancholia (4 patients), schizophrenia (3 patients), and mixed (3 patients). References to additional cases in the European literature can be found in Arieti and Bemporad.

Treatment is aimed at the basic disorder and the delusion resolves correspondingly. In its chronic form, the syndrome is generally associated with senile psychoses (Lehmann, 1975).

DE CLERAMBAULT'S SYNDROME

In 1942, G. G. de Clerambault published five cases of what he called "psychose passionelle," a delusional system that has come to bear his name and is also referred to as "erotomania." The essential features of the syndrome involve a female patient who comes to believe that a man, usually older and of higher social status than she, and often one whom she has never met, is in love with her. She may accept the fact that their situations interfere with realization of that love, or she may become convinced that the apparent disinterest of her supposed lover is only a pretense for some hidden motive. She is, at any rate, always cognizant of the paradoxical and contrary nature of his behavior toward her. She devotes her every thought and action to the delusional relationship and finds proof of the man's love in everything. Carried to its extreme, the delusion becomes dramatized in real life. As Enoch *et al.* (1967) pointed out, the patient can bring chaos to the life of her "suitor" and may become dangerous to him and his family, especially if she reaches a stage of resentment or hatred following repeated unrequited advances.

As with other syndromes discussed in this chapter, a nosological controversy exists. Arieti and Bemporad (1974) reported that de Clerambault's syndrome is considered a distinct entity in the French literature but is considered a symptom of a primary paranoid condition in the United States. Lehmann (1975) emphatically stated: "It would be advisable not to perpetuate the existence of this questionable syndrome in the literature." In the review article by Hollender and Callahan (1975), however, two forms of the disorder were distinguished: a primary form of sudden onset in which the delusion itself is the only psychopathology, and a secondary form of more gradual onset superimposed on a preexisting paranoid psychosis. Accordingly, a complete discussion of the syndrome will be presented here.

CASE REPORT

Miss J., a 27-year-old single Caucasian woman, was admitted to a university inpatient service after having presented herself to the walk-in evaluation unit on 3 consecutive days, claiming to be unable to provide food or shelter for herself. She had a history of two previous psychiatric hospitalizations since the age of 21, each time initiated by her father, who had found her withdrawn, inactive, and nonfunctional. From her second hospitalization she carried a diagnosis of paranoid schizophrenia.

She presented on this admission with the fear that her father was a sexual deviate who had incestuous intentions toward her and his own mother. She referred to her paternal grandmother, a crippled 80-year-old woman, as "criminally insane." She accused her grandmother of physically abusing her by "tearing off my clothes" and withholding food when she was sick. She claimed that in her first hospitalization she had been beaten, given massive doses of drugs, and sexually approached by one of the doctors.

She also described an intimate relationship over the past year and a half with a man, Mr. T. who had been the landlord of a building in which she had once rented an apartment. She referred to Mr. T. as her "husband," although admitting that she was not married to him and had never lived with him. She stated that his own mental illness had forced him to move back in with his own family and therefore made it impossible for him to provide for her needs at this time. She described him as her "dream man." She stated she had been overwhelmed by the intensity of his love and hadn't known how to respond.

History from Miss J.'s father indicated that Miss J. had harassed Mr. T. for several months following his having evicted her for failure to pay rent. Mr. T. eventually filed a complaint against Miss J. and had her jailed for 3 days. Miss J. herself explained this incident as a maneuver by Mr. T.'s family, who objected to their relationship on religious grounds. A private psychiatrist who had followed Miss J. for most of the previous year verified the delusional nature of the relationship with Mr. T. and added that the intensity of the delusion waxed and waned in proportion to the patient's own social adjustment.

During her hospitalization, Miss J. initially refused neuroleptics for fear of jeopardizing an impending pregnancy by Mr. T. She also refused a physical examination out of fidelity to Mr. T., who "would become insanely jealous if I had any physical contact with another man." She frequently telephoned or wrote letters to Mr. T. that went unanswered. On the ward, she was depressed, isolative, and secretive and manifested a thought disorder including looseness of associations, thought blocking, and distractability.

She finally agreed to begin thiothixene at an initial dose of 10 mg at night, and good results were achieved. She became angry over Mr. T.'s silence and admitted that the relationship might have been a "passing fancy." She considered seeking other male companionship and revealed an erotic interest in one of the male staff.

The patient was followed for 3 months after discharge and her de Clerambault delusion remained intact, although with variable intensity. She was continued on thiothixene, and a low dose of amitryptiline was added for elements of an agitated depression. At times whe was overtly delusional, with ideas of reference, claiming that Mr. T. drove by her home often to reassure her of his love, and that they communicated with each other through a radio announcer's voice. At other times she described Mr. T. as unreal, a fantasy, and allowed that she might have misperceived his feelings. She was eventually lost to follow-up, having moved to live with her father.

Etiological Considerations

The general consensus of the English-language literature is that the syndrome always occurs in the setting of paranoid schizophrenia or a paranoid state. Disorders of visual perception and recognition are not implicated, as with previous syndromes discussed in this chapter, and questions of organic contributions are therefore not treated in the literature. Hollender and Callahan have reviewed most of the case reports through 1975.

Two case reports deserve mention, if only for their colorful features. Pearce (1972) reported on a case of de Clerambault's associated with folie à deux. A 54-year-old spinster became convinced that a man she dated 30 years ago was sending her telepathic messages that he now planned to marry her. The patient's mother, with whom she lived, also came to share the delusion. The patient's history was one of sexual inhibition, social and emotional isolation, and excessive religiosity. Hence, Pearce felt she was undergoing an "eruption into consciousness of long repressed desires."

Sims and White (1973) described a 32-year-old divorced female who presented with a flagrant thought disorder, including several first-rank Schneiderian symptoms. In addition, she combined both the Capgras delusion directed at her mother and the de Clerambault syndrome directed at a former employer.

Psychodynamic Considerations

Hollender and Callahan (1975) stated that, dynamically, the delusion stems from feelings of being unloved or unlovable. The patient creates a grandiose fantasy against this terrible conviction. Other possible mechanisms include the denial and subsequent projection of self-love, or, more directly, projection of the patient's love for the man. The authors point out that this would be unusual for a paranoid disorder, where projected feelings are generally hostile. Another view of the mechanism involves the substitution of an intense heterosexual attachment for denied homosexual impulses.

Raskin and Sullivan (1974) described two cases in which female patients formed delusional attachments to their psychiatrists. In both cases, the delusional content peaked at the time of the patients' pending divorces and again at the termination of treatment. The symptoms were in part seen as adaptive in that they helped to ward off depression and loneliness. An interesting dynamic in these cases was the feeling on the part of both patients that their emotions, actions, and futures were controlled by their lovers, a situation that repeated an earlier relationship with an older parental figure—a grandfather in one case and a father in the other. In the case of Miss J., her relationship with her father was highly charged with erotic overtones, and it was her father who moved in to take control and provide protection in times of greatest need. The delusional relationship with Mr. T. could be seen as displacement of incestuous desires for her father, some of which were more directly evident in other delusional aspects of her thought content. Three of four cases described by Hollender and Callahan involved women who were unattractive, intellectually limited, and socially and sexually inhibited. The fourth was "pleasant and attractive." Miss J., while not physically attractive, was intelligent, artistically creative, and, by history, experienced sexually. In de Clerambault's syndrome there appear to be no consistent predisposing personality or developmental traits.

Treatment and Prognosis

All authors tend to agree that the de Clerambault delusion is relatively resistant to either pharmacotherapy or psychotherapy, and that the classic course is unremitting. In the case of Miss J., despite dramatic response of all other aspects of her thought disorder to antipsychotic medication, and her intermittent return of high levels of functioning, her delusion about Mr. T. lingered as something of a fallback position should her real-life situation threaten to deteriorate in any way. This probably reflects the often described intractability of fixed and circumscribed delusional systems, regardless of the underlying illness. It also may underscore the adaptive aspects of this particular delusion.

REFERENCES

Arieti, S., and Bemporad, J. R., 1974, Rare, unclassifiable and collective psychiatric syndromes, in "American Handbook of Psychiatry," 2nd ed., Vol. III (S. Arieti, ed.), p. 710, Basic Books, New York.

Bodamer, J., 1947, Die Prosopagnosie, Arch. Psychiatr. Nervenkr. 179:6.

Capgras, J., and Carette, P., 1924, L'illusion des sosies et complexe d'Oedipe, Ann. Med. Psychol. 82:48.

Capgras, J., and Reboul-Lachaux, J., 1923, L'illusion des sosies dans un délire systématisé chronique, Soc. Clin. Med. Psychol. 81:186.

Cavenar, J. O., Jr., Maltbie, A. A., and Petty, M., 1977, The Capgras syndrome: A review, Mil. Med. 142:617.

Charcot, J., 1883, Un cas de suppression brusques et isolée de la vision mentale des signes et des objects (formes et couleurs), Prog. Med. 11:508.

Christodoulou, G. N., 1977a, Dilusional hyper-identification of the Fregoli type: Organic pathogenetic contributors, Acta Psychiatr. Scand. 54:305.

Christodoulou, G. N., 1977b, The syndrome of Capgras, Br. J. Psychiatry 130:556.

Christodoulou, G. N., 1977c, Treatment of the syndrome of doubles, Acta Psychiatr. Belg. 77:254.

Christodoulou, G. N., 1978, Course and prognosis of the syndrome of doubles, J. Nerv. Ment. Dis. 166:68.

Cohn, C. K., Rosenblatt, S., and Faillace, L. A., 1977, Capgras syndrome presenting as post-partum psychosis, *South. Med. J.* 70:942.

Coleman, S. M., 1933, Misidentification and non-recognition, *J. Ment. Sci.* 79:42.

Coleman, S. M., 1934, The phantom double; its psychological significance, *Br. J. Psychol.* 14:254.

Courbon, P., and Fail, G., 1927, Syndrome d'illusion de Fregoli et schizophrénie, *Bull. Soc. Clin. Med. Ment.* 15:121.

Courbon, P., and Tusques, J., 1932, L'illusion d'intermétamorphose et de charmes, *Ann. Med.-Psychol.* 90:401.

Davidson, G. M., 1941, The syndrome of Capgras, *Psychiatr. Q.* 15:513.

de Clerambault, G. G., 1942, "Oeuvre Psychiatrique," Presses Universitaires, Paris.

Ellinwood, E. H., 1969, Perception of faces: Disorders in organic and psychopathological states, *Psychiatr. Q.* 43:622.

Enoch, M. D., 1963, The Capgras syndrome, *Acta Psychiatr. Scand.* 39:437.

Enoch, M. D., Trethowan, W. H., and Barker, J. C., 1967, "Some Uncommon Psychiatric Syndromes," pp. 1–12, John Wright and Sons, Bristol.

Fialkov, M. J., and Robins, A. H., 1978, An unusual case of the Capgras syndrome, *Br. J. Psychiatry* 132:403.

Gertsmann, J., 1958, Psychological and phenomenological aspects of disorders of body image, *J. Nerv. Ment. Dis.* 126:499.

Gluckman, J. K., 1968, A case of Capgras syndrome, *Aust. N.Z. J. Psychiatry* 2:39.

Hay, G. G., Jolley, D. J., and Jones, R. G., 1974, A case of the Capgras syndrome in association with pseudohypoparathyroidism, *Acta Psychiatr. Scand.* 50:73.

Hayman, M. A., and Abrams, R., 1977, Capgras syndrome and cerebral dysfunction, *Br. J. Psychiatry* 130:68.

Hollender, M. H., and Callahan, A. S., 1975, Erotomania or de Clerambault syndrome, *Arch. Gen. Psychiatry* 32:1574.

Hugonena, H., 1969, The illusion of doubles and postencephalitic Parkinson's disease, *Ann. Med.-Psychol.* 2:439.

Kimura, D., 1963, Right temporal lobe damage: Perception of unfamiliar stimuli after damage, *Arch. Neurol.* 8:264.

Larrive, E., and Jasienski, J., 1931, L'illusion des sosies une nouvelle observation du syndrome de Capgras, *Ann. Med.-Psychol.* 89:501.

Lehmann, H. E., 1975, Unusual psychiatric disorders and atypical psychoses, in "Comprehensive Textbook of Psychiatry" (A. M. Freedman, H. I. Kaplan, B. J. Sadock, eds.), pp. 1728–1729, Williams and Wilkins, Baltimore.

Leonhard, K., 1975, Prognosis of paranoid states in relation to the clinical features, *Acta Psychiatr. Scand.* 51:134.

MacCallum, W. A. G., 1973, Capgras symptoms with an organic basis, *Br. J. Psychiatry* 123:639.

Malliaras, D. E., Kossovitsu, Y. T., and Christodoulou, G. N., 1978, Organic contributions to the intermetamorphosis syndrome, *Am. J. Psychiatry* 135:985.

Merrin, E. L., and Silberfarb, P. M., 1976, The Capgras phenomenon, *Arch. Gen. Psychiatry* 33:965.

Mikkelsen, E. J., and Gutheil, T. G., 1976, Communication and reality in the Capgras syndrome, *Am. J. Psychother.* 30:136.

Moskovitz, J., 1972, Capgras symptom in modern dress, *Int. J. Child Psychother.* 1:45.

Moskovitz, J., 1973, Communicative meaning in Capgras syndrome, *Am. J. Psychiatry* 130:1297.

Moskovitz, J., 1975, Capgras syndrome in male siblings, *Am. J. Psychiatry* 132:86.

Murray, J. R., 1936, Case of Capgras syndrome in a male, *J Ment. Sci.* 82:63.

Nikolovski, O. T., and Fernandez, J. V., 1978, Capgras syndrome as an aftermath of chickenpox encephalitis, *Psychiatr. Opinion* 15:39.
Nilsson, R., and Perris, C., 1971, The Capgras syndrome, *Acta Psychiatr. Scand. (Suppl.)* 221:53.
Pearce, A., 1972, De Clerambault syndrome associated with folie à deux, *Br. J. Psychiatry* 121:116.
Raskin, D. E., and Sullivan, K. E., 1974, Erotomania, *Am. J. Psychiatry* 131:1033.
Rosenstock, H. A., and Vincent, K. R., 1978, Capgras syndrome: Case report of an adolescent and review of literature, *J. Clin. Psychiatry* 39:629.
Saavedra, V., 1968, The Cotard syndrome: Psychopathological and nosographic considerations, *Rev. Neuro-Psiquiatr.* 31:145.
Sims, A., and White, A., 1973, Coexistence of the Capgras and de Clerambault syndromes—A case history, *Br. J. Psychiatry* 123:635.
Siomopoulous, V., and Goldsmith, J., 1975, Two reports of the Capgras syndrome, *Am. J. Psychiatry* 132:756.
Stern, K., and MacNaughton, D., 1945, Capgras syndrome, a peculiar delusionary phenomenon, considered with special reference to the Rohrschach findings, *Psychiatr. Q.* 19:139.
Todd, J., 1957, The syndrome of Capgras, *Psychiatr. Q.* 31:250.
Todd, J., and Dewhurst, K., 1955, The double—Its psychopathology and psychophysiology, *J. Nerv. Ment. Dis.* 122:47.
Vogel, F., 1974, The Capgras syndrome in its psychopathology, *Am. J. Psychiatry* 131:922.
Waziri, R., 1978, The Capgras phenomenon: Cerebral dysfunction with psychosis, *Neuropsychobiology* 4:353.
Weston, M. J., and Whitlock, F. A., 1971, The Capgras syndrome following head injury, *Br. J. Psychiatry* 119:25.

8

Unusual Sexual Syndromes

RONALD F. REBAL, JR., ROBERT A. FAGUET, and
SHERWYN M. WOODS

Sexual behaviors differ from society to society and from individual to individual. Beliefs about which sexual practices are good, moral, and natural and which are wrong, immoral, and unnatural are mutable. Certain types of sexual behaviors are thought to be exhibited by only a small portion of the people of our society. Because of the presumed rarity and because of the difference between these practices and accepted sexual norms, these sexual behaviors are of interest to those who study human behavior. In this chapter we will attempt to review objectively the information available on the syndromes of necrophilia, vampirism, zoophilia, autoerotic asphyxia, coprophilia, rare types of incest, and hypersexuality. The intention is to provide the reader with a clear and objective view of the range of human sexual behavior.

NECROPHILIA

Necrophilia is an unusual and macabre paraphilia denoting sexual contact with the dead. Necrophilic activity has long been a subject of concern to society. The ancient Egyptians took steps to prevent its occurrence. As Herodotus writes (cited in Allen, 1962, p. 221): "The wives of men of rank, and such females as had been distinguished by their beauty or importance, are not immediately on their decease delivered to their embalmers; they are usually kept for three or four days, which is done to prevent any indecency being offered to their persons. An instance once occurred of an embalmer's gratifying his lust on the body of a female lately dead; the crime was divulged by a fellow artist." In modern

RONALD F. REBAL, JR., ROBERT A. FAGUET, and SHERWYN M. WOODS • Department of Psychiatry, University of Southern California Medical School, Los Angeles, California.

psychiatric literature, the term has been used to describe many different types of activities: sexual contact with corpses, sexual excitement in the act of murder (necrosadism or lust murder), mutilation of corpses (necrosadism), and devouring parts of a corpse (necrophagia), as well as fantasies involving corpses.

Sexual Contact with Corpses

Krafft-Ebing (1965) describes a case of necrophilia as follows: "He exhumed cadavers of females ranging from 3 to 60 years of age, sucked their breasts, practiced cunnilingus on them, but rarely coitus or mutilation. . . . he was caught after he had taken home the body of a child 3½ years of age which he secreted in the straw. On this he gratified his sexual desires even while the putrid body was falling to pieces. The stench filling the house betrayed him. Laughingly, he admitted to everything" (pp. 68–69).

Brill (1941a) reports the case of a young man who was in psychoanalysis predominantly for his homosexuality but in whom necrophilic activities were uncovered: "However, in the course of the analysis he confessed that it was his morbid desire to play with corpses which prompted him to work for the undertaker, and that he repeatedly attempted fellatio on the corpses" (p. 441). Brill believed that the corpse symbolized the patient's dead mother or the mother of his infancy whose breasts he still craved.

Rapoport (1942) notes the case of a 50-year-old adopted male whose necrophilic fantasies began 6 years after the death of his adoptive mother. "'It was in 1930 that I first began to masturbate. An aunt (maternal) died. She was laid out in a casket; looking at her caused an erection. I went into the bathroom, I spit on it (penis) and rubbed it with my right hand.' He would kiss the lips of the corpse or touch the breasts. If this was impossible, he would just look at the body. Any of these stimuli would cause an erection. He would then wait until he could go to a lavatory or until he returned home to masturbate" (pp. 278–279). Rappaport concluded that this patient's necrophilic desires served as a manic defense. They were an attempt to overcome the impact of the loss of his mother. These activities also enabled him to express his contempt and disparagement of the former loved object (mother). The corpse, being dead and passive, could not retaliate. In addition, his sexual needs were satisfied.

Ehrenreich (1960) uncovered necrophilic activities and a desire for sexual intercourse with corpses during the hypnotherapy of a 43-year-old soldier imprisoned for murdering a prostitute. In this case, again, it was thought that necrophilic acts were performed in an attempt to deny the emotional impact of the death of a loved one years earlier.

Klaf and Brown (1958) present a case of necrophilic fantasy being detected during a sodium amytal interview. In this case report, a 40-year-old male with the diagnosis of schizophrenia was reported to have related a sexual attraction to female corpses. "On some occasions he would hug the dead bodies or run home to masturbate while thinking of the corpse as if it were alive; or during sexual intercourse he would in imagination substitute the corpse for his wife" (p. 648). The authors speculated that corpses, funeral parlors, and funerals were a source of satisfaction to this individual, and that corpses were seen as dolls toward which sadistic scopophilic and incestuous forces were directed.

Foerster *et al.* (1976) provide a case report of a 17-year-old girl who was involved in necrophilic activities. This is the only report of a female performing necrophilic activities.

Preservation of the body of a loved one for continued sexual gratification after that loved one's death is unusual. Reminiscent of Faulkner's "A Rose for Emily" there is the report of the "Romantic Necrophiliac of Key West," as recorded by Foraker (1976). In this case report, an eccentric German immigrant stole the corpse of his young, prematurely deceased Cuban girl friend. He had created a bedroom for the corpse in his shack, where he reconstructed the face, breasts, arms, legs, trunk, and vagina of his deceased girl friend. A vaginal tube had been constructed so that intercourse could be performed. Unlike many other cases of necrophilia, the perpetrator was not interested in corpses in general but only in preserving his illusion of an unchanged relationship with his beloved girl friend.

Necrosadism and Lust Murder

The few case reports in the literature of necrophilia attest to its rarity. There are more reports of necrosadim. Krafft-Ebing (1965, pp. 67–68) details the infamous case of Sergeant Bertrand.

> ... by accident in a graveyard, he ran across the grave of a newly buried corpse. Then this impulse, with heavy palpitation of the heart, became so powerful that, although there were people nearby, and he was in danger of detection, he dug up the body. In the absence of a convenient instrument for cutting it up, he satisfied himself by hacking it with a shovel. ... he accidentally came across the body of a girl of 16, for the first time, he experienced a desire to carry out coitus on a cadaver.
>
> I covered it with kisses, and pressed wildly to my heart. All that one could enjoy with a living woman is nothing in comparison with the pleasure I experienced. After I had enjoyed her for about a quarter of an hour, I cut the body up, as usual, and tore out the entrails.

Brill (1941b) presents a case of necrosadism with elements of necrophagy. In this case report, the patient is a 32-year-old single male, almost blind from birth and totally blind from the age of 4, when his eyes were removed. "He had a great desire for a dead body, which he wished to mutilate, wallow in, and perhaps eat" (p. 53). Brill felt that this man's fantasies represented the gratification of unsatisfied pregenital impulses.

Smith and Braun (1979) report a case of lust murder in the late 1970s. The individual was charged with the partial strangulation of 20 women, the last of whom he murdered and then copulated with. Earlier he would often demand that his wife "play dead" during intercourse. If she refused to cooperate, he would strangle her until she lost consciousness and then would perform coitus on her unconscious body.

Krafft-Ebing (1965) describes eight cases of lust murder. It is often difficult to determine the motivation or reaction of the charged murderer, but in at least one case, the culprit, a young man in his 20s, admitted, "I had an unspeakable delight in strangling women, experiencing during the act erections and real sexual pleasure. The feeling of pleasure while strangling was much greater than I experienced while masturbating" (p. 65).

Krafft-Ebing (p. 64) presents another case of lust murder: "Berzeni finally confessed his deeds and their motive. The commission of them gave him an indescribable pleasant (lustful) feeling, which was accompanied by erection and ejaculation. As soon as he had grasped his victim by the neck, sexual sensations were experienced. It was entirely the same to him, with reference to these sensations, whether the women were old, young, ugly or beautiful. Usually, simply choking had satisfied him, and he had then allowed his victims to live; in the two cases mentioned, the sexual satisfaction was delayed, and he had continued to choke them until they died."

Krafft-Ebing also presents the case of Jack the Ripper (1965, p. 59). This case is typical of many reports of lust murder. The murderer mutilated the bodies of his young woman victims and often cut off the genitals and carried them away from the scene of the crime. Typical of many of the lust murders, the intent and desires of the murderer are unknown. It has been speculated that these mutilations are "equivalents of the sexual act."

Allen (1962, pp. 222–224) presents the case of the "Rillington Place Murders." The bodies of several women were found hidden in the home or the garden of a private dwelling. There was evidence of sexual intercourse having taken place at or shortly after the death of the victims. Very little is known about the murderer's motivation in these crimes. It was speculated that necrophilia was perhaps one way to avoid the intense guilt he associated with normal sexual relationships.

Lancaster (1978) reports the case of a gifted and otherwise seemingly psychologically healthy young adult male who twice, under the influence of alcohol, robbed mortuaries and had sexual intercourse with the corpses he stole. Again, under the influence of alcohol, he entered a neighbor's home and stabbed a young bride to death and allegedly had intercourse with her. No psychological motivation could be discerned for these crimes. Bartholomew *et al.* (1978) present the case of a 22-year-old male with long-standing homosexual desires who murdered a male friend. His statement was that this murder was solely to obtain a body on which to perform sexual acts.

Necrophilic Fantasies

Necrophilic fantasies, as distinguished from actual necrophilic acts, are said to be ubiquitous by Calef and Weinshel (1972). These putatively common necrophilic fantasies are said to be related to an unconscious wish to return to the mother's womb and to explore her interior. They are often accompanied by the wish to remove or replace an intrauterine rival. Reider (1976) reports that necrophilic fantasies are often present in those physicians who seduce or are seduced by frigid female patients. Such necrophilic fantasies do not necessarily represent sexual desire for a corpse but merely utilize the "corpse" to symbolize the "dead sexuality" of the frigid woman. Such individuals have the grandiose fantasy of bringing what is dead to life. The motivation underlying such a desire would vary with the individual. Segal (1953) reports a necrophilic fantasy that was uncovered only in the course of therapy, and the emergence of such unconscious fantasies is probably not rare. Karpman (1934) briefly reports a patient's necrophilic fantasy as follows: "'I imagined that I sat in a room where I had women in my power. After I had gratified myself by torturing them in every conceivable way, I imagined them to be dead, and committed on their bodies every sort of desecration'" (p. 604).

Lazarus (1968) presents a case of a 23-year-old male whose sex life was dominated by necrophilic fantasy. He was unable to have intercourse because of extreme anxiety: "Over the years his fantasies shifted from woman to woman—always beautiful, always dead, usually murdered by somebody else" (p. 114). This man enjoyed female company and an active social life. In Lazarus's evaluation, the necrophilic tendencies were based on anxieties about sexual arousal in front of a woman. Treatment consisted of the systematic desensitization that involved progressively imagining sexual arousal, first in front of corpses, then unconscious females, and so on, until the patient could imagine sexual arousal in front of a fully alert female without anxiety. Treatment was successful; the necrophilic fantasies abated and intercourse with live women ensued. Eleven months after termination of therapy there was no return of necrophilic desires.

In summary, we see that the term *necrophilia* covers a wide variety of sexual behavior. It denotes sexual contact with corpses instigated out of lack of opportunity for live sexual relationships, and also out of a true paraphilic desire for the dead. It is used to denote acts of lust murder, necrosadism, and necrophagia. Case reports suggest that paraphilic necrophilia is the result of either extreme anxiety over sexual activities with live persons, causing the displacement of sex drive to corpses, or the symbolic representation of the corpse as a substitute for a desired but unobtainable love object. The psychological etiology of lust murder cannot be generalized. Aside from the presumed sadistic element, there have been a variety of mental mechanisms described in the genesis of these activities. In contrast to true paraphilic necrophilia and lust murder, necrophilic fantasies are apparently widespread and are not necessarily an indication of serious psychiatric pathology.

VAMPIRISM

There is a tendency to equate vampirism with necrophilia. However, vampirism is more usefully viewed as sexual arousal during the act of drawing blood.

Krafft-Ebing (1965, p. 85) cites a man who reported that each time he wished to approach his wife, he first had to make a cut on his arm. His wife could then suck the wound and become sexually aroused. Predictably, the husband had numerous scars on both arms. In 1927 Havelock Ellis postulated that the "love bite" represented the unconscious desire to draw blood as part of sexual delight. He also described a young girl who had a lifelong fascination with the sight of blood. She often cut or scratched herself to see and suck the blood. She bit her husband during intercourse and sucked his blood (pp. 120–123). London (1957) describes a female patient who frequently bit her lover on the neck and shoulders in order to draw blood (p. 123). London and Caprio (1958, pp. 603–604) report another case of a female patient who became sexually excited by biting her roommate about the neck and shoulders in order to bring blood to the skin's surface during mutual masturbation. She was excited by the sight of blood once when a friend cut a finger. She tasted the blood and simultaneously experienced a pleasant vaginal sensation.

In a review of the literature, Vanden Bergh and Kelly (1964) cite two case reports of men who manifested vampirism.

In one case, a 28-year-old white male reported he first noted his interest in the flow of blood when, at the age of 8, he produced a series of nosebleeds by picking at the inside of his nose. The sight of blood dripping to the floor gave him the feeling of pleasure and excitement. On reaching puberty, he developed more pronounced vampiristic tendencies. He found erotic satisfaction by nicking a vein in his arm and watching the blood flow from it. Simultaneously he would masturbate with fantasies of puncturing the prominent neck vein of an adolescent with a long, slender neck. His activities did not necessarily involve sucking or drinking blood but merely watching it flow. However, at times he would catch his blood in glass jars and then drink it. Eventually he developed the ability to control arterial punctures to the degree that he was able to watch blood spurt from arteries or direct the blood from the artery in a stream to his mouth. During times of stress he increased the frequency of bloodletting. He came to medical attention when he developed a severe anemia and other medical problems secondary to his bloodletting activities. He was eventually hospitalized with a "schizophrenic break."

The second case involved a 20-year-old white male who was in prison for auto theft. He would trade homosexual favors for the opportunity of sucking other inmates' blood. He came under scrutiny when several prison mates began requesting iron tablets. This man had a history of physical abuse in childhood. He first felt excited at the sight of blood upon seeing dogs that had been run over by cars in the street. "During his late childhood he put his hands in the blood of a dog so killed, tasted the blood and felt definite sexual excitement." At the age of 14 he had his first heterosexual intercourse with a girl 14 years his senior. He obtained great satisfaction by sucking her breasts and neck and producing areas of reddening. At the age of 15 he had a brief homosexual relationship that involved mutual fellatio with an older man. He persuaded the older man to allow him to cut his chest and neck in order to "see the blood." As this occurred, the patient became very excited and began sucking the blood. He experienced a feeling of becoming very "powerful" and quickly reached orgasm. This type of bloodletting then became his primary sexual aim with both men and women. He also wished to obtain blood from the area around the groin but had never found a willing partner.

There is no one set of intrapsychic dynamics in vampirism. Oral sadism is presumed to be important. However, in the two case reports by Vanden Bergh and Kelly, neither patient obtained satisfaction from the actual pain inflicted on the partner, but only from the sight of blood. In the first case, it was felt that blood symbolized "an unobtainable object or forbidden fruit," e.g., the man's mother. In the second case, the individual left Vanden Bergh's treatment before adequate study could be completed, but it was felt that the blood symbolized to him a "highly powerful and highly sexualized" object.

Vampirism and vampiristic fantasies are not commonly reported in the psychiatric literature. How common such thoughts are is not known. Issues of sadism, aggression, power, and control figure prominently in many cases of vampirism but vary from case to case.The symbolic significance of blood and of causing blood to flow may also be highly individualistic.

ZOOPHILIA

Zoophilia, zooerasty, and bestiality all refer to sexual contact between humans and animals. The initial impression that such contact is both unusual and representative of significant psychiatric pathology is inaccurate. Kinsey and his co-workers (Kinsey *et al.*, 1948, 1953) investigated human–animal contact in great detail. Their survey revealed that in some locales in the western United States up to 65% of all farm boys have had sexual contacts with animals. In the total population, 1 male in 12 or 14 has had sexual contact with an animal. Kinsey speculates that the incidence would be higher if opportunities were present in the urban population. In males, vaginal coitus with an animal was the most common type of sexual contact, and inducing the animal to mouth the genitals was also common. Among adult females, Kinsey found that 3.6% of his sample population had had some sexual contact with animals during or after adolescence. Of 5940 adult females sampled about preadolescent sexual contact with animals, 2 had had actual coitus with dogs, and 29 had had the animals mouth their genitals. Likewise, in a sample surveyed about their adult contact with animals, 1 of 5793 admitted to actual coitus with an animal. Consequently, it may be inferred that human–animal sexual contact is not uncommon and may be considered within the spectrum of normal sexual conduct.

Bestiality has been documented as a part of human sexual experience in the earliest records of mankind, and societal reaction of this form of sexual experience has ranged from the prescription of death in biblical times—"Whoever lies with a beast shall be put to death" (Exod. 22:19), "If a man lies with a beast, he shall be put to death and you shall kill the beast. If a woman approaches any beast and lies with it, you shall kill the woman and the beast; they shall be put to death, their blood is upon them." (Lev. 19:15, 16)—to a quiet acceptance in many rural communities today.

A distinction can be made between human–animal contact that is motivated primarily out of lack of available human sexual partners and that which is the result of a paraphilic desire. DSM-III has specific diagnostic criteria for zoophilia. "The act of fantasy of engaging in sexual activity with animals as a repeatedly preferred or exclusive method of achieving sexual excitement" (page 270). For clarity the term *zoophilia* will be used to describe cases in which there is a preference for sexual contact with animals; the term *bestiality* will be used as a more all-inclusive term for all human–animal sexual contact.

Bestiality—Animals as Substitutes

There are many reported cases of bestiality in the medical and psychiatric literature. In one intersting case, sexual intercourse between a woman and a dog resulted in an anaphylactic reaction to the animal's seminal fluids (Holden and Sherline, 1973). The patient presented to her physician approximately 20 minutes following intercourse with her German shepherd. She complained of dizziness and light-headedness. The physician diagnosed an allergic reaction to the dog's seminal fluid and the patient was treated with adrenalin. The patient indicated that intercourse with her dog was a substitute for human contact and stated that she had had sexual intercourse with her dog without anaphylaxis twice before in the last 10 months. Psychiatric evaluation revealed that the patient was neither grossly neurotic nor psychotic.

Since most human–animal sexual contact is not physically injurious, it is seldom brought to the attention of medical specialists. Reports are more likely to appear in the psychiatric literature. Schneck (1974) describes the case of a 45-year-old man in hypnoanalysis therapy for depression, anxiety, and work inefficiency. In the course of therapy it was determined that a mare, with which he had frequent sexual intercourse as an adolescent, symbolized his mother, and it was this symbolic equivalence that was of significance to him as opposed to a specific sexual desire for animals. There was no indication that the acts of bestiality had either a negative or a positive effect on his psychological well-being.

Shenken (1964) reports other cases of bestiality. In these cases, intercourse with animals was seen as an alternative to anxiety-provoking human intercourse. For example, a 33-year-old married farmer was afraid of hurting his wife during intercourse and therefore resorted to sex with animals. In another case, a 41-year-old farmer used intercourse with animals as a method of reducing his sexual desire out of fear that, if unrelieved, he would molest women.

Krafft-Ebing (1965) reports several cases of bestiality. In one case, a 30-year-old man of "high social position" was caught in the act of having intercourse with a hen. His defense centered on the assertion that his genitals were so small that intercourse with women was impossible.

Medical examination determined that the man was mentally sound but that his genitals were indeed extremely small (p. 375).

Chee (1974) reports a case of bestiality that came to medical and psychiatric attention only because of the participant's hypochondriacal concerns. A 23-year-old Chinese male reported a 5- or 6-year history of sexual contact with hens, though human female contacts were more desired. After one sexual contact with hens, in which his penis was exposed to fecal droppings, he became fearful that he might have contracted a veneral disease. With this fear as an impetus, he presented himself for medical attention.

The stated preference for human sexual contact does not ensure that this preference does in fact exist. Many individuals without human sex partners do not resort to animals for sexual gratification. Nevertheless, many individuals apparently engage in sexual contact with animals without a pervasive preference for animals.

Zoophilia—A Sexual Preference

Many cases of apparent sexual preference for animals are recorded. Krafft-Ebing (1965, p. 377) reports the case of a 40-year-old male peasant: "The patient had inclinations neither for women nor for men, but for animals (fowls, horses, etc.). He had intercourse with hens and ducks, and later with horses and cows. Never onanism. . . . He always had an aversion for women. In a single attempt at coitus with a woman he was impotent, but with animals he was always potent. He was bashful before women; coitus with women he regarded almost as a sin."

Krafft-Ebing (1965, pp. 378–379) also presents a case in which there was sexual arousal by the sight or contact with animals: "One day when he mounted a mare for the first time, he experienced a sensation of lust; two weeks later, on a similar occasion, the same sensation with erection. During his first ride he had ejaculation. A month after, the same thing happened. . . . When he saw men on horseback, or dogs, he had erections. Almost every night he had pollutions accompanied by dreams on which he rode on horseback or was training dogs."

In an interesting treatment that seems to have presaged current psychotherapeutic techniques involving eidetic imagery, this patient was cured of his zoophilic impulses: "A further attempt at coitus was successful with images of riders and dogs, which stimulated erection. The patient grew more virile; his love for animals waned; erections at the sight of riders and dogs disappeared, nocturnal pollutions with dreams of animals becmme less frequent; he dreamed now of girls."

Krafft-Ebing (pp. 379–380) presents another case of treated zoophilia. A 47-year-old man requested help in changing his sexual practices:

"He was decidedly hypersexual, practiced masturbation with passion, and at the age of 14 forgot himself so far as to sodomize bitches, mares and other female animals.... The mere sight of animals excited him wildly. The society of ladies caused him ennui. When he went with a girl, she had to resort to all kinds of manipulation to prepare him for the act."

Once again, Dr. Krafft-Ebing's therapeutic acumen prevailed over zoophilia: "I made strong suggestions to be on his guard against masturbation and bestiality, and to seek more the society of ladies; prescribed anaphrodisiacs, advised frugality, slight hydrotherapy, plenty of open air, exercise, steady occupation, and had the satisfaction to learn that the patient at the end of ten months experienced a slight gratification in repeated sexual intercourse with a woman and that he was almost free from his former perverse desires."

Altogether, Krafft-Ebing reports seven cases of bestiality and one case of beast fetishism. No other investigator has as large a series of cases.

Allen (1962, pp. 211–214) presents the case of a 32-year-old man who was sexually preoccupied with horses: "His sexual interest in horses increased and led at first to masturbation and finally to actual intercourse. He realized that this was very dangerous and he might have lost his life, but said that he did not mind taking the risk and could sense whether the mare was receptive or not. He had had this sexual urge for 12 years when seen."

Allen makes these psychological etiologic assumptions: "It would seem, therefore, that this man was really fixated to his mother. He was able to have sexual intercourse with his wife but unconsciously desired his mother. This attachment to his mother came out in the longing for buttocks (as symbols for her breasts) and thence to mares. His intercourse with mares was therefore really intercourse with the mother."

More lengthy reports of cases of individuals with zoophilia treated with psychotherapy exist. Shenken (1964) reports the case of a single man in his late 20s treated for 21 months in psychoanalytic psychotherapy. He sought treatment for a pronounced sexual attraction for animals that had driven him to many acts of bestiality over several years. These acts of bestiality were pleasurable but were followed by severe guilt. The patient stated that he was interested in women but had never been able to develop satisfactory relationships. In the course of therapy, the patient achieved a full reorientation of sexual desire. It was the author's belief that for this patient the animal represented simultaneously the patient, his mother, and his father. Further, the author felt that the patient's libido functioned primarily at a pre-Oedipal level with problems involving anal eroticism and conflict over passive femininity.

In another case of zoophilia treated with psychoanalysis, reported by Rappaport (1968), a 20-year-old college graduate revealed a very unusual sexual practice involving animals:

> Habitually he sneaked or broke into stables where he knew he would find horses—he could get sexually excited merely from the smell of horses—and then would try to squeeze the neck of the horse between his legs, at the same time masturbating the horse's penis. Drawing forcefully on the horse's bridle, to pull its neck backward, he wanted the horse to get on its hind legs, or, best of all, to make it roll on its back, in either case for the purpose of making the penis point upward. Often, after he had sneaked into a stable, he tied up a stallion's legs, made it go on its knees, and then pushed the horse down, jumped on top of it and had "an emission" as he called it. At times he managed to insert his own erect penis into the foreskin of the stallion. . . . However, what he wanted most of all was to have the stallion mount the mare and then to jump on top of the stallion and then to ejaculate simultaneously with the stallion.

Rappaport's explanation of this paraphilia is lengthy and abstruse. He draws certain parallels between this case and Freud's case of Little Hans.

Bestiality has long been recognized as a part of human sexual expression. Despite social proscriptions against its practice, it persists as a not uncommon practice in our society. It is more frequent in males and in rural areas, but it is not unheard of in women and among city-dwellers. Its incidence may vary with opportunity. It often reflects the unavailability of human sexual contact. Zoophilia, defined as a specific preference for animal contact over human sexual contact, is presumably relatively rare, though its true incidence is unknown. The type of animal preference in zoophiliacs and the psychodynamics that determine the type of activity vary from case to case. Animal contacts often represent a displacement of sexual desire to an object that is a symbolic substitute for a forbidden, anxiety-laden sexual object or behavior. Once such behavior is established, it is presumably capable of self-perpetuation on the basis of its reinforcing properties. While case reports are few, the scant literature suggests that this paraphilia may respond to psychotherapeutic intervention.

As an interesting sidelight, Kinsey and his co-workers (Kinsey *et al.*, 1948, p. 677) report that some male dogs who have been masturbated during acts of bestiality develop a preference for human sexual contact over sexual contact with females of their own species.

AUTOEROTIC ASPHYXIA

VLADIMIR: What do we do?
ESTRAGON: Wait.
VLADIMIR: Yes, but while waiting?

ESTRAGON: What about hanging ourselves?
VLADIMIR: Hmm. It'd give us an erection.
ESTRAGON: With all that follows. Where it falls, mandrakes grow. That's why they shriek when you pull them up. Did you not know that?
ESTRAGON: Let's hang ourselves immediately!

Samuel Beckett, (*Waiting for Godot*, 1954, pp. 12–13)

The production of sexual excitement or even orgasm of self-induced asphyxia is an unusual but not uncommon sexual syndrome. It is estimated that over 50 deaths from autoerotic asphyxia occur in the United States each year (Litman and Swearingen, 1972). In Massachusetts, 25% of the reported suicides between 1941 and 1950 by individuals under 21 years of age were in retrospect thought to be due to autoerotic asphyxia (Stearns, 1953). Since one of the characteristics of this syndrome is repetitive self-asphyxiation without the apparent motive of suicide, most of these deaths are judged to be accidental.

This syndrome has been called the Kotzwarra syndrome, after the Czech bass player who died at the hands of a prostitute in 1791. Kotzwarra had apparently given the prostitute instructions to hang him by the neck for 5 minutes and then to release him. Following instructions faithfully, albeit with poor judgment, the prostitute released a dead man. The Marquis de Sade has also described the pleasure and orgasm caused by asphyxia. Interestingly, Eskimo children strangle themselves in play, probably to produce sexual pleasure, and various South American peoples practice partial strangulation to experience exhilaration (Resnik, 1972).

If death represents an accidental outcome of self-asphyxiation, then the true prevalence of those who pracitce this sexual syndrome without mishap must be much higher than the estimated 50 deaths per year would suggest. There are very few reports of living practitioners of this syndrome. Most of the information obtained on this syndrome has been about those who died practicing autoerotic asphyxia. For this reason, the bulk of the information we have on this syndrome may be from a select segment of its practitioners—those who were either careless enough or depressed enough to improperly plan and carry out this sexual practice and therefore died.

The following is a typical report of the syndrome. "A 21 year old single white male was found in a locked room at the foot of a bed. He was clad in a black brassiere, woman's bikini underpants, and high heeled shoes. Ropes were tied about his waist and legs and his hands were tied behind his back. In addition, a rope looped about his neck, protected by a towel, ran under the waist rope and was secured to the upper post of a double-decked bunk. A magazine was found on the floor showing a nude woman who was bound in a similar fashion to the victim. The manner of death was ruled accidental" (Walsh *et al.*, 1977, p. 164).

The presumed goal in such cases is asphyxia produced for erotic, not self-destructive purposes. Those who have died in this practice tend to be young white males who are naked or partially clothed, often with evidence of transvestite activity. In many instances there is evidence of other features of bondage (ropes, restraints, and chains). Mirrors, photographic equipment, or pornography and other sexual materials are often found. In keeping with the lack of suicidal intent, the contrivance used for producing asphyxia is usually padded to prevent bruising and allows quick release. It also often allows the participant to control the amount of asphyxia produced. Frequently there is evidence of penile engorgement and ejaculation. The act is usually solitary and often there is the suggestion that self-asphyxiation has been repetitively performed. Death results from faulty release mechanisms or when unconsciousness prevents manipulation of the asphyxiation device.

Methods of producing asphyxia vary greatly. The use of ropes, plastic bags, rubber sheets, and even heavy chains with padlocks or rubber scuba-diving helmets have been reported. Coe (1974) reports the instance of a victim who used a padded rope and electrically motorized lift to produce asphyxia.

Sass (1975) presents a rare case of autoerotic asphyxia in a female. The victim was a 35-year-old divorcee living with her 9-year-old daughter. There was no indication of depression, suicidal ideation, or emotional difficulty. The woman was found dead one morning in the rear of the closet in her bedroom.

> An electric vibrator connected to an extension cord was found running. The vibrator was positioned between her thighs with the hard rubber massaging head in contact with the victim's vulva. There was a spring type clothes pin on the nipple of the right breast, compressing the nipple, and another clothes pin of the same type found immediately below her left breast. . . . The victim had placed her head in the loop (of a nylon hose) and placed a hand towel between her neck and the nylon hose. . . . The victim intended to support her weight with her arms, as in a push-up, but passed out. This released her arms and the full weight of her body came to rest on the nylon stocking around her neck, causing the strangulation. (pp. 183–184)

Walsh *et al.* (1977) report on a series of 43 cases of autoerotic asphyxial deaths. They found that in all 43 cases, white males were the self-imposed victims. There was an age range of 14 to 75 years, but 28 of the 43 were below 25 years of age. Evidence of transvestism was present in over one-third of the cases. The cause of death was judged to be accidental in 35 of the cases, suicide in 3, and undertermined in 5.

There are a few descriptions of self-asphyxiation from living practitioners. Shankel and Carr (1956) present the case of a 17-year-old boy treated predominantly for transvestism who also admitted to episodes of self-hanging. The patient stated that his first self-hanging episode was at the age of 10 or 11 and was motivated primarily by the desire to kill himself. In the first hanging attempt he developed an erection and found the experience sexually arousing. Therefore, he engaged in the practice repetitively, accompanied by transvestism and masturbation. He denied subsequent suicidal intent. The authors speculate that the hangings represented a symbolic acting-out of castration fears. The body symbolized the genitals and the hanging symbolized threatened loss of the genitals. The patient gained control over the process by terminating the hanging short of physical harm.

Edmondson (1972) reports another case of autoerotic asphyxia in which death did not ensue: "John was referred at the age of 14½. He had been surprised in his bedroom by his mother, who found him lying on his back, clearly in the process of masturbating. He had rope passed around the end of his bed and then around his neck under his chin. He was blue in the face. The mother, distressed by this discovery, contacted the family doctor."

Edmondson determined that the hangings represented a form of self-punishment needed to combat the guilt associated with the sexual activity. He felt that the patient did not suffer from depression. The patient seemed to benefit from therapy by a marked lessening of his guilt surrounding sexual matters.

Litman and Swearingen (1972) placed an advertisement indicating their interest in talking to bondage practitioners in the *Los Angeles Free Press*. This ad generated nine face-to-face interviews with male practitioners of bondage. Of these, at least two had episodes of strangulation with masturbation. The authors concluded that these individuals manifested a death orientation and pervasive feelings of loneliness and isolation.

What motivates individuals to seek sexual gratification in this manner? In addition to sexual arousal, it has been speculated that the relative anoxia and hypercarbia caused by constriction of the neck produces a disinhibited state with light-headedness and exhilaration (Resnick, 1972). Resnik also hypothesizes that constriction of the neck represents an upward displacement of castration concerns, thereby explaining why this syndrome is most commonly seen in males, many of whom practice transvestism. Repeated constriction of the neck may be seen as a symbolic form of castration. Symbolic castration and near death may then serve to absolve guilt connected with Oedipal and incestual fantasies. Anxiety is also relieved by concurrent masturbation and sexual arousal, which verify the existence of a functioning penis. Resnick further hypothesizes that gambling with death is connected to fantasies of maternal reunion. Other theories suggest that repeated episodes of near death reduce anxiety and feelings of depression by giving the practitioner control and mastery over his life. For some, self-hanging may also be a punishment for the guilt-laden pleasures of sexual satisfaction.

COPROPHILIA AND RELATED PARAPHILIAS

Coprophilia is a rare paraphilia centering on the sexual arousal produced by excrement or the act of defecating. The most graphic description of coprophilia is found in the writings of Marquis de Sade.

> Having then adopted the most comfortable position, he glued his mouth to the object of his worship, and in less time than it takes to tell, I delivered a gobbet of shit the size of a pigeon's egg. He sucked it, turned it a thousand times about in his mouth, chewed it, savored it, at the end of three or four minutes I distinctly saw him swallow it; push again, the same ceremony is repeated, and as I had a prodigous charge to be rid of, ten times over he filled his mouth and emptied it, even after all was done, he seemed famished still. . . .
>
> "Oh, Great God, what pleasure you give me! I've never eaten more delicious shit, I swear to that before any jury. Give it to me, bring it hither, my angel, bring me your matchless ass to suck, let me devour it." (de Sade, 1957, pp. 90–91)

Case reports of coprophilia are very few. Krafft-Ebing (1965) briefly mentions one case: A Russian prince, who was very decrepit, was accustomed to having his mistress turn her back on him and defecate on his breast; this being the only way in which he could excite the remnant of libido" (p. 129).

He also reports the case of an individual with both coprophilic and urophilic desires: "It caused him the greatest pleasure if the prostitutes deposited their feces and urine on his mouth (or face). He would also pour wine over their bodies and as it flowed down over their vaginas, he would lap it up with his mouth. He was greatly pleased if he could suck the menstrual blood seeping from their genitals" (p. 129).

In Karpman's study of coprophilia (1948), he makes the following observation about the genesis of coprophilia: "The child's primitive method of evacuation brings the entire surface of its buttocks and lower extremities in contact with urine and feces. This contact seems unpleasant, even repulsive, to adults, whose repressions have removed them from the infantile reaction to these processes. They cannot appreciate the source of pleasure on which the libido of the infant can draw, in whom the stream of warm urine on the skin in contact with the warm mass of feces, produce pleasurable feelings" (p. 257).

In a later series of papers, Karpman (1949a, 1949b) presents the case of a young musician who had various sexual fantasies involving eating feces and playing with his own feces while masturbating.

> "Sometimes I get mad and just put myself in my place. Then I imagine myself lying way down in some sewer all the time, and living and lying in the sewage and urine and feces; and staying there and having no desire for anything else, and when I get hungry, just rolling over and eating of the feces that came along constantly, and when I wasn't eating, just otherwise enjoying the sensation of the feces. That would really be an ideal existence, with no worries of any kind, and I would be completely in my right place, for I've got a nerve trying anything else. I'd have everything right there— life, a bed, air, food, drink, and sex, and also defecation. That covers everything." (p. 170)

Karpman has no definite explanation for the patient's coprophilic fantasies but speculates that there was a historic association between the patient's attraction to his mother and a situation involving defecation or toilet functions.

Tarachow (1966) reports on two analyses in which coprophagic tendencies were uncovered. He described one case as follows: "He experienced strong pleasure in odors, in flatulence, in sweat, and in constipation. He had a strong interest in and an affection for his stool. He could not bear to flush the toilet, and would fondle and caress the stool in the bowl before, most reluctantly, permitting it to flush down. He had peculiar sensations in his mouth and had frequent fantasies and compulsive thoughts of eating his stool (p. 686). In Tarachow's second case he compares coprophagic impulses to the eating of nasal mucus, pulled hair, and other bodily secretions. These tendencies were related to both obsessional neurosis and depression.

Urolagnia

Urolagnia is also a rarely reported paraphilia. Pornographic publications and underground sex newspapers suggest that devotees of urolagnia or "golden stream" are not uncommon, especially among sadomasochistic homosexuals. However, there is a dearth of information about such individuals in the psychiatric literature. Krafft-Ebing (1965, p. 129) reports the case of a 45-year-old male who from his 16th year gained sexual satisfaction by drinking the urine of females. Bergler (1936) describes the case of a young man treated in psychoanalytic psychotherapy who manifested urolagnia: "If the girl wished him to have intercourse, he was potent. But he greatly preferred allowing the girl to urinate over him, and to drink the urine, while the girl uttered filthy expressions." Bergler feels that these activities allowed the patient to remain passive during the sex act and to avoid castration fears. Allen (1962) reports the case of a man prosecuted three times for loitering in public lavatories. The police arrested him on charges of attempting to procure homosexual prostitutes, but psychiatric examination revealed that he frequented these rest rooms because of his erotic interest in urine and urination.

Klismaphilia

Another form of paraphilia related to excretion and the excretory process is klismaphilia, sexual stimulation and even orgasm resulting from having an enema. Bieber (1970) states that the eroticization of enemas is caused by mothers who stimulate the genitals or the genital areas of their sons while giving them enemas. Nacht et al. (1956) report the case of a 30-year-old man, impotent with his wife, who can achieve orgasm when given an enema by a small boy. Denko (1973) presents two cases of individuals sexually stimulated by enemas. The first individual is a 27-year-old army officer who sought treatment because he found enemas more sexually stimulating than coitus. For years he had daily given himself an enema with which he experienced erection and usually ejaculation. Often this was accompanied by flagellating his buttocks with a hairbrush. In addition, he would at times attempt to induce his wife to administer an enema to him but would hide his arousal. The patient's amnesis revealed that in his family the young children were given daily enemas. At the age of 3 he attempted to sit on an oilcan with a spout to give himself an enema, or to produce the enema sensation. He admitted that throughout his marriage his true sexual interest had been in enemas, and he fantasized about them while having intercourse with his wife. Denko also reviewed the case of a 70-year-old disbarred lawyer who had klismaphilic tendencies. Intrigued by these first case reports, Denko (1976) placed an advertisement in a Cleveland underground newspaper asking for correspondence from those who used enemas for sexual arousal. From this advertisement she uncovered 13 additional klismaphiliacs. She divided these into three types. The first was an ego-alien compartmentalized type. The persons in this category did not accept their klismaphilic tendencies and felt that perhaps they were harbingers of some problem. The second were a monodeviant, egosyntonic type, who accepted their klismaphilic tendencies but did not involve themselves with other sexual deviations. The third group consisted of egosyntonic, pervasive, polydeviant individuals whose klismaphilia was only one of a number of other deviant sexual behaviors. Five of these newly discovered cases were females. One of these respondents reported that he had placed a similar advertisement in an underground newspaper and had received over 100 replies. He reported that 80% of his respondents were men and 20% were women. He also found that 50% reported engag-

ing in masochistic acts such as spankings, bondage, and compelled retention of the enema fluid. Twenty percent combined klismaphilia with
urine or excrement fetishes. Enema solutions used included ice water,
beer, soda water, coffee, vodka and water, wine, lemon juice and water,
soapy water and lemon juice, milk, and molasses.

Denko offers several explanations for this paraphilia, including
childhood conditioning, passivity, and masochism. She also suggests that
in some persons, "nerve endings in the rectum are capable of producing
reactions pleasurable and similar to those produced by nerve endings in
and around the genitalia, that is, in the cerebral connections and cortical
centers where orgasm is experienced" (p. 252).

While coprophilia and related paraphilias are not commonly
reported in the medical and psychiatric literature, it is likely that they
are not rare, given the volume of related pornographic literature. Apparently, practitioners of these sexual activities seldom come to psychiatric
attention and therefore the paucity of case reports does not reflect true
prevalence. Similarly, treatment outcomes of these unusual sex syndromes are for the most part unkown.

INCEST

Despite the fact that sexual contact between blood relatives is generally prohibited, it is found in virtually every culture. Almost every possible permutation of related partners has been reported. Father–daughter
incest is most frequently noted. Lukianowicz (1972) reports that of 650
psychiatric female patients in Northern Ireland, 26 cases of paternal
incest were found. This suggests that approximately 4% of these psychiatric patients had incestuous relationship with their fathers. Lukianowicz
also reviewed 700 unselected psychiatric patients (350 males and 350
females), uncovering 15 cases of brother–sister incest, 5 cases of grandfather–granddaughter incest, 4 cases of uncle–niece incest, 3 cases of
mother–son incest, and 2 cases of aunt–nephew incest. Meiselman (1979)
accumulated 58 cases of incest in an outpatient psychiatric clinic. Though
the majority were father–daughter cases, she found 1 case of father–son
incest, 1 case of mother–daughter incest, and 3 cases of mother–son
incest. We will review in greater detail the more unusual syndromes of
mother–son incest, father–son incest, and mother–daughter incest.

Mother–Son Incest

The Oedipus myth is the prototypic tale of mother–son incest. Oedipus was so concerned over the oracle's prophecy that he would kill his
father and marry his mother that he departed from his parents' home.

Unknown to him, he had been reared by adoptive parents. During his adventures after leaving home, he slew Laius, the king of Thebes, not knowing him to be his true father. Then, after solving the Sphinx's riddle, he was made the new king of Thebes, and given Jocasta (his natural mother) as his wife. Ultimately, the truth of his relationship to Laius and Jocasta became known to him and he blinded himself in a fit of remorse (Guirand, 1968, pp. 192–193).

The cultural proscription against mother–son incest appears to be relatively stronger and more widespread than the proscriptions against other forms of incest. The wide variety of case reports of mother–son incest reveal many diverse family patterns. Among the most unusual cases is one reported by Barry and Johnson (1958) wherein a marriagelike arrangement developed between a mother and son as a misperception of their family physician's advice. When the alcoholic father deserted the family, the physician encouraged the son to assume the paternal duties. The mother and son interpreted this in a more global sense than the physician had intended and engaged in sexual relations. Neither mother nor son manifested feelings of guilt, nor were they reported to have any psychiatric disorder.

Other cases, however, suggest pathology in the involved son. Bender and Blau (1937) report the case of a 6-year-old Puerto Rican boy who slept with his mother following her divorce. Repeatedly during the night he would attempt to mount her and place his penis in her vagina. After the mother remarried, the child shared the conjugal bed. His sexual behavior now included attempting to insert his foot into his mother's vagina. At the instigation of the stepfather the case was brought to psychiatric attention. The boy spent 5 years in treatment facilities. He then returned home (Bender and Grugett, 1952). Little is said about the psychological makeup of the family members. It was noted that, subsequent to the boy's return, everyone made a normal adjustment. Lukianowicz (1972) briefly reports three cases of mother–son incest. In one case, the son was diagnosed as schizophrenic and the mother was reported to have subsequently developed a delusional depression. In the second case, the mother was diagnosed as schizophrenic and the son was thought to be educationally subnormal. In the third case, the mother was termed neurotic and the son was thought to be normal.

In many instances the mother is the instigator. Yorukoglu and Kemph (1966) describe the case of a 13-year-old boy whose mother had been playing with his penis and instructing him to use his hand and mouth on her genitalia. At times the mother would have her son suck one breast and use a vibrator to stimulate her genitalia, while having her daughter suck on the other breast. She also instigated sexual intercourse with her son. The mother engaged in these activities when she was intoxicated. The child admitted to guilt feelings about these activities but otherwise had a positive relationship with his mother and desired to remain with her. The boy had a history of fire setting and of making sexual advances to both boys and girls. The mother's history included having been raped by her brother-in-law. She had been severely berated by her own father for many years over this incident. In the first of her two marriages she had been emotionally and physically abused.

Meiselman (1979) reports the case of a mother who intiated mother–son intercourse. The mother, a prostitute, was thought to suffer from both psychosis and alcoholism. Often she would have intercourse with her customers in front of her son and then beat him with a strap if she felt angry with the customer. "When Earl was about 4, she took him into her bed one night and rubbed her genital organs against his in order to masturbate; after obtaining sexual gratification, she found some excuse to beat him. These incidents occurred many times in the next two or three years and seemed to have been the only occasions on which Earl received any warmth or emotional involvement from his mother. . . ." (p. 304).

Though the son made a fair adjustment, he became a voyeur and would later delight, after becoming intoxicated, in picking up prostitutes. He would have them undress and then laugh sadistically as he said that he had no intention of paying them. He did, however, graduate from college, marry, and at least superficially maintain a facade of competence.

Meiselman presents another case of mother–son incest in which the son, now in his mid-40s, sought psychotherapy. He was intermittently depressed, often drank heavily, and had made several suicide attempts. At times he would dress in his wife's lingerie and had pedophiliac tendencies, with a special attraction to prepubescent girls. He had married at age 33 to a quiet but undemonstrative wife. His father was described as an alcoholic who ignored his wife and the children most of the time. The patient's contact with his mother was described as follows: "When Dale was three years old, she began to regularly manipulate his genitals while bathing him, and this behavior continued throughout his childhood. She would explain from time to time that their family doctor had told her to play with his penis so that it would not become diseased. He also recalled many instances of seeing his mother nude and becoming sexually excited by the sight of her body."

This provocative behavior continued throughout the patient's childhood: "She presented Dale with many opportunities to have sexual intercourse with her, but the incestuous affair was not fully consummated for three more years because he would become impotent at the last minute. Finally his mother took him out to dinner on the occasion of his 19th birthday, he became intoxicated, and she suggested that he try to think of her as a girl his age, just for the evening. He then succeeded in having intercourse with her and repeated the experience on several occasions until he left home at the age of 23" (pp. 307–309).

In a case of mother–son incest recorded by Berry (1975), the son had always seen himself as the mother's special confidant in the struggle with a distant, hostile father. Throughout his childhood the mother had periodically inspected her son's penis to see if "it's growing properly." Also, on more than one occasion she insisted that he examine her genitalia. Though intercourse was never consummated, she at times made seductive advances to him. As an adult, the patient had entered treatment because of his fears of homosexuality.

Wahl (1960) reports two cases of mother–son incest. In the first case, the son was thought to be schizophrenic and the mother was an alcoholic who was often vulnerable to sexual abuse while intoxicated. In the second case, the son was also thought to be schizophrenic. In this case the mother was overtly seductive and was even observed to play with her son's genitals in the psychiatric hospital.

Based on these two case reports, Wahl presents 11 possible predisposing factors to mother–son incest. These include the mother's physical or psychological absence during childhood, the absence of a strong father, overt maternal seduction, loss of maternal control, slight age discrepancy between parent and child, the witnessing of the primal scene, incestual experiences with other family members, lack of sexual outlets, low intelligence, undue physical manipulation of the child by the parent, and nonconsanguinous parental relationships.

Raphling *et al.* (1967) describe the case of a 29-year-old married man referred for psychiatric evaluation because of incestuous relationships with his daughters. His history revealed a complex series of incestual relationships. The patient had been incestuously involved with his own sister and had been overtly seduced by his mother. His father and his sister were also involved in an incestuous relationship. Later the patient had frequent intercourse with his 16- and 17-year-old daughters and had encouraged his 14-year-old son to have intercourse with the mother. The patient had also attempted a sexual relationship with his 10-year-old daughter but desisted when she protested. Interestingly, his only acknowledged feeling of guilt was in regard to the sexual contact with his own mother.

There are multiple etiological factors in the reported cases of mother–son incest. The strong cultural prohibition against incest necessitates that several permissive factors be present before such incest can be consummated. In most instances the mother either actively or covertly encourages the relationship, often in association with weakened behavioral controls secondary to alcoholism or severe psychopathology. The father is usually either absent or emotionally uninvolved with the family. In most of the families there is a weakened incest taboo, often secondary to psychopathology or to prior incest experiences of the patient.

Father–Son Incest

Father–son incest has been thought to be a relatively uncommon occurrence. Dixon *et al.* (1978) questions its rarity after finding 6 cases of father–son incest in 1300 male psychiatric patients. Reichenthal (1979) cites 33 reported cases and adds 4 of his own discovery. Many of the fathers involved in this form of incest are reported to have severe psychological problems and often exhibit alcoholism or abusiveness.

Dixon *et al.* (1978) describe a case of a 5-year-old male, the eldest of two children, who presented to a psychiatric clinic with hyperactivity, aggressive behavior, and poor peer relations. His IQ scores were on the borderline mental retardation range. After he had been in treatment for a year and a half, he spontaneously reported that his father had tried to put his "ding-dong where I go poo-poo. . . . It didn't fit." The father, known to be physically abusive, had since left the family. It was thought that this incestuous act occurred while the mother was in the hospital. In another case reported by the same authors, a 6-year-old boy, the eldest of three children, was hospitalized for evaluation of child abuse by the father. The patient had complained to his mother that the father had been touching his genitals and putting his mouth on the boy's penis. Some of these incidents had been witnessed by the mother and sister, and earlier bite marks had sometimes been found around the patient's penis. The father was known to abuse alcohol and the mother had a history of prostitution and psychiatric hospitalization. In another of the six cases presented, Dixon describes a 15-year-old boy who was seen in a psychiatric consultation for abdominal pain, anorexia, withdrawal, depression, insomnia, and self-mutilation. During the course of the examination, it was uncovered that the father was sexually abusing all six children in the family. The 13- and 14-year-old daughters, as well as four sons, aged 8, 10, 12, and 15, had all suffered sexual abuse over the preceding 10 years. In another case report, an 18-year-old boy reported a homosexual involvement with the father. Apparently the mother had suspected this for more than 6 years but had never protested or reported the occurrence, a finding often reported in families with father–daughter incest. The father was a fifth-grade dropout, unemployed for several years. He was "disabled due to nerves," drank excessively, and was physically abusive to the children.

Reichenthal (1979) presents four cases of father–son incest. He describes one as follows: "John had been sexually used by his father from the time he was 8 until age 13 when his father suicided while psychotic. The almost daily activity involved masturbation and fellatio performed upon the boy whose reaction was a mixture of pleasure, excitement and shameful disgust" (p. 122).

Rhinehart (1961) describes an 18-year-old male who had been involved in father–son and brother–brother incest since the age of 12. The father was noted to be an alcoholic and was supposed to have initiated the homosexual acts. At the time of psychiatric intervention the patient felt that the only thing that could be done for him was to turn him into a woman. He became involved in homosexual relations with a "father surrogate" and made several suicide attempts when separated from this man.

Awad (1976) writes of father–son incest that occurred while the father was intoxicated. The mother was aware of the activity but said nothing. The author's interpretation was that the father had been struggling against latent homosexuality over a long period of time and that the disinhibiting effect of the alcohol allowed its expression.

Not all cases suggest that aggressive, alcoholic fathers are a prerequisite for father–son incest. Raybin (1969) reports a case of father–son genital contact initiated by the father when the son was 20. It appears that the son, after reporting a homosexual episode to the father, was subsequently propositioned by him. Their encounter consisted of the son having his genitals passively manipulated by the father. The father admitted that his own father had periodically manipulated his genitals when he was 5 to 10 years of age, and that he had had sexual relationships with his brother and cousin.

Langsley *et al.* (1968) commented on an 18-year-old youth who ingested LSD and during the subsequent psychotic episode reported multiple homosexual experiences with his father. The father confessed to initiating mutual masturbation, beginning when the son was 12 and continuing for about a year and a half. The father had himself been involved in an incestuous affair consisting of mutual masturbation with a 19-year-old uncle when he was 12. At the age of 25 he began to mutually masturbate with a male cousin. His heterosexual adjustment was tenuous. At the age of 36 he married a woman 10 years his junior. During their first year of marriage he had difficulty ejaculating during intercourse. On one occasion the wife had observed her husband and son exercising in the nude, but she said nothing and later denied the incident.

Medlicott (1967) cites three cases of father–son incest. He concludes that the fathers symbolically castrate their sons by homosexual assault as a reaction to the son's rivalry. He also believes that the fathers feel inadequate with their wives.

As yet another example of father–son incest, Berry (1975) describes the case of a 24-year-old man who presented concerns over his limited sexual and social experience with women. His amnesis revealed that between the ages of 3 and 8 he frequently showered with his father. During these showers the father inserted his finger into the child's anus under the pretext of washing the child.

The case of reports of father–son incest demonstrate etiologic factors and family dynamics similar to those found in other forms of incest, including the frequent failure of the mother to intervene. In many cases, the father abuses alcohol and is impulsive and aggressive. Often the father has a lifelong homosexual orientation. In all instances recorded, the incestuous activity has been initiated by the father. The ultimate psychological effect on the child is difficult to determine. Meiselman (1979) suggests that the sons in these cases become disturbed and anxious about the possibility of becoming homosexual when they approach adolescence. She further notes that most victims of father–son incest become either heterosexual or bisexual as adults.

Mother–Daughter Incest

Mother–daughter sexual relationships are extremely rarely reported. Meiselman (1979) reports a case that might be considered covert mother-daugher incest: "When Carol was about 8, her mother went through a period of extreme suspiciousness about the possibility that her husband was sexually molesting the children and insisted on conducting frequent pelvic examinations, inspecting Carol's vagina for any sign of irritation" (p. 321–322). Medlicott (1967) cites the case of a student he saw in psychotherapy for tension headaches, sexual fears, and academic underachievement. This woman admitted that during her adolescence her mother insisted on sleeping with her to avoid the father and often seduced her into sexual play.

Weiner (1964) describes the case of a daughter separated from her mother by foster home placement until she was 26 years of age. Upon reuniting, they had a brief homosexual affair. Neither was felt to be psychotic, but the daughter had a later psychiatric hospitalization for depression following the breakup of another homosexual affair.

There are too few cases to enable one to make generalizations regarding the etiology of this rarely reported condition.

The long-range effects of the rare forms of incestuous couplings on the psychological well-being of the participants is difficult to predict.

Many children involved do not escape without some emotional scarring, but the severity is variable. Additionally, it is difficult to separate the long-term effects of the act of incest from the long-term effects of the conditions that allowed or caused the incest to occur.

HYPERSEXUALITY

More than any of the other sexual syndromes discussed in this chapter, "hypersexuality" is a concept without clear definition. Don Juanism, satyriasis, nymphomania, and compulsive sexuality have all been used synonymously with hypersexuality. Kinsey *et al.* (1948) suggest that individuals who exhibit an extremely high orgasmic frequency are simply on a continuum with individuals who have a lower frequency, and that hypersexuality does not exist as a specific syndrome. As an example, they cite the case of a "scholarly and skilled lawyer" who averaged over 30 ejaculations per week for a period of 30 years, and suggest that there was nothing in this individual's history to indicate that this rate of sexual activity was pathological. In contrast, Cooper *et al.* (1972) describe a 40-year-old "hypersexual" whose "coital needs" averaged five to seven times per week. Episodes of loss of control and "sexual assaults" on his 15-year-old daughter brought this man to legal and psychiatric attention. In this case, the term *hypersexual* was apparently used not to denote the relatively increased frequency of sexual activity but to indicate deviant sexual activity. Brotherton (1974) provides a tautological definition of hypersexuals as "those who have been discovered by the police because of abnormal hypersexual behavior or because they were a sexual nuisance." To further confound our notions of the meaning of hypersexuality, Noy *et al.* (1966) apply the term *Don Juan* to a group of impotent males. In this instance, the term is used to describe a specific attitude toward women and not toward actual sexual activity. Several reports on the endocrinologic treatment of hypersexuality (with cyproterone acetate) do not specifically identify the exact sexual behavior being treated (Brotherton and Harcus, 1973; Unger, 1977; Van de Merwe, 1979).

Davies (1974) divides a group of 50 hypersexual males into six categories: men who have been convicted of sexual assault or of indecently exposing themselves on several occasions, men who complain of vivid sexual fantasies and are distressed by them, oligophrenics whose sexual behavior is contrary to accepted social convention, homosexuals, individuals with chromosomal abnormalities, and elderly men accused of sexual misbehavior.

Orford (1978) compares the difficulty in defining hypersexuality to the difficulty involving the operational definitions of alcoholism and excessive gambling. Despite these difficulties and ambiguities, the term *hypersexuality* is generally used to denote a condition in which there is a relative increase of sexual desire or frequency of sex acts (either as a change in an individual or between an individual and an arbitrarily accepted norm) and in which this sexual behavior causes a problem either for society or for the individual.

Hypersexuality Without Known Etiology

Krafft-Ebing (1965) divides what could be termed hypersexuality into hyperesthesia, and nymphomania and satyriasis. He makes the now-controversial statement: "Since woman had less sexual need than man, a predominating sexual desire in her arouses a suspicion of its pathological significance" (p. 48). Whether one shares his assumption or not, the case of Mrs. V. (pp. 323–324) describes a highly sexually active individual: "Mrs. V., from earliest youth had a mania for men. Of good ancestors, highly cultured, good natured, very modest, blushed easily, but always the terror of the family. Indeed, when she was alone with a member of the opposite sex, irrespective of whether he was a child, in the prime of life, or an old man, or whether he was handsome or ugly, she would immediately remove her clothes and urgently request that he satisfy her desire by inserting his penis or hand. Marriage was resorted to as a cure. She loved her husband most ardently, but nevertheless was unable to restrain herself from demanding intercourse with any man, if she happened to catch him alone, whether he was a friend, a paid gigolo or a schoolboy."

Moore (1980) presents a case of satyriasis in a 24-year-old man. He finds no organic etiology or convincing psychodynamic rationale for this man's relatively high sexual activity. This patient came to psychiatric attention after being charged with frotterism by a young female. The patient complained, "I'm horny twenty hours a day." He noted that he had intercourse two to three times every day, and in addition would masturbate three to four times every day. He experienced wet dreams approximately twice a week. This man's history revealed that he had been totally preoccupied with women and sex since the seventh grade. His sexual activities outside of intercourse with his wife involved the use of vacuum cleaners, inflatable dolls, and rope and chain for carrying out sadomasochistic fantasies. He was treated with medroxyprogesterone acetate, 40 mg intramuscularly, every other week, and with insight-oriented psychotherapy twice weekly. On this regimen his libido decreased and he desired intercourse only once daily. After 4 months, the medroxyprogesterone acetate was discontinued and the patient's libido increased to its pretreatment level. This was unacceptable to the patient and he requested that the drug be resumed.

Hypersexuality in Manic-Depressive Illness and Schizophrenia

Increase in sexual desire and the frequency of sexual acts is a common, though not invariable, component of different phases of mania (Tsuang, 1975). The hypersexuality ranges from thoughts and statements to sexual behavior, and often causes social and economic disruption. Sexual activity between episodes is not necessarily increased.

Akhtar and Thompson (1980a, 1980b) report that the early phase of the schizophrenia is often accompanied by heightened sexual drive with increased masturbation, intercourse, touching of other persons, and temptation to become involved in frequent sexual affairs. They report that prodromal schizophrenics engage in behaviors such as masturbation, autofellatio, autocastration, overt homosexual behavior, anal intercourse, oral intercourse, and mutual masturbation. However, Woods (1981), in reviewing sexuality associated with mental illness, found that few consistent generalizations could be made regarding sexual activity and mental illness except for the increased sexuality associated with manic and hypomanic episodes.

Hypersexuality in Temporal Lobe Epilepsy

Temporal lobe epilepsy is most often associated with hyposexuality, although occasionally, increased sexual activity occurs associated with this seizure disorder. Currier *et al.* (1971) report two cases of ictal hypersexual behavior in temporal lobe epilepsy. Freeman and Nevis (1969) report a case of a 38-year-old woman whose seizures were accompanied by unusual sexual behavior. "'The patient would spread her legs apart, beat with both hands on her chest, verbalize her sexual needs, often in vulgarities, and place her hand over her perineum." Mohan *et al.* (1975) present a case of a 20-year-old female who manifested hypersexuality and limbic system dysfunction (temporal lobe epilepsy). Premorbidly she was noted to be sexually naive and shy. After onset of traumatic epilepsy, she began to have frequent intercourse with a number of men. Her behavior returned to normal when she was treated with anticonvulsants.

Blumer (1970a, 1970b) reports on 50 individuals treated for temporal lobe epilepsy. In 3 individuals hypersexual behavior during postictal periods was discovered. For example, one patient's wife stated that her husband would demand intercourse immediately following his attacks, even when his attacks occurred several times a day. Another patient reported experiencing orgasms during seizures. Blumer also reports the case of a 66-year-old man whose temporal lobe seizures were successfully treated by medications. Relatively hyposexual before treatment, he began to desire intercourse twice each day.

Shukla *et al.* (1979) review 70 cases of temporal lobe epilepsy and compare them with 70 cases of grand mal epilepsy. They report only one case of hypersexuality (as defined by the excessive indulgence in sexual activity leading to social or other domestic problems, embarrassment to others, etc.) and this case was in a temporal lobe epileptic. Taylor (1969) reports a sample of 100 individuals with temporal lobe epilepsy. In only one instance did he find hypersexuality.

Sexual automatisms and increased frequency of sexual behavior may accompany temporal lobe seizures or be manifest in the postictal state, but hyposexuality is a more typical concomitant of temporal lobe epilepsy. Hypersexuality is rarely found to accompany temporal lobe epilepsy.

Other Neurologic Abnormalities Resulting in Hypersexuality

The Klüver-Bucy syndrome is characterized by visual agnosia, oral behavior, hypermetamorphosis, emotional changes, and hypersexuality. It was experimentally produced in rhesus monkeys by the removal of the temporal lobes and the rhinecephalon (Klüver and Bucy, 1937). Instances of unilateral or bilateral temporal lobe damage have been thought to create partial Klüver-Bucy syndromes in man (Dahlmann and Shaefer, 1979; Terzian and Ore 1954). The ensuing hypersexuality is often not as pronounced as other cases of hypersexuality described. In the Shoji *et al.* (1979) case report, "The patient acted erotically toward the nurses, but this was temporary. When they counted his pulse, the patient tried to touch the nurses on the thigh."

Bulmer (1970a, 1970b) describes 42 temporal lobe epileptics who were treated with unilateral temporal lobectomy for control of refractory seizures. Two of these individuals reported transient hypersexuality. One, a 41-year-old male, had been married at the age of 37. During the first 4 years of his marriage, he had sexual relations with his wife only three times, despite his wife's encouragement. After the lobectomy, he became increasingly preoccupied with sex. He demanded frequent intercourse with his wife and also demanded that she masturbate him. He manifested incessant obscene language and was almost constantly genitally-sexually aroused. Hill *et al.* (1957) describe 27 individuals who had undergone temporal lobectomy for temporal lobe seizures. Fourteen patients evidenced increased intensity in libido. One patient was noted to become hypersexual and "perverse." He masturbated openly on the hospital ward as many as 20 times a day, exhibited himself to nurses, and made homosexual advances.

Increased sexual behavior has been noted in association with the presence of a brain tumor in the parabasocentral portions of the right frontal lobe (Lesniak *et al.* 1972) and with a tumor in the right parietal lobe (Erickson, 1945). Levine and Albert (1951) reported that 4 of 40 patients with frontal lobotomies in a 4-year follow-up developed sexual behavior that caused them social difficulties. It should be noted that three of these individuals had had difficulty modulating their sexual behavior before the operation. Dewhurst *et al.* (1970) report on 102 patients with Huntington's disease. Of the 55 males, 12 were noted to have hypersexual behavior, and 7 of the 47 females were noted to have hypersexual behavior.

Hypersexuality and Drugs

L-Dopa, an accepted treatment for Parkinson's disease, is an exogenous precursor of the neurotransitter dopamine, and has been implicated in the production of hypersexual behavior. O'Brien *et al.* (1971) report that 7 of 12 males treated with L-Dopa noticed an increase in libido with spontaneous penile erections. Shapiro (1973) reports one case of hypersexual behavior, consisting of persistent advances toward the nursing staff, in a 76-year-old patient treated for Parkinson's disease with L-Dopa.

Hormones and Hypersexuality

Though androgynic hormones are a necessary prerequisite for normal sexual functioning in both males and females, in men no relationship has been found between elevated testosterone levels and hypersexuality. Kraemer *et al.* (1976) found that testosterone in males was higher in sexually less active individuals. Dorner *et al.* (1975) discovered no difference in average testosterone levels between normal and hypersexual men. Goodman (1976) reports on six girls who had been exposed to virilizing hormones either *in utero* or in childhood. He felt that they manifested both hypersexuality and delinquency. However, his definition of hypersexuality is not explicit and his sample size is small and not randomly selected.

Kleine-Levin Syndrome and Hypersexuality

There are two case reports of hypersexuality accompanying the rare Kleine-Levin syndrome (periodic hypersomnia and megaphagia, usually in adolescent males). In one case, there were episodes of sexual assault and exposure (Yassa and Nair, 1978). In the other case, a female with Kleine-Levin syndrome displayed hypersexuality by exposing herself and publicly scratching her genitals (Duffy and Davison, 1968).

Hypersexuality of Psychogenic Etiology

This etiology encompasses the great majority of cases of hypersexuality. Sex and hypersexuality can be used as a defense against depression (Martin, 1976); as a device to ease one's insecurity over sexual prowess, as a method of degrading or debasing another, as a way of living forbidden incestuous fantasies, as an attempt to find a satisfying relationship, as an act of rebellion against parental or other authorities, as a defense against the fear of death (Shainess, 1973), or as one defense against homosexual or pseudohomosexual anxiety (Oversey and Woods, 1980). Hypersexuality can result from many different psychological conflicts.

In summary, hypersexuality, as currently used, does not refer to an absolute frequency of sexual activity or to a specific behavior. Rather, it is variably used to denote increased desire, increased sexual capacity, or sexual behavior that produces difficulties for the individual or for society. A high frequency of sexual activity is not in itself an indication of psychopathology. We have reviewed many diverse conditions that have produced hypersexuality.

REFERENCES

Akhtar, S., and Thomson, J. A. Jr., 1980a, Schizophrenia and sexuality: A review and a report of twelve unusual cases—Part I, *J. Clin. Psychiatry* 41:134.

Akhtar, S, and Thomson, J. A. Jr., 1980b, Schizophrenia and sexuality: A review and a report of twelve unusual cases—Part II, *J. Clin. Psychiatry* 41:166.

Allen, C., 1962, "A Textbook of Psychosexual Disorders," University Press, London.

American Psychiatric Association, 1980, "Diagnostic and Statistical Manual of Mental Disorders" 3rd ed., American Psychiatric Association, Washington, D.C.

Awad, G. A., 1976, Father–son incest: A case report, *J. Nerv. Ment. Dis.* 162: 135–139.

Barry, M. J., Jr., and Johnson, A. M. 1958, The incest barrier, *Psychoanal. Q.* 27:485–500.

Bartholomew, A. A., Milte, K. L., and Galbally, F., 1978, Homosexual necrophilia, *Med. Sci. Law* 18:35.

Beckett, S., 1954, "Waiting for Godot," Grove Press, New York.

Bender, L., and Blau, A., 1937, The reaction of children to sexual relations with adults, *Am. J. Orthopsychiatry* 7:500.

Bender, L., and Grugett, A. E., Jr., 1952, A follow-up report on children who had atypical sexual experience, *Am. J. Orthopsychiatry* 22:825.

Bergler, E., 1936, Obscene words, *Psychoanal. Q.* 5:226.

Berry, G. W., 1975, Incest: Some clinical variations on a classical theme, *J. Am. Acad. Psychoanal.* 3:151.

Bieber, I., 1970, Enemas and sex, *Med. Aspects Hum. Sexuality* January: 89.

Blumer, D., 1970a, Hypersexual episodes in temporal lobe epilepsy, *Am. J. Psychiatry* 126:1099.

Blumer, D., 1970b, Changes of sexual behavior related to temporal lobe disorders in man, *J. Sex. Res.* 6:173.

Brill, A. A., 1941a, Necrophilia—Part I, *J. Crim. Psychopathol.* 2:433.

Brill, A. A., 1941b, Necrophilia—Part II, *J. Crim. Psychopathol.* 3:53–73, 1941b.

Brotherton, J., 1974, Effect of oral cyproterone acetate on urinary and serum FSH and LH levels in adult males being treated for hypersexuality, *J. Reprod. and Fertil.* 36:177.

Brotherton, J, and Harcus, A. W., 1978, Effect of oral cyproterone acetate on urinary FSH and LH levels in adult males being treated for hypersexuality, *J. Reprod. Fertil.* 33:356.

Calef, V., and Weinschel, E. M., 1972, On certain neurotic equivalents of necrophilia, *Int. J. Psychoanal.* 53:67.

Chee, T. K., 1974, A case of bestiality, *Singapore Med. J.* 15:287.

Coe, J. I., 1974, Sexual asphyxias, *J. Life-Threatening Behav.* 4:171.

Cooper, A. J., Phanjoo, A. L., and Love, D. L., 1972, Antiandrogen (cyproterone acetate) therapy in deviant hypersexuality. *Br. J. Psychiatry* 120:59.

Currier, R. D., Little, S. C., Suess, J. F., and Andy, O. J., 1971, Sexual seizures, *Arch. Neurol.* 25:260.

Dahlmann, W., and Schaefer, K.-P., 1979, Klüver-Bucy syndrome and primitive motor reflexes after heavy brain trauma, *Arch. Psychiatr. Nervenkr.* 226:229.

Davies, T. S., 1974, Cyproterone acetate for male hypersexuality, *J. Int. Med. Res.* 2:1159.

Denko, J. D., 1973, Klismaphilia: Enema as a sexual preference, *Am. J. Psychother.* 27:232.

Denko, J. D., 1976, Klismaphilia; amplification of the erotic enema deviance, *Am. J. Psychother.* 30:236.

de Sade, D. A. F., 1959, "The 120 Days of Sodom" pp. 90–91, Olympia Press, Paris.

Dewhurst, K., Oliver, J. D., and McKnight, A.L., 1970, Socio-psychiatric consequences of Huntington's disease, *Br. J. Psychiat.* 116:255.

Dixon, K. N., Arnold, L. E., and Calestro, K., 1978, Father–son incest: Underreported psychiatric problem? *Am. J.Psychiatry* 135:835.

Dorner, G., Stahl, F., Rohde, W., Halle, H., and Schott, G., 1975, Elevated free testosterone in the plasma of early pregnant women bearing male fetuses and of hypersexual men, *Endokrinologie* 65:224.

Duffy, J. P., and Davison, K., 1968, A female case of the Kleine-Levin syndrome, *Br. J. Psychiat.*, 114:77.

Edmondson, J. S., 1972, A case of sexual asphyxia without fatal termination, *Br. J. Psychiatr.* 121:437.

Ehrenreich, G. A., 1960, Headache, necrophilia and murder; a brief hypnotherapeutic investigation of a single case, *Bull. Menninger Clin.* 24:274.

Ellis, H., 1927, "Studies in the Psychology of Sex" 2nd ed., Vol. 3, F. A. Davis, Philadelphia.

Erickson, T. C., 1945, Erotomania (nymphomania) as an expression of cortical epileptiform discharge, *Arch. Neurol. Psychiatry* 53:226.

Faulkner, W., 1967, A rose for Emily, in "The Portable Faulkner" (M. Cowley, ed.), pp. 435–449, Viking Press, New York.

Foerster, K., Foerster, G., and Roth, E., 1976, Necrophilia in a 17 year old girl, *Schweiz. Arch. Neurol. Nerochir. Psychiatr.* 119:97.

Foraker, A. G., 1976, The romantic necrophiliac of Key West, *J. Fla. Med. Assoc.* 63:642.

Freemon, F. R., and Nevis, A. H., 1969, Temporal lobe sexual seizures, *Neurology* 19:87.

Goodman, J. D., 1976, The behavior of hypersexual delinquent girls, *Am. J. Psychiatry* 133:662.

Guirand, F. (ed.)., 1968, "The New Larousse Encyclopedia of Mythology," Hamblyn Publishing Group, New York.

Hill, D., Pond, D. A., Mitchell, W., and Falconer, M. A., 1957, Personality changes following temporal lobectomy for epilepsy, *J. Ment. Sci.* 103:18.

Holden, T. E., and Sherline, D. M., 1973, Bestiality, with sensitization and anaphylactic reaction, *Obstet. Gynecol.* 42:138.

Karpman, B., 1934, The obsessive paraphilias (perversions), *Arch. Neurol. Psychiatry* 32:601.
Karpman, B., 1948, Coprophilia: A collective review. *Psychoanal. Rev.* 35:253.
Karpman, B., 1949a, A modern Gulliver: A study in coprophilia (parts I–III *Psychoanal. Rev.* 36:162.
Karpman, B., 1949b, A modern Gulliver: A study in coprophilia (parts IV–XII), *Psychoanal. Rev.* 36:260.
Kinsey, A. C., Pomeroy, W. B., and Martin, C. E., 1948, "Sexual Behavior in the Human Male," pp. 667–678, W. B. Saunders, Philadelphia.
Kinsey, A. C., Gebhard, C. E., Pomeroy, W. B., and Martin C. W., 1953, "Sexual Behavior in the Human Female," pp. 502–509, W. B. Saunders, Philadelphia.
Klaf, F. S., and Brown, W., 1958, Necrophilia, brief review and case report. *Psychiatr. Q.* 32:645.
Klüver, H., and Bucy, P. C., 1937, "Psychic blindness" and other symptoms following bilateral temporal lobectomy in rhesus monkeys, *Am. J. Physiol.* 119:352.
Kraemer, H. C., Becker, H. B., Brodie, K. H., Doering, C. H., Moos, R. H., and Hamburg, D. A., 1976, Orgasmic frequency and plasma testosterone levels in normal human males, *Arch. Sex. Behav.* 5:125.
Krafft-Ebing, R. von, 1965, "Psychopathia Sexualis," Bell, New York.
Lancaster, N. P., 1978, Necrophilia, murder and high intelligence: A case report, *Br. J. Psychiat.* 132:605.
Langsley, D. G., Schwartz, M. N., and Fairbairn, R. H., 1968, Father–son incest, *Compr. Psychiatry* 9:218.
Lazarus, A. A., 1968, A case of pseudonecrophilia treated by behavior therapy, *J. Clin. Psychol.* 24:113.
Lesniak, R., Szymusik, A., and Chrzanowski, R., 1972, Multidirectional disorders of sexual drive in a case of brain tumor, *Forensic Sci.* 1:333.
Levine, J., and Albert, H., 1951, Sexual behavior after lobotomy, *J. Nerv. Ment. Dis.* 113:332.
Litman, R. E., and Swearingen C., 1972, Bondage and suicide, *Arch. Gen. Psychiatry* 27:80.
London, L. S., 1957, "Sexual Deviations in the Female" Rev. ed., Julian Press, New York.
London, L. S., and Caprio, F. S., 1958, "Sexual Deviations," Linacre Press, Washington.
Lukianowicz, N., 1972, Incest: Part I—Paternal incest, *Br. J. Psychiatry* 120:301.
Martin, M. J., 1976, Impulsive sexual behavior masking insidious depression, *Med. Aspects Hum. Sexuality* 10:45.
Medlicott, R. W., 1967, Parent–child incest, *Aus. N.Z. J. Psychiatry* 1:180.
Meiselman, K. C., 1979, "Incest," Jossey-Bass, San Francisco.
Mohan, K. J., Salo, M. W., and Nagaswami, S., 1975, A case of limbic system dysfunction with hypersexuality and fugue state, *Dis. Nerv. Syst.* 36:621.
Moore, S., 1980, Satyriasis: A case study, *J. Clin. Psychiatry* 41:279.
Nacht, S., Diatkine, R., and Favreau, J., 1956, The ego in perverse relationships, *Int. J. Psychoanal.* 37:404.
Noy, P., Wollstein, S., and Kaplan-De-Nour, A., 1966, Clinical observations on the psychogenesis of impotence, *Br. J. Med. Psychol.* 39:43.
O'Brien, C. P., DiGiacomo, J. N., Fahn, S., and Schwarz, G. A., 1971, Mental effects of high dosage Levodopa, *Arch. Gen. Psychiatry* 24:61.
Orford, J., 1978, Hypersexuality: Implications for a theory of dependence, *Br. J. Addict.* 73:299.
Oversey, L., and Woods, S. M., 1980, "Homosexual Behavior: A Modern Reappraisal" J. Marmor, ed.), Basic Books, New York.
Raphling, D. L., Carpenter, B. L., and Davis, A., 1967, Incest, a geneological study, *Arch. Gen. Psychiaty* 16:505.
Rapoport, J., 1942, A case of necrophilia, *J. Crim. Psychopathol.* 4:277.

Rappaport, E. A., 1968, Zoophily and zoerasty, Psychoanal. Q. 37:565.

Raybin, J. B., 1969, Homosexual incest, report of a case of homosexual incest involving three generations of a family, J. Nerv. Ment. Dis. 148:105.

Reichenthal,J. A., 1979, Correcting the underreporting of father–son incest (Letter), Am. J. Psychaatry 136:122.

Reider, N., 1976, On a particular neurotic equivalent of necrophilia, Psychoanal. Q. 45:288.

Resnik, H. L. P., 1972, Erotized repetitive hangings: A form of self-destructive behavior, Am. J. Psychother. 26:4.

Rhinehart, J. W., 1961 Genesis of overt incest, Compr. Psychiatry 2:338.

Sass, F. A., 1975, Sexual asphyxia in the female, J. Forensic Sc. 20:181.

Schneck, J. M., 1974, Zooerasty and incest fantasy, Int. J. Clin. Exp. Hypn. 22:299.

Segal, H., 1953, A necrophilic phantasy, Int. J. Psychoanal. 34:98.

Shainess, N., 1973, Nymphomania and Don Juanism, Med. Trial Techniques Q. 1:1.

Shankel, L. W., and Carr, A. C., 1956, Transvestism and hanging episodes in a male adolescent, Psychiatr. Q. 30:478.

Shapiro, S., 1973, Hypersexual behavior complicating levodopa (L-dopa) therapy. Minn. Med. 56:58.

Shenken, L. I., 1964, Some clinical and psychopathological aspects of bestiality, J. Nerv. Ment. Dis. 139:137.

Shoji, H., Teramoto, H., Satowa, S., Satowa, H., and Narita, Y., 1979 Partial Klüver-Bucy syndrome following probable herpes simplex encephalitis, J. Neurol. 221:163.

Shukla, G. S., Srivastava, O. N., and Katiyar, B. C., 1979, Sexual disturbances in temporal lobe epilepsy: A controlled study, Br. J. Psychiatry 134:288.

Smith, S. M., and Braun, C., 1979, Necrophilia and lust murder: Report of a rare occurrence, Bull. Am. Acad. Psychiatry Law 6:259.

Stearns, A. W., 1953, Cases of probable suicide in young persons without obvious motivation, J. Maine Med. Assoc. 44:16.

Tarachow, S., 1966, Coprophagia and allied phenomena, J. Am. Anal. Assoc. 14:685.

Taylor, D. C., 1969, Sexual behavior and temporal lobe epilepsy, Arch. Neurol. 21:510.

Terzian, H., and Ore, G. D., 1954, Syndrome of Klüver and Bucy, Neurology 5:373.

Tsuang, M. T., 1975, Hypersexuality in manic patients, Med. Aspects Hum. Sexuality 9:83.

Unger, H. R., 1977, Cyproterone and hypersexuality (Letter), N. Z. Med. J. 86:39–40, 1977.

Van de Merwe, T. J., 1979, Cyproterone and hypersexuality (Letter), S. Afr. Med. J. January 27, 1979.

Vanden Bergh, R. L., and Kelly, J. F., 1964, Vampirism, a review with new observations, Arch. Gen. Psychiatry 11:543.

Wahl, C. W., 1960, The psychodynamics of consummated maternal incest, Arch. Gen. Psychiatry 3:188.

Walsh, F. M., Stahl, C. J., III, Unger, H. T., Lilenstern, O. C., and Stephens, R. G., III, 1977, Autoerotic asphyxial deaths: A medicolegal analysis of forty-three cases, in "Legal Medicine Annual: 1977" (C. H. Wecht, ed.), pp. 155–182, Appleton-Century-Crofts, New York.

Woods, S. M., 1981, Disordered sexuality in psychiatric illness, in "Human Sexuality," American Medical Association, Chicago.

Yassa, R., and Nair N. P. V., 1978, The Kleine-Levin syndrome—A variant? J. Clin. Psychiatry March: 254.

Yorukoglu, A., and Kemph, J. P., 1966, Children not severely damaged by incest with a parent, J. Am. Acad. Child Psychiatry 5:111.

Weiner, I. B., 1964, On Incest: A Survey, Excerpta Criminology 4:137.

9

Koro (Shook Yang)
A Culture-Bound Psychogenic Syndrome

ROBERT T. RUBIN

INTRODUCTION

Koro, or shook yang, is a culture-bound psychogenic disorder occurring predominantly in men of the Chinese race who live in southern China and the countries of Southeast Asia to which the southern Chinese have migrated. The syndrome has three cardinal manifestations: first, delusions of retraction of the penis into the body with a fear of impending death; second, an intense panic with feelings of collapse, palpitations, sweating, nausea, breathlessness, visual blurring, bodily spasms, pain, and paresthesias; and, third, generally minor complications arising from patients' idiosyncratic remedial measures to physically prevent the ostensible disappearance of the penis into the abdomen (Koro Study Team, 1969). The strength of the delusory belief determines the degree of fear and panic, which in turn determines the vigor with which remedies are attempted, leading to various degrees of physical damage to the genitals.

The syndrome has names both in Malay *(koro)* and in Chinese *(shook yang)*. The origin of the word koro is not definitely known; it might have been a Javanese word meaning "tortoise" (Yap, 1965a). The Chinese have a tendency to refer to the glans penis as a tortoise head; *coitus reservatus* is likened in ancient Chinese writings to the retraction of a tortoise's head. However, it may be more likely that the word koro arose from Malay terms like *keruk*, meaning "to shrink" (Gwee, 1968).

The Chinese term shook yang (*suk yeong* in Cantonese) means

ROBERT T. RUBIN • Department of Psychiatry, University of California at Los Angeles School of Medicine, Harbor General/UCLA Medical Center, Torrance, California.

"shrinking penis." The Chinese language uses the word "yin" to denote both male and female genitalia, and shrinking of the penis (shook yin) had been described in several very old Chinese medical texts (Gwee, 1968). For example, Pao Sian-Ow, in his treatise "New Collection of Remedies of Value," written in 1834, stated that "during intercourse, the man may be seized suddenly with acute abdominal pain. The limbs become cold and the complexion dusky, the penis retracts into the abdomen. If treatment is not instituted at once and effective, the case will die. The disease is due to the invasion of cold vapors and the treatment is to employ the 'heaty' drugs" (Gwee, 1963). Another remedy suggested by Pao Sian-Ow is the powdered ash produced by the burning of female undergarments (Gwee, 1968).

A number of early Chinese medical writings described this condition, mentioning, in addition to retraction of the genitals, muscle spasm, sunken chest, poor hair color, blurred vision, and impotence, with death following frequently (Gwee, 1968). These accounts may have been of male patients with peritonitis and abdominal wall edema, which was regarded as a sign of certain death in ancient Chinese medicine (Gwee, 1963). It also has been considered in several writings as a sequela of intercourse when a person is ill, or of exposure to wind and cold, or of the ingestion of raw or cold food (Gwee, 1968). These accounts are all considered to be of shook yin; the term yang has been used to refer to the penis only in the last 100 or so years.

Koro appears as a culture-bound disorder of southern Chinese males most likely because of the long tradition in Chinese culture of attaching great importance to the preservation of sexual function. For example, Chinese medicine states that ten grains of rice form a drop of blood, ten drops of blood form a drop of spermatic fluid, and a man's health can be seriously jeopardized if he suffers an excessive loss of spermatic fluid (Gwee, 1963). Thus, guilt over excessive masturbation, unsatisfactory intercourse with one's wife, promiscuity, and consorting with prostitutes frequently have been psychological precipitants of an acute koro attack. Most of the men suffering such an attack have not been highly educated, and they generally adhered to popular Chinese medical beliefs. Gwee (1963) stated that "it would appear that the disease is probably a result of the free play of imagination of a physician on top of a culture which links fatality with genital retraction and sexual activity with risk to life." In fact, as recently as 1967, the Chinese Physician Association of Singapore still accepted the classical entity of shook yin, although no authenticated cases of that condition, as described in the early Chinese medical literature, had been reported (Gwee, 1968) (cf. section on Singapore koro epidemic). Thus, in a susceptible individual, hearsay information about koro, along with preexisting sexual fears and subjective sensations in the genitalia associated with such phenomena as sexual intercourse, urination, defecation, or trauma, leads to the vicious circle of the delusion of genital shrinkage, attendant panic, and enhanced fears of a delusory nature, with even greater panic and crude attempts to prevent the disappearance of the penis. While the vast majority of koro patients are men, women also may suffer analogous symptoms, including delusions of retraction of the nipples and vulva.

In their anxiety to prevent the fantasied disappearance of the penis, or of the labia majora in women, patients may hold onto the penis or labia to prevent the supposed retraction; they may enlist willing family members to do this for them; or they may use a clamp, a loop of string, or even a safety pin (Gwee, 1963). On occasion, the pans of a small jeweler's weighing instrument *(lie teng hok)* have been used to clamp the penis (Figures 1–3). A few cases of koro have been reported in very young children, where the child actually was the victim of a delusion held by family members, who also physically held the child's penis or labia while bringing him or her to medical attention. As mentioned, damage to the genitalia, while generally minor, has been produced by vigorous home remedies for this syndrome. The following case reports will serve to illustrate the features of koro.

TYPICAL KORO CASES IN ASIANS

Case 1 (Gwee, 1963). An 8-year-old Chinese schoolboy suffered an insect bite on his penis. A couple living in the house inspected the penis and detected some retraction occurring. The penis was held, and vigorous local applications of balms were begun. The child was fed some brandy, considered to be a "heaty" medicine. The condition diminished within an hour, but during the next evening the boy again thought his penis was retracting, whereupon it was anchored with string, and he was brought to the hospital. He improved after several injections, but two evenings later the child woke up with the same complaint. Again balms were applied, and the penis was clamped with chopsticks. The following day he had another attack, with hypogastric pain, and was again brought to hospital. When seen by the doctor, the boy held a loop of string tied around the mid-shaft of his penis, which was mildly bruised. Both he and his parents appeared quite alarmed. After several hours of persuasive reassurance, his symptoms abated. He remained symptom-free for the next 7 years.

Case 2 (Gwee, 1963). A 34-year-old single Chinese man desired to urinate while attending a cinema. While in the lavatory, he suffered loss of feeling in his genital region, had the immediate thought that he was

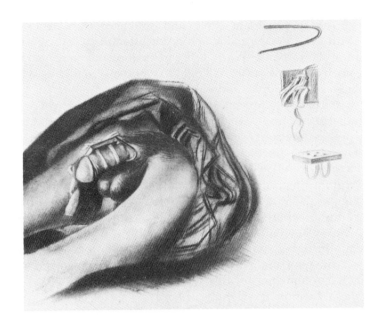

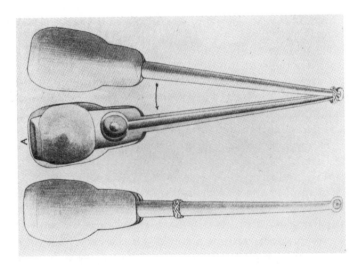

FIGURE 1. Drawings of a penis clamp and a lie teng hok, used by koro patients to prevent "retraction of the penis into the abdomen." Reproduced from van Wulfften Palthe (1934).

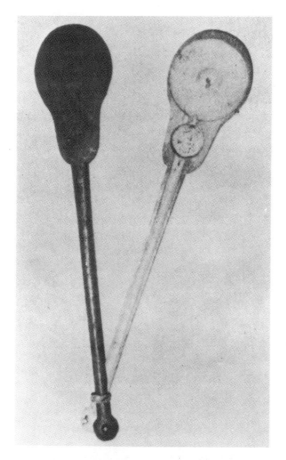

FIGURE 2. Photograph of a lie teng hok (jeweler's
clamp). Reproduced from Koro Study Team (1969),
with permission of Dr. Gwee Ah Leng, team chairman, and the *Singapore Medical Journal*.

going to get penile retraction, and then noticed that his penis was getting
shorter. With great alarm he held onto his penis and cried out for help;
however, the lavatory was deserted. He then felt cold in his limbs and
weak all over, and his legs gave way. He sat on the floor for about 30
minutes, holding onto his penis, after which the attack abated. He was
prescribed some pills by a doctor, but he subsequently became nervous
and jittery, particularly when meeting women. He had been of a nervous
disposition during his school years, and at age 15 he had had his first
nocturnal emission, after which he felt quite weak. These continued with
some regularity. At age 24 he had visited a prostitute and contracted gon-

orrhea; he apparently had no further sexual encounters after that. He had been aware of the condition of koro from friends. His treatment consisted of strong reassurance and education on sexual anatomy, after which no further attacks occurred during a 7-year follow-up period.

Case 3 (Gwee, 1963). A 38-year-old Chinese man, married for 16 years and with seven children, had his first attack of koro at age 18 following a strong dose of purgative, which caused some retraction of his penis. The episode was transitory and did not frighten him unduly. In the 2 years prior to examination he had complained of feeling weak, and during defecation he worried about penile retraction. He had regular inter-

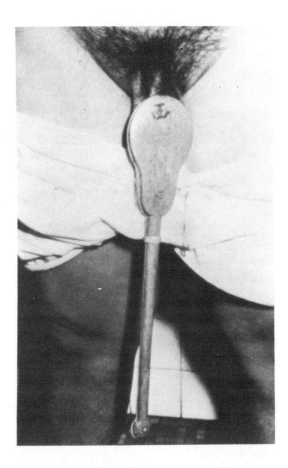

FIGURE 3. Photograph of a koro patient using a lie teng hok. Reproduced from Koro Study Team (1969), with permission of Dr. Gwee Ah Leng, team chairman, and the *Singapore Medical Journal.*

course with his wife, but he felt weakened physically by it. He had no extramarital sexual contacts. He had heard about koro during his school days and believed it to be very dangerous and likely fatal. His most recent attack had occurred during intercourse some months prior to examination, and he recovered spontaneously after holding onto his penis for 20 minutes. He did not dare to have intercourse after that. Following several reassuring talks and education about sexual anatomy, he began once again to have a normal sex life, with no attacks during an 8-year follow-up period. He did decrease his frequency of intercourse and believed he felt better for it.

Case 4 (Rin, 1963, 1965). A 32-year-old single cook from central China sought psychiatric help for complaints of panic attacks and somatic symptoms including palpitations, breathlessness, dizziness, and numbness of his limbs. For several months he had visited herb doctors, who diagnosed his disease as a "deficiency in vitality" and prescribed the drinking of boys' urine and eating of human placenta to supply energy and blood. During this time the patient also noticed that his penis was shrinking and withdrawing into his abdomen; this occurred usually a day or two after intercourse with a prostitute. He became anxious about his penis and ate excessively to relieve sudden hunger pangs.

The patient was brought up in a small town and had a rather disturbed childhood, having been beaten by his stepfather when he was unruly. He spent most of his earned money on gambling and in brothels. According to him, he became emaciated and jaundiced because of excessive masturbation at age 18; many kinds of herbal medicines offered him no relief, which came only after he began drinking his own urine. He had his first attack of somatic symptoms at age 32, consisting of breathlessness, palpitations, dizziness, nausea, etc. He recovered from this attack, began visiting brothels again, and had another attack within a few days. His attacks became more frequent and of longer duration, and in a constant panic he went from doctor to doctor receiving vitamin injections. One doctor told him he had a sexual defect and would eventually die if he continued visiting prostitutes, and he thought that his symptoms were caused by poisons secreted in the uterus and that penetrated his penis. Although almost irresistible sexual desire seized him whenever he felt somewhat better, he experienced strange feelings in his abdomen after intercourse, at which time he often found his penis shrinking into his abdomen. He would become very anxious and hold onto his penis in terror, experiencing severe vertigo, palpitations, and fainting spells. At night he would find his penis shrunk to about 1 centimeter in length, and after pulling it out he would be able to go to sleep. He believed that his anus, as well, was withdrawing into his abdomen. He tried to prevent nocturnal emissions by holding his penis, as he was afraid of losing "vital essence." He made frequent trips to the clinic, in a state of panic, and described his symptoms in an exaggerated manner: "hands tremble, anguish in the abdomen, penis withdrawing, heart pounds kag-kag, kazu-kazu, I am scared . . . my body trembles at night, it moves, blood does not come up, my body stops moving, my lung gets hot and my head too, my mouth will dry up so that I drink a cup of tea and then I have to urinate . . . I cannot breathe at night, my heart pounds; my head aches if I talk too much, my heart sounds kok, kok-kok, my head sounds zuzu-zuzu." The patient had several periods of psychotherapy, during the last of which he attempted to find a light job. He avoided prostitutes to save his strength.

Case 5 (Rin, 1963, 1965). A 39-year-old married man from central China was admitted to the hospital presenting with ideas of reference, delusions of being poisoned, and hypochondriacal complaints. Some months prior to admission he began complaining of back, leg, and facial pain, became insomnic, and began to suspect that someone was hiding in the ceiling to spray poisons. He then experienced a number of strange sensations, including retraction of his penis; loosening of his scrotal skin (which he thought would make his testicles drop off); a dull pain in his left testicle; a sharp pain in his perineum; and an expanding feeling in his penis at night: these sensations were accompanied by a great deal of anxiety.

The patient grew up in a troubled and economically burdened small-town family. At age 16 he moved to Shanghai, where he lived in a dormitory with several boys who taught him to masturbate. He masturbated two or three times a week but felt guilty about it; he stopped this practice 2 years later. He married when he was 23, over the strong objections of his wife's family. After he and his wife had a baby girl, they lost interest in sexual relations and eventually lived apart, having intercourse only once every other month or so. He felt lonely and drank heavily. He got back together with his wife after the Sino-Japanese War, separated again from his wife and child, and then reunited with them, migrating to Taiwan. At the time his symptoms began he was chief accountant for a college office and had been blamed by the dean for not supervising his workers properly, one of whom was dismissed for dishonesty. He felt very ashamed and worried about his future. He also had some difficulty with the local police concerning some construction on his home, and shortly thereafter his salary was stolen from his home. At this time he became insomnic, hypochondriacal, and developed overt paranoid delusions. Over the ensuing months these became severe enough to require his hospitalization. He smelled gunpowder in the toilet and felt that his tonsils and throat were swollen. His eardrums and lungs were painful, he said, and his heart pounded violently. He believed that his scrotal skin was so loose that semen was leaking out and was making the surrounding skin gelatinous, and that his entire skin was getting loose, his buttocks were sinking down, and his penis was withdrawing into his abdomen.

In the hospital, this patient received a course of insulin shock treatment, which relieved his various somatic symptoms. However, he continued to believe that his previous excessive masturbation had damaged a particular nerve, which caused his penis to shrink. Subsequently, he gradually became aware of the emotional stresses of the past few years of his life and of his dissatisfaction with his wife.

These five cases illustrate the variety of ages, premorbid personalities, life histories, ancillary symptoms, and underlying psychiatric illnesses in patients presenting with the triad of koro symptomatology. It appears that koro may be a component of both psychotic and neurotic illnesses, becoming manifest in those individuals who continue to believe in traditional Chinese medical concepts, have heard of the occurrence of the disease, and are frightened by it; who are not highly educated, and who have some conflict and guilt concerning sexuality. Yap (1965a, personal communication), over a 15-year period in Hong Kong, collected 19 typical cases of koro, 6 cases in which koro features occurred against a background of schizophrenia, and 1 case each in which koro symptoms presented against a background of general paresis and heroin withdrawal. All Yap's patients were from the working class, with some education, and none had a family history of psychosis or neurosis. The patients generally were described as slow, shy, self-effacing, of nervous temperament, not endowed with a great deal of intelligence, and of a decided immaturity of personality. Many of the patients had a history of sexual conflicts and maladjustments and were troubled by sexual deprivation, because of their shy personalities, their fear of venereal disease, their lack of money to visit prostitutes, their being single, or their having wives who were not sexually cooperative. Yap (1965a) indicated that all his patients were gravely worried over what they imagined to be sexual excesses. He treated his patients with psychotherapy aimed at the presenting symptoms and appropriate pharmaco- and somatic therapies when an underlying psychiatric illness was diagnosed. Most of his cases had either a complete or an almost–complete reversal of symptoms, but some were still subject to occasional bouts of anxiety.

The aforementioned reports are of patients who had considerable premorbid psychological conflicts, very often of a sexual nature, which were long-standing and which conferred a special vulnerability for the development of koro. In several cases the koro syndrome was superimposed upon a more serious psychiatric illness, e.g, paranoid psychosis. However, there was an epidemic of koro in Singapore in 1967, in which hundreds of persons developed the koro syndrome in what can be described best as a contagion of mass hysteria, spreading rapidly on the basis of predisposing cultural beliefs rather than predominant individual psychopathology. This epidemic of koro will be described next.

THE 1967 SINGAPORE KORO EPIDEMIC

In October 1967 there was an outbreak of koro in Singapore that lasted approximately 10 days (Mun, 1968; Ngui, 1969; Koro Study Team, 1969). Because a total of 469 cases was recorded during this epidemic, and because the presentation of these cases to hospitals and clinics followed a newspaper report about the syndrome, an examination of the public events preceding the outbreak and the demographic and psychosocial characteristics of the patients is of interest.

For some years, the Singapore population had been concerned about the use of implants of estrogenic hormones into chickens to increase their growth rates (Gwee, 1968). There had been reports that some of the chickens were sold before the hormone implants were completely absorbed, so that people eating the necks of the chickens, where the implants were placed, got a strong dose of estrogens.

Some cases of gynecomastia in men developed, and some men in the community stopped eating chicken. Thus, in this predominantly Chinese community there was a general knowledge that some foods may contain injected chemicals that produce sexual changes.

On the background of this general community awareness, the newspapers in October 1967 reported that some people developed koro after eating the meat of pigs that had been inoculated with anti-swine-fever vaccine. Some months earlier there had been an outbreak of swine fever in Singapore, and the inoculation of pigs with vaccine had been publicly announced as a control measure. Following the initial newspaper report, there was a further report a few days later alleging that an inoculated pig had died with penile retraction. Rumors spread that the flesh of inoculated pigs was unwholesome and would cause koro, which could be a lethal disease. Pork sales declined, reports of more koro cases appeared in the news, and physicians emphasized that the disease should be treated quickly and effectively with injections, acupuncture, and so on. The Singapore government issued a statement that swine fever itself and the vaccine were harmless to man. However, the number of reported koro cases increased rapidly in the next few days, with 97 male cases being seen in a single day, 5 days after the initial newspaper report. After public announcements by the Singapore Medical Association and the Ministry of Health were given wide exposure on television and in the newspapers stating that koro was a result of fear, not a physical disease

with fatalities, and that meat from inoculated pigs was completely harmless to human beings, there was an immediate decline in the incidence
of koro. Several days after these public announcements there were only
a few cases reported, and within a month koro was not being reported
in Singapore at all. The following two cases are illustrative of the presenting symptomatology of this epidemic.

Case 6 (Mun, 1968). A 16-year-old schoolboy dashed into the clinic
with his parents, shouting for medical attention because he had "shook
yang." The boy was frightened and pale, and he was pulling hard on his
penis to prevent it from disappearing into his abdomen. He had heard
about koro in school, and that morning he had eaten pork for breakfast.
While urinating, he noticed that his penis was small as he finished, and,
frightened, he grasped his penis and rushed to his parents for help. He
and his parents were reassured at the clinic, and he was given a 2-day
supply of chlordiazepoxide. He had no recurrence.

Case 7 (Mun, 1968). A young mother rushed into the clinic holding
the penis of her 4-month-old baby and asking that the baby be treated
quickly for koro. For 2 days the baby had suffered from a cold, with some
diarrhea. While the mother was changing the child's diaper and cleaning
him, he had some intestinal cramping and screamed. His mother saw his
penis getting smaller and thought he had koro, as she had heard rumors
about the epidemic. The mother was reassured and the baby's cold and
diarrhea treated.There was no recurrence.

Of the total of 469 koro cases reported during the 1967 epidemic,
95% were males and 5% were females. Of the 454 men, 95% were Chinese;
the rest were Malaysian and Indian. Of the females, all cases were
Chinese. Among the men, ages of patients ranged from 4 months to 70
years, with the greatest number of patients being between 16 and 30
years of age. The fact that 6 male cases were under 6 years of age and 14
cases were between the ages of 6 and 10 suggests the important role of
family members in deciding that a young boy has this disease. Among
the female cases, there was only 1 younger than 10 years, with most
being between the ages of 11 and 30 years. The majority of the total of
469 cases came from about ten postal areas clustered near the center of
Singapore. Few of the patients were completely uneducated, most having finished either Chinese or English primary or secondary schools;
only 3 patients had higher education beyond secondary school (Koro
Study Team, 1969).

The predominant symptoms in this epidemic were fear (90%), delusions of shrinking of the genitals (74%), delusions of retraction of the

penis (61%), and palpitations (41%); other symptoms included breath-lessness (11%), collapse (10%), body pain (7%), blurred vision (7%), etc. (Ngui, 1969). The principal remedies were manual restraint by the afflicted individuals (72%) and placebo medications and reassurance (74%). Only 17% of the cases had further attacks, and in only 7% was there a feeling that sexual power had been affected.

Of particular note were the symptoms presented by the female patients, six of whom were interviewed by the Koro Study Team. Of these six cases, five complained of retraction of the nipples and one complained of retraction of the vulva. The latter patient, a girl 12 years of age, had heard of koro at school and developed a sudden fear with a feeling of retraction and shrinkage of her vulva. Her mother pulled at her labia majora and brought her to the hospital. The general complex of symptoms seen in the female cases was similar to that seen in male cases, except for the anatomical site of the sensation of retraction.

Compared to the isolated cases of koro reported in the earlier liter-ature, there was, to a degree, less desperation among the patients in the 1967 koro epidemic, suggesting that the beliefs surrounding koro were no longer so fixed among the Chinese population and that koro as an illness syndrome was declining. That the vast majority of cases occurred among the Chinese population of Singapore again highlights the cul-ture-relatedness of koro. The very rapid rise and fall of the number of cases presenting daily to the hospitals and clinics (the bulk of the epi-demic having occurred within a 10-day period following the aforemen-tioned newspaper report) and the frequency of cases rapidly subsiding after appropriate public reassurance from governmental agencies suggest that this koro epidemic was a phenomenon of mass hysteria in a cultur-ally susceptible population. The low incidence of repeated attacks and the virtual lack of lingering symptomatology, such as persistent loss of sexual power, argue against more serious psychiatric illness in the pop-ulation affected during this epidemic. The mass hysteria of koro certainly was accompanied by delusions concerning the genitals, but it was not accompanied by the psychological indifference to symptoms usually attendant to conversion reactions. Rather, fear and anxiety were promi-nent features.

While koro, at least in its intensity of symptomatology, may be on the decline, it is interesting to note that the Chinese Physicians Associ-ation of Singapore held a seminar during the 1967 epidemic and con-cluded that it was caused by fear, rumors, climatic conditions, and an imbalance between heart and kidneys, and that, furthermore, it was in no way similar to the classical entity of shook yin. Thus, the Chinese Physicians Association still accepted the possibility of the occurrence of a syndrome of penile retraction with high risk to life, although no authentic, verified cases had ever been reported (Gwee, 1968). This attests to the strong psychological cathexis of the penis in Chinese culture, which (in fact, and not surprisingly) is a phenomenon of all cultures. Koro syndromes and elements of the syndrome, notably delusions of shrinkage or disappearance of the genitals, have been reported in Westerners as well, usually superimposed on a major psychiatric disorder. The following six case reports will highlight the occurrence of these phenomena in non-Asian patients.

KORO AND KORO-LIKE CASES IN WESTERNERS

Case 8 (Bychowski, 1952). A 46-year-old Orthodox Jewish man presented with symptoms of profound depression. Six years earlier the patient's much beloved wife had died. Before her death he promised that he would not remarry until their sons were grown. For 6 years he did not think of remarrying and was able to deny himself any sexual gratification. However, he then met a woman to whom he became quite attached. He began to think about marriage but developed feelings of remorse, thinking that his sons were not quite yet grown up (in fact, his youngest child was 17 years old). Another conflict was that his intended wife was liberal in her religious beliefs, which contrasted with his own orthodoxy. He therefore decided not to marry this woman, and he became depressed. One of his complaints was a feeling of estrangement from his genitals, such that at times he could not feel their presence. The patient would grab his genitals frequently to make sure they still were there. In time, the feelings of estrangement spread to other organs. The depersonalization of the genitals in this very depressed man was considered to be a psychological defense against forbidden sexual impulses toward his intended mate, and also as a symbolic realization of a castration wish.

Case 9 (Yap, 1965b). A 43-year-old British bookkeeper had suffered three bouts of depression since age 22, during which times he complained of neck, back, and testicular pain, and paresthesias in his legs. One depression coincided with his engagement. The most recent episode had lasted 2 months, during which he had been tense, with loss of libido and impotence, but still with occasional nocturnal emissions. On one particularly cold morning he felt his penis shrinking to about 1 centimeter in length, although it did elongate during urination. This feeling lasted about 24 hours; the patient thought it was a unique physical illness, although he apparently had never heard of koro. His past history included having a worrying, nervous disposition, stuttering during his youth, experiencing guilt over masturbation, with fears of insanity, and chronic worrying and shame over what he thought was a somewhat small penis.

Case 10 (Edwards, 1970). A 40-year-old American man, born in Greece but raised since infancy in the United States, developed a chronic schizophrenic illness at age 22. At various times over the ensuing 18 years he manifested a formal thought disorder with blocking of thoughts, flattening and incongruity of affect, delusions, and auditory hallucinations. He said he wanted to forget his past life and asked everyone to call him "Nameless." On one occasion, when accidentally called by his real name, he experienced sudden acute anxiety and a feeling of shrinking of his penis. This lasted for approximately 1 hour, and for several weeks afterward he felt he could get only a partial erection. Subsequently being called by his real name never reproduced these feelings. When the patient was 18 years old he became preoccupied with the small size of his penis and dreamed that there was a vagina where his penis should have been. He had never previously heard of koro and apparently had not encountered other patients with genital symptoms.

Case 11 (Lapierre, 1972). A 55-year-old man had been in good health until 4 months earlier, at which time he had a lobectomy for bronchial carcinoma. Three days after surgery, while having a bath, he felt that his penis had twisted upon itself and curved back into his abdomen. This made him anxious, whereupon he pulled on his penis, temporarily relieving his anxiety. The feeling recurred intermittently during his hospital stay, during which times he was convinced that his penis was withdrawing, and that if this were allowed to happen, he might not survive. However, when calm he believed that this impression was indeed imaginary. When presenting for psychiatric evaluation he was depressed and anxious and pulling at his penis. A course of antidepressant medication relieved his depression and lessened the severity of his anxiety about his genitals. Some weeks later he developed an organic brain syndrome, and an inoperable metastasis was discovered in the left frontal-temporal region. His tumor was irradiated, but marked deterioration of his mental faculties persisted, and he died 5 months later. The patient's sexual life had never been satisfactory, and he had been impotent on many occasions, which did not particularly displease his wife. She considered him to have been a weak, immature, and irresponsible husband and father, although his work record had been quite good. He had never heard of koro, nor of any cases with symptoms similar to his own.

Case 12 (Dow and Silver, 1973). A 20-year-old Canadian youth came to the hospital complaining of vague aches, feelings of depersonalization, and panic over a feeling that his penis was shrinking. He stated he had taken six Benzedrine tablets and one methadone tablet in the preceding 24 hours; he denied any drug intake for several days prior; and he gave a 5-year history of intermittent amphetamine, cannabis, and LSD abuse.

There was no evidence for any precipitating factor other than the taking of the Benzedrine. On mental status examination he was very anxious, hyperactive, and complaining of feelings of depersonalization, derealization, and a shrinking penis. His thinking was tangential, but he denied hallucinations or ideas of reference. He was oriented but showed a decreased attention span and concentration ability. His symptoms responded rapidly to diazepam and reassurance, and within 12 hours he was asymptomatic. He had no recurrence over a 2-month follow-up, although it appeared that he was still abusing drugs.

Case 13 (Barrett, 1978). A 33-year-old British engineer, who recently had become engaged, awakened at 3:00 A.M. with a feeling of impending doom and an awareness that his penis was shrinking into his body. He rapidly developed palpitations, sweating, nausea, and other symptoms of a panic attack. The feeling that he was about to die was linked to the shrinking of his penis, which he sought to alleviate by pulling it. The attack lasted about 20 minutes. The next day he was given diazepam by his physician, who told him he had a case of "nerves." Over the following year, beginning at the same time of morning, the patient experienced 12 to 15 similar attacks, though their intensity and duration decreased. The antianxiety agent helped relieve the attacks, as did his forcing his mind to other things, especially to erotic thoughts. He subsequently married and thereafter had only mild, nonspecific anxiety attacks and was sexually well adjusted. He had no previous psychiatric history or particularly pathologic premorbid personality features.

These six cases in Westerners of various components of the koro syndrome presented as acute episodes superimposed on a prominent depressive or schizophrenic illness, on an organic brain syndrome, or as part of a severe anxiety attack. These Occidental patients had never heard of koro, nor had they been exposed to other patients with genital delusions, as far as their examiners knew. Thus, the predisposing factor of culturally transmitted beliefs concerning the prevalence and life-threatening severity of koro was absent in this group of patients. They were individual, isolated cases, and they all had a profound psychiatric disturbance that developed from predisposing intrapsychic conflicts. In this regard they were more like the five individual cases of koro in Orientals described above than the hundreds of cases of koro occurring in the Singapore epidemic. As mentioned earlier, the koro cases in Singapore most likely represented a mass hysteria, the illness being quite benign in the vast majority of patients and responding quickly to simple reassurance.

Thus, the koro syndrome, or major components of it, has been clinically manifest both in Orientals and in Occidentals. While most patients have been Chinese men, a sufficient number of cases has been reported

in Westerners to cause some generalizations about the universal psychodynamic origins of this illness syndrome to be made. The psychodynamics, diagnostics, and treatment of koro will be examined next.

PSYCHODYNAMICS, DIAGNOSTICS, AND TREATMENT OF KORO

The psychodynamics of koro are rooted in two major areas: traditional Chinese beliefs about sexuality, and the primacy of psychosexual
dynamics and conflicts in the psychologies of all cultures. Yap (1965a)
indicated that traditional Chinese ideas of sex physiology are founded
on the theory of a harmonious equilibrium between *yin* and *yang*, the
female and male principles. The traditional belief is that during normal
intercourse there is a healthy exchange of yin and yang humors, but with
masturbation and nocturnal emission in men there is an unbalanced loss
of yang (the male principle). Traditional Chinese medicine also recognizes a neurasthenic state associated with sexual excesses which includes
symptoms of giddiness, physical and mental debility, aching of the loins,
and excessive shivering at the completion of urination. Thus, worry and
guilt over excessive or unsatisfactory sexual practices have been powerful psychological precipitants of koro in culturally susceptible Chinese
and other ethnic groups. Yap pointed out that the koro belief is not just
pathoplastic but actually pathogenic in that it can help bring about the
clinical manifestations of the syndrome. That is, the coherence of the
syndrome is dependent upon the patient's having learned a certain set
of beliefs that not only mold the form of the illness but also contribute
to its occurrence. Yap (1965a) referred to koro as a "culture-bound depersonalization syndrome," placing central emphasis on the proprioceptive
perceptual distortion of a part of the body image, rather than having considered it a pure delusion without a sensory basis.

Gwee (1963, 1968) and Rin (1963, 1965) also emphasized the importance of traditional Chinese beliefs about sexuality in the pathogenesis
of koro. They pointed out that patients who developed koro had conflicts
about masturbation, nocturnal emissions, prostitutes, promiscuity, and
often had unfulfilling sexual relations with wives who themselves were
not kindly disposed toward intercourse. Again, the underlying cultural
theme is the importance of preserving yang, the vital essence of the male,
the inappropriate loss of which is believed to lead to the koro syndrome
with its potentially fatal consequences.

In a more general sense, the importance of sexual conflicts in human
psychodynamics has been appreciated formally since the writings of
Freud. Sexual conflicts are often a prominent component of neurotic processes, which can include fantasies and dreams of genital mutilation

analogous to the koro symptom of the shrinking penis (Devereux, 1954). Concern about the size of one's penis may be a specific expression of general feelings of masculine inadequacy and inferiority. It is of interest to note that the visual angle subtended by one's own penis on casual self-inspection is less than that of the view of another man's genitals, which may be the basis of a general regard of one's own genital apparatus as smaller than another's. Under normal circumstances this remains but a fleeting impression, being counteracted by one's adequacy of sexual performance and competence in other areas of life. However, in men with predisposing sexual conflicts or with the aforementioned culturally determined beliefs, an otherwise innocuous phenomenon such as the normal retraction of the penis after a bath or on a particularly cold day may serve to trigger the koro fear of the penis completely shrinking into the abdomen, with the attendant panic over a supposedly fatal outcome.

As illustrated in the case reports, the koro syndrome can be super-imposed on a major psychiatric illness of an affective (depressive) or schizophrenic nature, or as a component of an organic brain syndrome. Gittleson and Levine (1966) compared the incidence of subjective ideas of sexual change in 70 male schizophrenics to 45 control subjects, the latter group consisting of patients with mania, endogenomorphic and reactive depressions, and personality disorder. Each subject was asked whether his illness was associated with a change in his interest in women, a change in the power of his erection, genital feelings of an unusual or abnormal type (hallucinations), a belief that the size or shape of his genitals had altered, a belief that he was changing or had changed into a neuter being or eunuch, or a belief that he was changing or had changed into a woman. Genital hallucinosis (pulling, drawing, electricity, etc.) and delusions of sex change occurred in approximately 30% of the schizophrenic patients, with a close but not complete association of these two symptoms. Delusions of sex change were more common in the unmarried patients. These symptoms were completely absent in the control subjects. Thus, about one-third of schizophrenic men may experience psychotic symptoms referable to their genitalia, and, as noted, the koro syndrome has occurred in conjunction with schizophrenic illnesses in both Oriental and Occidental patients.

From a diagnostic standpoint, koro has been considered a peculiar manifestation of an obsessive-compulsive illness, an unusual form of anxiety neurosis, an imaginary organic illness based on folk belief, an acute castration anxiety neurosis, a psychotic delusional state, a state of acute anxiety with partial depersonalization, and a psychic hysteria (Yap, 1965a; Gwee, 1963, 1968; Rin, 1963, 1965; Marks and Lader, 1973). Indeed, the aforementioned case reports of koro support all of these possibilites. It appears, then, that koro is a syndrome in the strict sense—a coherent collection of symptoms stemming from diverse etiologies. The range of effective therapies has included antidepressant medication for an underlying depressive illness, benzodiazepines for generalized anxiety, somatic treatments for underlying schizophrenia, psychotherapy for those patients with chronic neurotic conflicts, and simple education and reassurance for many of the culturally induced cases presenting during the Singapore epidemic. Koro thus remains a fascinating, predominantly culture-bound syndrome, which may be decreasing in incidence in its classic form. However, anxieties and delusory beliefs about genital inadequacy that are reminiscent of koro will undoubtedly continue to occur in individual patients because of the primacy of sexuality in human psychodynamics.

REFERENCES

Barrett, K., 1978, Koro in a Londoner, *Lancet* 2:1319.

Bychowski, G., 1952, "Psychotherapy of Psychosis," pp. 109–110, Grune and Stratton, New York.

Devereux, G., 1954, Primitive genital mutilations in a neurotic's dream, *J. Am. Psychoanal. Assoc.* 2:484.

Dow, T. W., and Silver, D., 1973, A drug induced koro syndrome, *J. Fla. Med. Assoc.* 60(4):32.

Edwards, J. G., 1970, The koro pattern of depersonalization in an American schizophrenic patient, *Am. J. Psychiatry* 126:1171.

Gittleson, N. L., and Levine, S., 1966, Subjective ideas of sexual change in male schizophrenics, *Br. J. Psychiatry* 112:779.

Gwee, A. L., 1963, Koro—A cultural disease, *Singapore Med. J.* 4:119.

Gwee, A. L., 1968, Koro—Its origin and nature as a disease entity, *Singapore Med. J.* 9:3.

Koro Study Team, 1969, The koro "epidemic" in Singapore, *Singapore Med. J.* 10:234.

Lapierre, Y. D., 1972, Koro in a French Canadian, *Can. Psychiatr. Assoc. J.* 17:333.

Marks, I., and Lader, M., 1973, Anxiety states (anxiety neurosis): A review, *J. Nerv. Ment. Dis.* 156:3.

Mun, C. T., 1968, Epidemic koro in Singapore, *Br. Med. J.* 1:640.

Ngui, P. W., 1969, The koro epidemic in Singapore, *Aust. N.Z. J. Psychiatry* 3:263.

Rin, H., 1963, Koro: A consideration on Chinese concepts of illness and case illustrations, *Transcult. Psychiatr. Res.* No. 15:23.

Rin, H., 1965, A study of the aetiology of koro in respect to the Chinese concept of illness, *Int. J. Soc. Psychiatry* 11:7.

van Wulfften Palthe, P. M., 1934, Koro, eene eigenaardig angstneurose, *Geneesk. Tijdschr. Ned.-Indie* 74:1713.

Yap, P. M., 1965a, Koro—A culture-bound depersonalization syndrome. *Br. J. Psychiatry* 111:43.

Yap, P. M., 1965b, Koro in a Briton, *Br. J. Psychiatry* 111:774.

10

Amok

JOSEPH WESTERMEYER

INTRODUCTION

History

Amok—a Malay term referring to homicidal assault—has been reported to the Occidental world by travelers to India and the Malay Archipelago from the 16th century up to today (Norris, 1849; Oxley, 1849; Spores, 1976). Amok (also written "amuk" or "amuck") has long been known in Malay and Indian folklore as a special type of violent behavior, either common enough or important enough to acquire a specific term for it. Over the last several decades, British physicians in Malaysia and Singapore (Ellis, 1893; Gimlette, 1901; Abraham, 1912; Galloway, 1923) and Dutch physicians in Indonesia (Van Loon, 1926–27; van Wulffton-Palthe, 1933) have described the amok phenomenon in great detail, usually including case histories.

While perhaps originally an Indian word (see Spores), the term *amok* has been restricted to cases of violence in Malaysia and Indonesia until recent years. Separated by the Strait of Malacca, Malaysia and Indonesia share many characteristics. Their inhabitants are predominantly paddy rice farmers and fishermen, Moslem, and racially similar, and they speak languages that are dialects of each other. Art forms and literature are alike, and in former times the men in both areas went about their daily occupations armed with a *kris*, or short sword.

In recent decades the term *amok* has been applied—primarily by psychiatrists—to sudden outbursts of violence among other peoples. Such reports have originated from the Philippines (Zaguirre, 1957), Papua-New Guinea (Burton-Bradley, 1968), Laos (Westermeyer, 1972,

JOSEPH WESTERMEYER • Department of Psychiatry, University of Minnesota, Minneapolis, Minnesota.

1973a), the United States (Lion *et al.*, 1969), and the Arctic (Kloss, 1923). Similar forms of sudden assault, but with a different label, have been described among medieval Scandinavians *(berserk)*.

As the term *amok* has been used to describe sudden and unexpected assault in regions outside the Malay Archipelago, an interesting paradox has arisen. One Occidental writer (Carr, 1978) has argued that the amok form of violence is specific to Malaysia, and that the term *amok* should be reserved for Malay cases alone. And an Oriental writer—himself a citizen of Malaysia—has emphasized that amok is not restricted to Malaysia, as "senseless killings" occur in all countries (Teoh, 1972).

CLINICAL DESCRIPTION

Typically, the Malay person afflicted with amok has been described as undergoing a particular series of behavioral, psychological, and social changes, with the attendant stereotyped assaultive behavior. This "classical" picture generally began with a period of social withdrawal. After some hours or days of quietude and isolation, the amok person (or *pengamok* in Malay) suddenly attacked any and all within reach: family, acquaintances, strangers. These assaults persisted for minutes, hours, or—rarely—days, until the amok person was killed or restrained. If he survived, the pengamok fell into a profound sleep, stupor, or comatose condition for a period of hours to a few days. Upon awakening he continued to be withdrawn and noncommunicative. He ordinarily showed some emotional disturbance (depression or hostility) but was amnesic for the assaultive period. These characteristics are noted in a report from 1891 regarding a Malay case:

> . . . it appears that Imam Mamat . . . had been at work fencing his land all day, and about 4 to 5 P.M. he entered the house of Bilal Abu [his brother-in-law] with a spear and a *golak* [bladed weapon] in his possession. On entering he took the hand of Bilal Abu and asked for pardon; he then shook hands with his [own] wife Alang Resak and said the same thing, but immediately stabbed her in the abdomen with the *golak*. She immediately fell, and received two more superficial wounds . . . Bilal Abu rushed to the rescue, and received for his trouble a deep wound in the region of the heart and a superficial wound on the right side: he fell never to rise again. At this moment Ngah Intan, wife of Bilal Abu, followed by four of her children, rushed to the door and jumped out, her eldest son Kassim receiving a stab in the back as he jumped out. Imam Mamat jumped out [houses are on stilts], and, with two more spears picked up in the house, gave chase to Ngah Intan, who was followed by the three youngest children . . . One little girl, Si Teh, received two wounds in the back, not dangerous ones; a boy, Mumin, received a deep wound in the side . . . his recovery being doubtful (he subsequently died); and the second little girl, Si Pateh, received a severe wound in the stomach, from which she died the next day. Having satisfied himself with the children, he followed up the mother, catching her 100 yards off,

and killed her on the spot by a stab in the abdomen. . . . It appears that Imam then walked down stream some 200 yards, and met a friend, Uda Majid, who was coming to stop him, but unarmed. Uda Majid saluted him respectfully, and asked him if he recognized him, and not to make a row; he replied "Yes, but my spear doesn't know you," and immediately stabbed him twice in the breast and stomach.

Imam killed yet another village man who sought to restrain him and then disappeared into the jungle. Search parties were organized against him, and people in the region prepared for an assault by him. The next evening he tried to attack another family but was repulsed, receiving wounds in the face and thigh. He died the following day after reporting that "he did not know what he was doing, only his head went round and the devil told him to do it." At the inquest, fellow villagers could give no reason for it, stating he was "on most friendly terms with everyone." He had killed six people in his assaults and wounded four others. Two of the fatalities were pregnant women whose almost-term infants died (Spores, 1976)

Another "classical" element was the use of bladed instruments, such as the Malay short sword, or *kris*. The *pengamok* were all men, ranging from early adulthood through middle age. Most were illiterate farmers/fishermen/peasants, although merchants, soldiers, skilled workmen, and at least one prince were reported. Prior to colonization by the English and Dutch, Malay and Indonesian *pengamok* who survived presumably returned to their former personalities and social existence. Rarely was there a recurrence of their amok behavior.

REVIEW OF CASE STUDIES

Most amok studies have been written by general physicians and psychiatrists, and more recently by a few behavioral scientists in collaboration with psychiatrists. Cases have been reported for over a century. Sampling methods have varied, with subjects being identified in jails, prisons, mental institutions, and community surveys. Methods of collecting information have included the following: interviews with *pengamok* themselves, and sometimes with their relatives and acquaintances; physical and/or mental status examinations; historical reconstructions of the person's former personality and/or social existence; descriptions of the amok behavior, the weapons, and the victims; and subsequent outcomes for the *pengamok*.

As one might expect, this variability in examiners, historical context, sampling procedures, and method for collecting data has resulted in diverse observations. Studies done 50–100 years ago by general physicians, at a time when psychiatric method and theory were just beginning, emphasized biomedical causal factors. Theories by psychiatrists in the first half of the 20th century stressed psychodynamic factors and amok as a "cultural manifestation" of generic psychiatric disorders. Investigators over the last decade have depicted amok as a behavioral syndrome or "final common pathway" with diverse historical, biomedical, psychodynamic, psychopathological, social, and cultural origins.

Demographic Characteristics (see Table I)

Review of case series with 20 or more amok persons from the Malay Archipelago and Southeast Asia has indicated a somewhat younger age than given in classical descriptions. Amok has infrequently occurred before age 20 or after age 45. The mean age of institutionalized Malay *pengamok* was found to be in the early 30s by two investigators. The earlier mean age of 26.2 years in the Laotian sample could be attributed to real cultural differences. This age gap may also be due to different sampling methods, since the Malay samples consisted of amok survivors in hospitals, whereas the Laotian sample included those who died or escaped.

In these combined cases only one woman was labeled as "running *amok.*" Her case is not a typical one since there were no deaths and the assault was not indiscriminate. Schmidt *et al.* (1977) report the case as follows:

> L. A. N. is the only female in our series who has exhibited a behavior pattern which was called by those around her running *amok*, and which certainly bears most of its characterisation. She is 31 years old and lives alone, although she said she had been married several times for a short while, fifteen years prior to the event. She taps her own rubber. She is an Iban and lives in an Iban longhouse. She is said to have had four husbands who all divorced her after a few months. During her last marriage, she was exhibiting signs of mental instability which led to the break-up. She had always been suspicious and complaining that people were talking badly about her. One day she grabbed a *parang* (machetelike knife) and attacked those whom she believed to be against her, four people, two men and two women without mortally wounding them. She was overpowered and in the fight received some wounds herself. She was diagnosed as a case of paranoid schizophrenia and was discharged as much improved after five months.

Despite this exception, amok has been overwhelmingly a male phenomenon in past centuries as well as recently (Spores, 1976). Students of psychopathology in Malaysia have argued that *latah* (the sudden yelling of obscene or vulgar epithets) may be the female counterpart to male amok, since most latah individuals have been women (Abraham, 1912).

Amok persons from throughout the region have been predominantly farmers (at paddy rice, rubber tapping), laborers, and unskilled workmen (e.g., driver, soldier). Other occupations have been represented, including skilled workmen (e.g., tailor, carpenter), salaried per-

TABLE I. Demographic Characteristics

	Author and year of publication		
	Schmidt et al., 1977	Tan and Carr, 1977 / Carr and Tan, 1976	Westermeyer, 1972
Number of subjects	24	21	20
Region	Sarawak, Malaysia	West Malaysia	Vientiane province, Laos
Sampling method	Mental institution	Mental institution	Community survey
Age			
Range	20–43 (9 subjects)[a]	21–43 (17 subjects)[a]	17–35 (20 subjects)
Mean	32.0 years	33.6 years	26.2 years (SD = 5.95)
Sex			
Male	23	21	20
Female	1	0	0
	24	21	20
Education	12 illiterate / 6 literate / 18[a]	Not mentioned	9 illiterate / 5 1–3 years education / 6 4–6 years education / 20
Occupation	13 farmer/rubber tapper / 9 laborer/skilled/salaried / 22[a]	Rural-related, mercantile, unemployed or marginally employed	15 soldiers / 5 farmer merchant / 20
Ethnicity	Malay, tribal, Chinese	14 Malay / 5 Chinese / 2 Indian / 21[a]	16 Lao / 4 tribal / 20
Religion	Not mentioned	Not mentioned	Buddhist, animist
Marital status			
Single	2	Not mentioned	8
Married	5		8
Divorced	1		3
Widowed	0		1
	8[a]		20
Current residence	Not mentioned	11 town / 10 rural / 21[a]	5 same location as birthplace / 15 different / 20

[a]Data not known for all subjects.

sons (e.g., civil servants), and merchants. Education has been uniformly low in all reports. Many amok persons have been illiterate, and few have education at even the secondary school level. As with occupation, these relatively low educational levels have been common throughout the region.

Residence of amok persons has included urban centers, towns, and rural villages. All religions common throughout the area have been represented, including Islam, Buddhism, and animism.

Marital status of the *pengamok* has been variable, with somewhat more than half of them married. The proportion of single, divorced or separated, and widowed among them has been higher than would be expected for this age group and for the region.

Time, Place, Weapon, and Victims (see Table II)

Most Malaysian cases reported by Schmidt *et al.* took place early in the day, with 12 out of 14 occurring at noon or earlier. By contrast, the Laotian cases occurred mostly in the evening. The cause for this discrepancy is not obvious, although cultural factors and/or sampling differences may be operating.

Both in Malaysia and in Laos, sudden assault was more apt to occur at public gatherings and in homes rather than in isolated or remote locations. The location of the violence enhanced the likelihood of a large number of victims, and a public rather than a secretive assault.

Bladed weapons constituted the most common weapon in Malaysia. As pointed out by Tan and Carr (1977), however, a wide variety of weapons were employed by Malaysian *pengamok*, ranging from the naked fist to guns to a truck. Rifles have been used by amok persons in Indonesia (Van Loon, 1928). Bladed weapons were widely used in Papua-New Guinea (Burton-Bradley, 1968). Among Filipino veterans going amok, Zaguirre (1957) noted a high frequency of military ordnance, especially carbines and submachine guns. For a time in Laos, grenades (widely available among village militia and sometimes used to stun and catch fish in rivers) were used by those suddenly exhibiting violence (Westermeyer, 1972). In both the Philippines and Laos studies, bladed weapons were also reported.

Victims have included predominantly family members, relatives, neighbors, and acquaintances of the amok person. Especially in towns and cities, some strangers were also involved. Most victims belonged to the same ethnic group as the *pengamok*, but cross-ethnic violence was present, particularly in Malaysian towns, which are often multiethnic. Tan and Carr (1977) observed that Malay *pengamok* had more victims (mean of 4.3 victims in 10 amok cases) as compared to Indian or Chinese *pengamok* (mean of 2.2 victims in 5 cases).

TABLE II. Timing, Location, Weapons, and Victims

	Author and year of publication		
	Schmidt et al., 1977	Carr and Tan, 1976 Tan and Carr, 1977	Westermeyer, 1972
Time of day	10 "dawn to noon" 1 "noon" 1 9:00 P.M. 1 "evening" 1 "night" $\overline{14^a}$	Not mentioned	2 midnight to 6:00 A.M. 1 6:01 A.M. to noon 4 noon to 6:00 P.M. 11 6:01 P.M. to midnight $\overline{18^a}$
Location	3 home 1 work camp dormitory 1 army sick quarters $\overline{5^a}$	Not mentioned	1 forest 8 home 11 (public place, temple festival, army camp, public street, theater) $\overline{20}$
Weapons	5 parang, knife 1 truck 1 blunt object 1 fists only $\overline{8^a}$	Kris, parang, gun, scissors, meat cleaver, hoe	18 grenade 2 bladed weapons $\overline{20}$
Victims' identities		32 Malay 30 Chinese 7 Indian	9 cases—relatives, friends, and/or neighbors only 6 cases—strangers only 3 cases—strangers and relatives/friends/neighbors $\overline{18^a}$
Average numbers	0.8 injuries/case 1.25 deaths/case (N = 24 cases)	3.5 "victims"/case (N = 15 cases)[a]	6.23 injuries/case (range 0–30) 4.22 deaths/case (range 1–16)

[a]Data not known for all subjects.

The number of victims also varied as a result of the authors' differing criteria. Some included cases where a person suddenly and publicly began to assault others, but in which no death, or even injury, was inflicted. These were all cases from Malaysia in which the local people labeled the violence as amok. Larger numbers of victims, with injury or death a *sine qua non* for inclusion in the study, have been noted in non-Malaysian studies in which the investigators applied the term *amok* to the violent behavior. This suggests that the prevalence of amok among the Malay may reflect more inclusive criteria among the Malay folk, rather than a true higher prevalence of amok.

Biopsychosocial Concomitants (See Table III)

Older writers emphasized the role of various medical disorders in the genesis of amok, including malaria and neurosyphilis. This may reflect the character of the amok syndrome at that time, the higher prevalence of malaria and neurosyphilis in previous decades, and/or diagnostic bias among physicians describing early cases. Even in more recent cases, however, neurosyphilis and other organic brain syndromes have been noted in a few patients. A few recent observers have noted the frequent association of alcohol use with amok in regions outside Malaysia (Burton-Bradley, 1968; Westermeyer, 1972).

Psychiatric assessment has been primarily performed on subjects in mental institutions. This approach has indicated that psychosis, emotional disturbance, and personality disorder occur commonly among surviving *pengamok*, but no one diagnostic entity prevails. Functional psychosis (schizophrenia and manic depression) has been most commonly diagnosed, but virtually any and all psychiatric labels have been applied. In studies using prison or field survey samples, psychiatric diagnoses have not been so widely applied, perhaps reflecting the sampling method or the difficulty of careful psychiatric assessment in those settings.

Psychological reconstruction of the prodromal period among one series of Malay *pengamok* did support the notion of "classical" amok psychological concomitants (Schmidt *et al.*, 1977). Social withdrawal and emotional disturbance were present in 17 out of 20 subjects. Postmorbid amnesia for the amok event was present in 15 cases to a total extent, and in 5 to a partial extent. As with the matter of bladed weapons, however, the "typical" prodrome and postviolence amnesia were not inevitably present.

Particular attention to social concomitants has appeared only in the last score of years, although some earlier case studies included information regarding recent social events. Several themes have recurred as precipitating social events: migration from one location to another (usually

TABLE III. Biopsychosocial Concomitants

	Author and year of publication		
	Schmidt et al., 1977	Carr and Tan, 1976 / Tan and Carr, 1977	Westermeyer, 1972
Biomedical	2 neurosyphilis 1 epilepsy $\overline{3^a}$	1 neurosyphilis	15 drinking context 5 not drinking context $\overline{20}$
Psychiatric diagnosis	9 schizophrenia ? paranoid schizophrenia 3 endogenous depression 2 anxiety reaction 1 epilepsy 1 involutional depression 1 manic depression 1 paranoid reaction 1 paranoid personality $\overline{22^a}$	14 schizophrenic 1 manic depression 1 general paresis (neurosyphilis) $\overline{16^a}$ Later mental status: 16 "normal" 5 psychotic $\overline{21}$	1 psychotic 2 character disorder $\overline{3^a}$
Social	1 rural-to-town migration 6 none 2 separated from family $\overline{9^a}$	Not mentioned	Occupational mobility: 2 occupation same as father 18 occupation different from father Educational mobility: 0 less than father 9 same as father 11 greater than father $\overline{20}$
Outcome	Not systematically studied	Prolonged psychiatric hospitalization	11 suicide 5 imprisonment 4 escape $\overline{20}$

[a]Data not known for all subjects.

rural to town or urban), separation from family, loss of face or prestige, loss of spouse or a romantic relationship, loss of money or material goods. Those individuals for whom no associated social event could be discerned tended to be diagnosed as psychotic, usually schizophrenic.

THEORIES

Folk Theories

Among the Malay, amok has been considered an illness in recent decades (Tan and Carr, 1977; Carr, 1978), although it may have had different connotations in former centuries (Spores, 1976). More specifically, it is considered a form of mental illness or insanity. The formal term in the folk nomenclature is *gila mengamok* or "running-amok insanity" (Chen, 1970; Resner and Hartog, 1970). At least in former times, the folk theory for its genesis was spirit possession and/or soul loss. Within the folk cosmology, such preternatural events could be brought about by human disrespect for the spirits, by a broken taboo, or by a malevolent spirit who needed to be mollified or controlled magically. Fever, magic, threat, or anger have also been reported as causes by Malay people, especially in recent times.

Carr and Tan (1976) asked a series of 21 amok patients at a psychiatric hospital in West Malaysia about their ideas regarding amok and its role in their behavior. Ten patients—all Malay—were familiar with the amok concept, were able to provide in-depth opinions about its characteristics and etiology, and viewed themselves as *pengamok*. Six patients—all Chinese or Indian—were not familiar with the concept of amok and gave personal reasons for their violent behavior. Five other patients were incoherent or totally noncommunicative and provided no information or opinion.

Biological Theories

During the 19th century biomedical explanations for amok predominated. Malaria, dengue, paratyphoid, typhoid, and vague gastrointestinal maladies were implicated (Ellis, 1893; Gimlette, 1901; Spores, 1976). Neurosyphilis, leprosy, and epilepsy have been occasionally mentioned as causes (Spores, 1976; Schmidt et al., 1977; Tan and Carr, 1977). Although alcohol is religiously proscribed for Moslem Malay and Indonesians, acute intoxication has been frequently associated with amok-like cases in Papua-New Guinea (Burton-Bradley, 1968) and Laos (Westermeyer, 1972). The latter is not unexpected in view of the common association between violence and alcohol use (Spain et al., 1951; Jones, 1967; Nicol et al., 1973; Taylor et al., 1976).

Psychological Theories

Some authors—including Tan and Carr (1977)—have reported all amok persons as psychotic upon admission to a psychiatric institution. This finding has not been replicated by others, although psychosis has been commonly noted among amok psychiatric patients studied by Schmidt et al. (1977), Burton-Bradley (1968), and others. In general, the diversity in psychiatric diagnosis among various investigators is a more striking finding than is any universality: Virtually all major diagnostic groups have been represented.

Certain psychodynamic characteristics, while not present in all cases, have been frequently noted by investigators of amok. One of these is projection, the blaming of others for one's own difficulties—a theory supported by the prevalence of paranoia and paranoid schizophrenia among *pengamok* (Schmidt et al., 1977). Another is extraordinary sensitivity to hurt (O'Brien, 1883). A third is overinvestment in control and decorum, such that the failure of these rigid and overdetermined defenses results in a total abandonment of restraint in an orgy of slaughter and selfdestruction (Wilkinson, 1928). While careful psychological testing of amok persons has not yet been conducted in Asia in order to validate or invalidate these theories, a study of "sudden murderers" has been conducted in the United States. It showed that such people have difficulty forming close relationships, do not directly express hostility, and commonly use projection as a defense (Lamberti et al., 1958).

Social Theories

Loss of social standing—via insult, loss of employment, financial loss—has been posited as a precipitating event for amok. Loss of important social relationships, especially lovers or spouses, has also been a frequent premorbid finding. Migration from rural home villages to work camps, the military, towns, and cities has been frequently associated with amok. (See Burton-Bradley, 1968; Schmidt et al., 1977; Westermeyer, 1972, 1973a, for case examples from various cultures.) In other studies, violent behavior has similarly been noted in association with the following: rejection by a lover, fiancee, or spouse (Tanay, 1976), and childhood, occupational, marital, and parental loss (Humphrey, 1977).

As has been noted by Holmes and Rahe (1967) and Rahe et al. (1967), the effect of major life change over a period of 1 or 2 years appears to be cumulative and may be causal in precipitating illness. Attneave (1969) and Pattison et al. (1975) have shown that a stable, intact social network serves a protective function in crisis, enabling the individual to survive and resolve the difficulty. Major loss and migration—frequent concomitants of amok—may be important causal factors in such violence, as well as in the physical illness and psychiatric disorder that sometimes predate amok violence.

Cultural Theories

As one might expect with a "culture-bound" syndrome, theories focusing on cultural dimensions of amok are most numerous. One of these regards child raising. Certain factors have been implicated as subsequently favoring amok phenomena among Malay men: a "highly protected environment," indulgence or reward of children that is not connected to expectations or requirements, emphasis during socialization on social duty rather than individual enjoyment, and constraint from expressing aggression (Carr, 1978).* These child-raising strategies theoretically shape the following personality characteristics often noted among amok persons in Malaysia and elsewhere: projection as a predominate defense, helplessness in the face of frustration or adversity, difficulty expressing hostility, and the assignment of responsibility for adversity or failure onto the community rather than onto oneself.

Cultural values, attitudes, and customs may support or elicit violent outbursts. Carr and Tan (1976) have shown that the concept of amok is well known to Malay *pengamok* but not to those from other ethnic groups in Malaysia, indicating that the amok entity has a degree of cultural validity, perhaps even acceptance, among the Malay. Within Malay society, where balance and distribution of power are informal and social rather than written and legal, amok may have functioned over the centuries as a means for limiting the power of hereditary rulers, since arbitrary dictums might elicit amok violence (Gullick, 1958).

A low suicide rate among the Malay has been noted (Hassan, 1970; Teoh, 1974). This suggests that members of the group might be less likely to blame themselves for failure or frustration, and perhaps more apt to act against others in such circumstances (Carr, 1978). Malay cultural and religious strictures may assign suicide as a more taboo or noxious behav-

---

*Theoretical formulations are not just the province of academicians in ivory towers. Similar ideas regarding etiology are readily obtained in the course of field work from thoughtful villagers. For example, during field studies on amok-like violence in Laos, I was interviewing a village headman regarding a person who had gone amok in the village. We were considering events that had preceded the violence. A village matriarch, on her way to a market, stopped to join our group. After listening for a time, she volunteered the following: "You Americans do not go crazy and kill people like that because you speak your anger openly. I know, I see you in the market and I see the manner that you speak to each other. We Lao are different. We seldom show anger, and when we do there is loss of face *(seah naa)*. So the anger builds and can suddenly come out in killing. When we can show anger like you, the killing will not be so common." This soliloquy was unexpected, since the Lao viewed the strong, public expression of feelings by Caucasians as indicating their lack of civility and cultural inferiority.

ior than assault. Consequently, the individual seeking his own destruction arranges his end indirectly, and in a more socially acceptable manner, by assaulting and killing others so that he himself is then killed by others. As support for this theory, ethnic groups with high suicide rates—the Japanese, Northern Europeans, Euroamericans in the United States—tend to have relatively low rates of homicide.*

Historical and institutional factors within a culture may also support amok as a behavioral alternative. Among the Malay, military attacks and assaults were reportedly once accompanied by yelling, "Amok" (Shaw, 1972), in the same fashion that attacking Japanese soldiers more recently yelled, "Banzai." Five hundred years ago Islam, for a time, taught that infidels should be slain, and there have been instances in which violence has served as a form of religious fanaticism (such as the Juramentado of the Philippines).

Proximity of weapons may play a role in the frequency of amok violence. Malay men carried the bladed *kris* or *parang* with them virtually at all times. Similarly, the peasant/farmers elsewhere in Southeast Asia and the Malay Archipelago carried spears and machetelike knives for their work, as well as for self-defense against jungle animals and bandits. Use of guns by amok Indonesians and Malay soldiers (Van Loon, 1928; Schmidt et al., 1977) and by Filipino veterans (Zaguirre, 1957) also underlines the importance of weapon availability in amok, as does the use of grenades by Laotian soldiers and militia (Westermeyer, 1973a).

CURRENT ISSUES CONCERNING AMOK

Contagion

Amok has been widely considered a Malay-Indonesian syndrome. However, virtually all of the ethnic groups living among or close to Malays and Indonesians have had cases of amok. Case reports from

---

*At least one study, that by Franke et al. (1977), does not support the inverse correlation between suicide and homicide. However, their data were drawn exclusively from the United States. Data from Laos, where grenade-*amok* was prevalent for a time in the mid-1960s, do support the "indirect suicide" theory. As Buddhists, the Lao had religious strictures against killing. Tribal animists or Thai Moslems were often hired to slaughter animals. Lao often rationalized that catching fish was not actually a killing procedure, since all the fisherman did was remove the fish from water to air without directly killing the fish. As soldiers, the Lao employed a similar rationalization. They were fervent users of artillery, bombs, mortars, and grenades, since death indirectly came to an enemy who was "in the wrong place at the wrong time" and the Lao soldier did not perceive himself as directly willing his enemy's death. By contrast, the killing of an enemy by gunfire or knife was considered direct killing. Thus, the adaptation of the grenade to a traditional form of violence had numerous ideological and moral advantages, since it indirectly killed others, and frequently oneself also.

Malaysia have included numerous non-Malay individuals from China and India, as well as from indigenous tribal groups (i.e., sea and land Dayak, Kayan, Punan, Melanau, and Iban). Schmidt *et al.* (1977) have shown that amok in West Malaysia is most common among the Malay (i.e., those with societal supports for amok), intermediate among tribal groups of Malaysia (i.e., those who have had close contact with the Malay for thousands of years), and least common among those with more recent contact (i.e., the Chinese in Malaysia).

Sudden, widespread popularity of automatic weapons for amok in the Philippines (Zaguirre, 1957) and grenades in Laos (Westermeyer, 1973a) further support a "contagion" or "learning" hypothesis for amok. Such "contagion" is not only a characteristic of amok violence. Berkowitz and McCauly (1971) have documented unusual increases in violent crimes following spectacular murders in the United States (e.g., Kennedy assassinations, Whitman and Speck mass murders).

Endemicity versus Epidemicity

During the period 1945-1968, Schmidt *et al.* (1977) noted a fairly constant number of amok cases by 3-year intervals in Malaysia. Tan and Carr's cases from Malaysia (1977) also fail to show much fluctuation by 10-year intervals. Thus, amok in that country appears to follow an endemic pattern, at least for the years since World War II.

By contrast, amok violence in Laos, the Philippines, and Thailand has followed an epidemic pattern during the same period (Westermeyer, 1973b). Several social factors may be correlated in time with increased amok; these include rapid culture change, political unrest, increased geographic mobility, and increased social mobility. Unlike the persistence of bladed weapons in many amok cases in Malaysia, other weapons (especially guns and grenades) have outnumbered the traditional bladed weapons in these amok "epidemics."*

Other problematic behaviors have been noted to follow an epidemic periodicity. One of these is narcotic addiction in the United States (Hughes *et al.*, 1972). By contrast, opium addiction in Laos—a tradition for generations and probably centuries—is an endemic phenomenon (Westermeyer, 1974). Suicide by immolation was epidemic for a time in the Western world (Bourgeois, 1969). These observations, together with

---

* "Grenade-amok" cases reached their zenith in Laos during 1966. A common site for such violence was Buddhist temple festivals or *boun*, where money was raised to meet expenses for temples and adjacent monasteries. So frequent were amok outbursts during this time that Souvanna Phouma, prime minister of Laos, placed a moratorium on all *boun* during the remaining festival season in 1966-67. Subsequently, *boun* were resumed in their traditional fashion without a recurrence of amok violence.

those regarding amok, suggest that a problematic behavior is apt to be "endemic" in a society where the phenomenon is integrated into the society, is relatively frequent, and has been present for a long time. A problematic behavior is more apt to be "epidemic" in a society where it functions as a response to a transient crisis, has been relatively infrequent, and does not have a lengthy tradition.

Changes Over Time

Students of amok in Malaysia have argued that amok has changed over the centuries (Murphy, 1972; Tan and Carr, 1977). Originally it may have been chosen as a response to crisis by various religious fanatics, indentured warriors, and political dissidents among whom psychopathology played little role. Cases in Malaysia and Indonesia over recent decades have reportedly been increasingly associated with severe mental illness, especially schizophrenia, affective disorder, and paranoia. Military, religious, and political themes have reportedly diminished among these latter-day cases, or have been either minor or tangential.

Amok may have been more frequent in Malaysia and Indonesia prior to the arrival of English and Dutch colonizers. Decrease in amok violence following colonization has been attributed to the colonizers' new methods for handling *pengamok* (Murphy, 1972; Spores, 1976). Rather than kill them directly or eventually return them to full status in their communities, the English and Dutch kept them alive but committed them for decades or a lifetime to prison or to mental institutions. Another possible explanation for this decrease is that the colonizers brought a period of relative socioeconomic, cultural, and political stability and peace—conditions perhaps inveighing against amok (Westermeyer, 1973b).

Connor (1970) has hypothesized that the change from a simple "role-self" in traditional society to multiple roles in modern societies might reduce the risk of amok when a loss is experienced. This view is supported by the opinion of various investigators who believe that amok has been decreasing in the urban settings of Malaysia (Murphy, 1959; Carr and Tan, 1976; Schmidt et al., 1977).

Semantics

The disagreement regarding what constitutes amok was mentioned earlier. Some would restrict the term only to "classical" cases of amok perpetrated by Malays and Indonesians. Other investigators have extended the term to sudden violence among non-Malays when it occurs in Malaysia and is identified by Malays themselves as amok. And still other writers have applied the term *amok* to cases that involve sudden and unexpected public violence but that occur in societies having no special term for such violence.

At the base of this semantic issue is a real paradox: Such cases both resemble one another and differ from one another across cultural boundaries. For example, the "sudden murders" studied in the United States (Lamberti *et al.*, 1958; Blackman *et al.*, 1974; Ruotolo, 1975) and the "mass murderer" Wagner in Germany (Bruch, 1967) show many features typical of Malay amok. These include difficulties expressing anger, premorbid eccentricity or personality disorder, a high rate of various types of mental illness, paranoia, the public nature of the violent acts, and an apparent (often explicit) wish to be executed. At the same time, there are numerous differences. Even among Malay amok cases, atypical features occur, such as the use of nonbladed weapons (guns, a truck, blunt objects), lack of a "brooding" prodrome, or absence of postmorbid amnesia. The differences become greater as one considers non-Malay *pengamok* in Malaysia: Tan and Carr (1977) noted that they had fewer victims, used a greater variety of weapons, and were even unfamiliar with the amok entity. Differences are further accentuated when cases outside Malaysia are considered, such as the epidemic aspect and use of military ordnance in reports from Southeast Asia and elsewhere in the Malay Archipelago.

How might this semantic dilemma be resolved? One approach might be to further expand the term *amok* to include all related cases of sudden, mass assault. Plainly, some students of the syndrome will not accept this alternative, as they wish to maintain the emphasis on the unique or culture-bound aspects of the syndrome. Another alternative would be to employ a more generic term, such as *mass murder* or *amok-like murder* to cases from all cultures, while restricting the use of the Malay term *amok* for Malays themselves.

For those choosing the latter alternative, I suggest the term *SMASH: sudden mass assault syndrome, with homicide*. In order to lend some commonality to the cases, persons included in the category should manifest the following: (1) sudden outburst of violent behavior (the violence may have been thought about or planned for some time, but the actual violent behavior should be sudden and unexpected); (2) a public display of the violence, so that the perpetrator allows himself/herself to be readily identified to the community; (3) the injurious behavior should not be specifically aimed at only one or a few people but should occur against all present; (4) the community should not support the violence, so that the perpetrator is restrained, executed, exiled, or imprisoned (communities may support certain assaults such as assassinations, lynchings, or violence during riots and allow person(s) to resume normal existence); (5) at least one or more homicides ensue from the assault (this arbitrary criterion will limit the cases to those most dangerous and serious).

Use of a more generic term would allow us to learn more about this problematic and frightening behavior, which occurs in virtually all societies, albeit with rates that may vary widely. As we learn more about the core aspects and rates of this violence in various societies, we will perforce also learn more about its culture-bound and culture-independent aspects.

REFERENCES

Abraham, J. J., 1912, Latah and amok, Br. Med. J. 1:438.
Attneave, C. L., 1969, Therapy in tribal settings and urban network intervention, Family Proc. 8:192.
Berkowitz, L., and McCauly, J., 1971, The contagion of criminal violence, Sociometry 34:238.
Blackman, N., Lum, J. T., and Vanderpearl, R. J., 1974, Disturbed communications: A contributing factor in sudden murder, Ment. Health Soc. 1:345.
Bourgeois, M., 1969, Suicides by fire in the bonze manner, Ann. Med. Psychol. 2:116.
Bruch, H., 1967, Mass murder: The Wagner case, Am. J. Psychiatry 124:693.
Burton-Bradley, B. G., 1968, The Amok syndrome in Papua and New Guinea, Med. J. Aust. 1:252.
Carr, J. E., 1978, Ethno-behaviorism and the culture-bound syndromes: The case of amok, Culture, Med. Psychiatry 2:269.
Carr, J. E., and Tan, E. K., 1976, In search of the true amok: Amok as viewed within the Malay culture, Am. J. Psychiatry 133:1295.
Chen, P. C., 1970, Classification and concepts of causation of mental illness in a rural Malay community, Int. J. Soc. Psychiatry 16:205.
Connor, J. W., 1970, A social approach to an understanding of schizophrenic-like reactions, Int. J. Soc. Psychiatry 16:136.
Ellis, W. G., 1893, The amok of the Malays, J. Ment. Sci. 39:325.
Franke, R. H., Thomas, E. W., and Queenen, A. J., 1977, Suicide and homicide: Common sources and consistent relationships, Soc. Psychiatry 12:149.
Galloway, D. J., 1923, On amok, in "Far Eastern Association for Tropical Medicine: Transactions of the Fifth Biennial Congress, Singapore," Vol. 5, pp. 162–171, John Bale Sons and Danielson, London.
Gimlette, J. D., 1901, Notes on a case of amok, J. Trop. Med. Hyg.4:195.
Gullick, J. M., 1958, Indigenous political systems in western Malaysia, in "London School of Economics Monographs on Social Anthropology," No. 17, Athlone Press, 1958.
Hassan, R., 1970, Some sociological aspects of suicide in Singapore, in "Mental Health Trends in Developing Society" (M. Yap and P. Ngui, eds.), Roche Far East Research Foundation, Singapore.
Holmes, T., and Rahe, R., 1967, The social readjustment rating scale, J. Psychosom. Res. 11:213.
Hughes, P. M., Barker, N. W., Crawford, H. A., et al., 1972, The natural history of a heroin epidemic, Am. J. Public Health 62:995.
Humphrey, J. A., 1977, Social loss: A comparison of suicide victims, homicide offenders and non-violent individuals, Dis. Nerv. Syst. 38:157.
Jones, F. D., 1967, Experiences of a division psychiatrist in Vietnam, Mil. Med. 132:1003.
Kloss, C. B., 1923, Arctic amok, J. Malaya Branch R. Asiat. Soc. 1:254.
Lamberti, J. W., Blackman, N., and Weiss, J. M. A., 1958, The sudden murderer: A preliminary report, J. Soc. Ther. 4:2.

Lion, J. R., Bach-y-Riat, G., and Ervin, F. R., 1969, Violent patients in the emergency room, *Am. J. Psychiatry* 125:1706.

Murphy, H. B. M., 1959, Culture and mental disorder in Singapore, *in* "Culture and Mental Health" (M. Opler, ed.), Macmillan, New York.

Murphy, H. B. M., 1972, History and the evolution of syndromes: The striking case of latah and amok, *in* "Psychopathology: Contributions from the Social, Behavioral and Biological Sciences" (M. Hammer, K. Salzinger, and S. Sutton, eds.), Wiley, New York.

Nicol, A. R., Gunn, J. C., Gristwood, J., Foggitt, R. H., and Watson, J. P., 1973, The relationship of alcoholism to violent behavior in long-term imprisonment, *Br. J. Psychiatry* 123:47.

Norris, W., 1849, Sentence of death upon a Malay convicted of running amuck, *J. Indian Archipelago* 3:460.

O'Brien, H. A., 1883, Latah, *J. Straits Branch R. Asiat. Soc.* 11:143.

Oxley, J., 1849, Malay amoks, *J. Indian Archipelago* 3:532.

Pattison, E. M., DeFrancisco, D., Wood, D., Frazier, H., and Crowder, J., 1975, A psychosocial kinship model for family therapy. Presented at annual meeting, American Psychiatric Association.

Rahe, R. H., McKean, J. D., and Arthur, R. J., 1967, A longitudinal study of life-change and illness patterns, *J. Psychosom. Res.* 10:355.

Resner, G., and Hartog, J., 1970, Concepts and terminology of mental disorder among the Malays, *J. Cross-Cult. Psychol.* 1:369.

Ruotolo, A. K., 1975, Neurotic pride and homicide, *Am. J. Psychoanal.* 35:1016.

Schmidt, K., Hill, L., and Guthrie, G., 1977, Running amok, *Int. J. Soc. Psychiatry* 23:264.

Shaw, W., 1972, Amok, *Fed. Museums J. (Malaysia)* 17:1.

Spain, D. M., Bradess, V. A., and Eggston, A. A., 1951, Alcohol and violent death: A one year study of consecutive cases in a representative community, *J. Am. Med. Assoc.* 146:334.

Spores, J. C., 1976, Running amok: A sociological analysis. Doctoral Dissertation, Xerox University Microfilm, Univ. of Mich., Ann Arbor.

Tan, E. K., and Carr, J. E., 1977, Psychiatric sequelae of amok, *Culture, Med. and Psychiatry* 1:59.

Tanay, E., 1976, The Dear John syndrome during the Vietnam War, *Dis. Nerv. Syst.* 37:165.

Taylor, S. D., Gammon, C. B., and Capasso, D. R., 1976, Aggression as a function of the interaction of alcohol and threat, *J. Pers. Soc. Psychol.* 34:938.

Teoh, J. I., 1972, The changing psychopathology of amok, *Psychiatry* 35:345.

Teoh, J. I., 1974, An analysis of completed suicide by psychological post-mortem, *Ann. Acad. Med.* 3:117.

Van Loon, F. H. G., 1926–27, Amok and latah, *J. Abnorm. Soc. Psychol.* 21:434.

Van Loon, F. H. G., 1928, Protopathic instinctive phenomena in normal and pathologic Malay life, *Br. J. Med. Psychol.* 8:264.

van Wulffton-Palthe, P. M., 1933, Amok, *Med. J. Geneesk.* 77:983.

Westermeyer, J., 1972, A comparison of amok and other homicide in Laos, *Am. J. Psychiatry* 129:703.

Westermeyer, J., 1973a, Grenade-amok in Laos: A psychosocial perspective, *Int. J. Soc. Psychiatry* 9:251.

Westermeyer, J., 1973b, On the epidemicity of amok violence, *Arch. Gen. Psychiatry* 28:873.

Westermeyer, J., 1974, Opium smoking in Laos: A survey of 40 addicts, *Am. J. Psychiatry* 131:165.

Wilkinson, R. J., 1928, "Papers on Malay Subjects," Federated Malay States Government Press, Kuala Lampur.

Zaguirre, J. C., 1957, Amuck, *J. Philipp. Fed. Priv. Med. Pract.* 6:1138.

11

Cargo Cult Syndromes

BURTON G. BURTON-BRADLEY

INTRODUCTION

Crisis cults have been reported from many different countries since Greco-Roman antiquity. They appear under a multitude of different names and guises, such as (1) the Taiping ("Great Peace") Rebellion, whose leader, Hung Hsiu-chuan, had a psychotic episode, claimed to be the younger brother of Jesus Christ, and under the influence of Protestant Missionary tracts tried to set up a new order in China (Yap, 1954); (2) the Kikuyu maumau in Kenya, whose goal was the acquisition of ancestral land (Kenyatta, 1937; Carothers, 1954, 1972); (3) the Ghost Dance of the Plains Indians of North America, who fantasied that a new skin would slide over the earth, covering all the whites and their material appurtenances, and leaving the great buffalo herds to themselves alone (Mooney, 1896; La Barre, 1972); (4) the movement associated with the Mad Mullah of Somaliland (Guillaime, 1956); (5) the prophetic movement of the Xhosa in South Africa in the 1850s, who believed that their ancestors would return with cattle as numerous as the stars in the sky and quantities of milk more abundant than water (Wallis, 1943); and (6) the Vailala Madness, which was characterized by mass hysteria, tremors, and trances associated with a belief in the return of ancestors bearing abundant riches (Williams, 1923, 1934).

Central to all these cults are marked feelings of inferiority, conflict, and anxiety among the members, and an attempt to renovate their self-image. Underlying these nonlogical magicoreligious endeavors (Pareto, 1935) is a strong wish for a resolution of the social, economic, and political problems, and for a new and better way of life like that thought to be present in other cultures. The widespread distribution of this phe-

BURTON G. BURTON-BRADLEY • Honorary Professor of Psychiatry, The University of Papua New Guinea; Clinical Associate Professor of Psychiatry, The University of Hawaii; Mental Health Services, P.O. Box 1239, Boroko, Papua New Guinea.

nomenon, both geographically and historically, lends little support to the Rousseauian view of Bodley (1975) that tribal cultures are well-integrated, self-contained, and satisfying systems.

The crisis cult occurring in Papua New Guinea is known as a cargo cult. It does not occur outside Melanesian countries and is characterized by (1) a two-way person–spirit interrelationship through visual and auditory hallucinations, a trait said to be uncommon to other cults (Brown, 1966); (2) intense individualism, forthrightness, and a great concern with wealth and status among the members, both in their customary display (in the form of symbolic bones, pieces of bamboo, or other insignialike decorations worn around the neck) and in conspicuous consumption; (3) locally devised expressions of prestige (such as the number of pigs or wives one has, the size of one's yams, or one's fertility); (4) the usual confinement of the cult to one language group (among the more than 700) and the occasional spread of the cult via Melanesian pidgin or other *linguae francae* of the area, such as Hiri Motu or Bahasa Indonesian; and (5) the use of the term *cargo*, a word that appeared among public servants, missionaries, and traders around 1935 and signifies wealth (Mair, 1948). From its original restricted meaning of goods, baggage, and other material belongings on ships and aircraft, it has now acquired a broader connotation to include anything of a spiritual or symbolic character that the traditional individual in Papua New Guinea intensely desires and that he believes his ancestors' spirits will convey to him (Mihalic, 1971). High in the priorities of such desired acquisitions is spiritual power, whether it be directed to the fall of rain and the success of food gardens or to the control of people.

In earlier views, cults and movements of these kinds were seen as aberrations, as parallels of mental disorder. Virchow (1849) believed that psychic epidemics are indicative of gross disturbance within a group. Similar views were contained in Le Bon (1879), Martin (1920), MacKay (1932), and Strecker (1940). More modern viewpoints have tended to understand such behavior as purely social in nature, as a collective effort by a large number of people to solve a common problem (Smelser, 1962; Toch, 1965). Yet both views are restricting. It is becoming increasingly apparent, through work of Lipowski (1977) and Wilson (1978), that to achieve a comprehensive understanding of people in groups it is necessary to study them as individuals ceaselessly interacting with their physical, psychological, social, and cultural environments. Group behavior cannot be adequately assessed without reference to all its component parts, including the physical disease processes and mental disorders of individuals.

It is to be noted in passing that (1) crisis cults are not by any means always constructive and can at times become stressors beyond the capacities of vulnerable individuals; (2) persons with already existing mental disorders are often attracted to, rewarded by, and consolidated in prestigious roles within the cargo system, and this perpetuates and elaborates their disturbances; and (3) outside the cult system, mental disorders of many kinds show clear evidence of simplistic cult thinking.

CARGO THINKING

Cargo thinking is endemic in the country, as it is indeed in many other geographical locations in different manifestations, technological cultures not excluded.

In Papua New Guinea cargo thinking does not occur *de novo*. It has the myths related to the return of heroes as precursors. It is widespread in latent form and becomes manifest when group expectancies are intensified—for example, when there is some precipitating factor, or when a leader, prophet, or messiah arises to exploit discontent.

Although there can be much divergence in the overt expression of individual cults, a basic nucleus is common to most of them. Cargo thinking is an anxiety-reducing device. It meets psychological needs, and the style of cult development allows a variety of options, albeit in fantasy form, away from the superimposed alien (i.e., European) economic system. It may occur in an isolated individual or, following interactions with others, find expression in group activity. It is associated with a desire for speedy acquisition of material goods, usually by preternatural means. The cardinal symptom of the initiator is status anxiety. The leader is often a mediocrity as measured by different cultural standards and sometimes by those of his own people as well. The leader is not averse to the use, or threatened use, of sorcery in bringing nonbelievers into line. He may, or may not, be suffering from an overt mental disorder, defined as such not only by the technological culture in contact (heteropathology) but by his own people as well (autopathology) (Ackerknecht, 1943). The fantasy-based solution he offers his followers is initiated by a dream or a hallucination, both powerful agents in effecting conversion. He announces a great future event, or a millennium, and may even supply the specific date for its advent. The people prepare for the anticipated happenings, new moral and legal codes are introduced, often with severe punishments (including death) for transgression, and new and elaborate clothing, a most important status-renovating device, may be adopted. Godowns, airstrips, helipads, or roads are built in preparation for the arrival of ancestral spirits who will bring in the highly prized cargo. Pigs are killed, food gardens neglected, and money destroyed in the belief that they will be unnecessary. The cult subsides with the failure of cargo to arrive, but it may reemerge in virulent form

at a later date in response to some new stimulus. The nonarrival is sometimes attributed to the fraud and deceit of the whites, and sometimes to
a lack of faith and full commitment by some of the followers; in short,
by an *ex post facto* rationalization.

THE LITERATURE

There is a mountain of information on the subject of cargo cults from
the anthropological-sociological point of view, but very little from the
medical and psychological perspective. The former is contained in geographically limited ethnographic studies by Burridge (1960) on the
Tangu of the Bogia region, Maher (1961) on the Tommy Kabu movement
in the Purari delta, Schwartz (1962) on the Paliau movement in Manus
Province, and Lawrence (1964) on Yali of the Rai Coast. General evalua-
tions of these phenomena from a sociological point of view are included
in Wallace (1956), Worsley (1959), Thrupp (1962), Jarvie (1964), Christiansen (1969), Cochrane (1970), and Steinbauer (1971), and cult bibliog-
raphies have been prepared by Leeson (1952) and Worsley (1968). Most
of these authors are primarily interested in group phenomena and social
structure, but it is interesting to note that they have all reported briefly
en passant on compulsive twitchings, shaking fits, trances, hysterias,
bizarre behavior, revolutionary destructiveness, psychological margin-
ality, deprivations in childhood, and auditory and visual hallucinations.
My own interpretations of these phenomena are contained in Burton-
Bradley (1973, 1975).

In her study of these psychological states, Inglis (1957) pointed out
that there is a remarkable similarity among all cults, particularly among
the leaders, who are both exceptional and unusual men and often mentally disturbed. A related viewpoint is supported by De Bruyn (1949) in
his description of the Mansren cargo cults of Biak in the Indonesian
Province of Irian Jaya (West Melanesia).

Kennedy (1893), Abel (1902), and Chinnery and Haddon (1917) gave
a classic description of the mad Prophet of Milne Bay. Kennedy was mag-
istrate in Samarai at the time and described in the Annual Report on British New Guinea a young man named Tokerua who asserted he was in
communication with a spirit who resided in a traditionally sacred tree.
This hallucinatory experience was associated with a dissociative reaction
in which the subject's face was transfigured; following this, he pro-
claimed the advent of a gigantic tidal wave that would engulf the whole
coast. Believers would be saved, he said, if the people heeded his message
to eat their pigs, abandon their food gardens, and build new houses in
the interior.

F. E. Williams (1923, 1934) spent 20 years in fieldwork as the government anthropologist for Papua, and early on he evaluated the significance of psychological factors in cargo cults. His account of the Vailala Madness was the first systematic study of what was eventually to be categorized as cargo cult. He described mass hysteria and psychological contagion, and emphasized the importance of a psychologically dominant leader.

Finally, Mair (1948), Firth (1951), Cohn (1957), and Muhlmann (1961) all stressed the importance of envy and were of the opinion that cultism contains significant psychological phenomena not to be ignored. Stanner (1953) pointed to the prominence of hallucinations in Melanesian cargo cults, where they are much more in evidence than in any other adjustment cults.

DREAMS AND HALLUCINATIONS

Dreams and hallucinations are highly significant events in the life of the nonliterate individual. They are prominent in the precipitation of cargo cults, and a common feature in the symptomatology of those patients among whom cargo thinking is prevalent. The dream or hallucination is said to reflect reality. For example, if one person transgresses a code against another in a dream, it may be mandatory to take payback (vendetta) action in real life according to customary law, and this has led to acts of violence and homicide (Burton-Bradley, 1967).

CULT LEADERS AND THEIR FOLLOWERS

Cult Leaders

It is among the leaders or potential leaders that most pathology is found, although not all leaders are mentally ill. Well-defined diseases have made their appearance among them, including schizophrenia, affective psychosis, paranoia, folie à deux, head injury, thyrotoxic psychosis, chronic syphilitic meningoencephalitis, starvation ketosis, hysteria, epilepsy, and arecaidine intoxication. Physical illnesses and deformities are not uncommon, including obesity, narcolepsy, gonorrhoea, tuberculous spondylitis, chronic dermatitis, and chronic poliomyelitis. The leaders are of three main kinds: the prophet, the messiah, and the practically motivated leader. The prophet is the one who initiates a cult through a dream or a hallucination, the messiah type is believed to have the capacity to bring the cargo millennium to pass, and the practically motivated leader endeavors to guide the cult in a realistic direction. Kwekmarin et al. (1971) gave a very interesting account of the Yangoru cargo cult of that period in which the leader was described as a recluse who locked himself in his house for long periods and whose deputy was involved in frequent fighting and suffered from epilepsy. Some examples follow.

The so-called Lyndon B. Johnson Cult arose on New Hanover Island, in what was then the New Ireland District, in 1964, on the first day of polling for elections to the House of Assembly. Three hundred people took part in a demonstration in which they insisted that they wanted to vote for President Johnson of the United States. One young cult leader had collected a large sum of money to buy Lyndon B. Johnson. Our patient attempted a speech, largely incomprehensible to bystanders, but clearly directed toward promoting the movement. As he delivered his oration, he repeated himself many times, exhibited thought blocking, and worked himself into a frenzy. He was subsequently shown to be suffering from schizophrenia.

A man from Porgera River in the remote Highlands region had been working in unskilled jobs in Port Moresby for some years. He was liked by his employers and considered normal in every way until he suffered two upsetting events. He was knocked down by an automobile and 1 week later was kidnapped and brutally beaten. He suffered head and neck injuries, followed by 6 weeks' hospitalization and 4 months' outpatient treatment. On discharge from the hospital ward, on attempting to cross the street, he pressed the pedestrian button at the main traffic crossing and suddenly felt that power went up his arm. At that point he realized that he possessed power that no one else had, and henceforth he believed that the power in the traffic lights came from him. He directed the traffic by coordinating his directions with the change of the lights from green to red and vice versa, and he continued to do this for a number of years, to the great amusement and approval of everyone. He reinforced his delusional state by dressing in florid and ostentatious clothing, by giving Kung Fu-like performances in an adjacent park (about which he had learned in popular magazines), and by recruiting a deputy to assist him. He believed that his power also prevented accidents and that his actions protected many people from danger. He stated that within 2 years, 10,000 Kina (Papua New Guinea money) would be given to him from a Higher Source. Melanesians enjoyed his performance and were impressed by his charismatic personality, but did not share his beliefs. They assigned to him a *longlong* (insane) status. Nonetheless, he had a proven capacity to recruit a following, which was growing at the time of his enforced repatriation to his own village.

A 25-year-old male from the Northern Province argued with his European manager in Port Moresby over the introduction of a new mode of work. He was fired and attacked his employer, biting him on the buttock. His intent was clear, as another employee had to release the bite by forcing a stick between his teeth. At this stage an ancestral spirit appeared before him and told him to return to his village cemetery. He did this and dug a deep hole there, with the intent of finding a big snake with a skin like a white man to lead him to paradise and solve all problems. In addition, the snake would provide a thousand dollars, an enormous sum in this area. He gathered an enormous following, as the area was well known for its earlier Baigona and Taro cults, but after the digging failed to produce results when 20 feet deep, the followers started to fall away, although he was never at any time without followers. Even later, when confined to a mental (state) hospital, he escaped and walked the 70 kilometers back to his village and resumed the digging. He assassinated a woman who laughed at his endeavors by cutting her five times with an ax. He was arrested, convicted of murder, and referred to a psychiatrist for assessment. Examination showed thought disorder, affective incongruity, and a grandiose delusional state. The history showed that he had dug the hole for 3 years. He was dressed in his brother's army uniform and was wearing a Japanese army steel helmet from the Second World War, pieces of red cloth and feathers, and three pairs of socks. His condition was consistent with paranoid schizophrenia.

An elderly mission catechist from the Madang Province had for decades discussed with a friend the discrepancy between the people's way of life and that of the white expatriates. They came to the conclusion that Christianity was responsible for the wealth and conspicuous abundance of material things and supposedly superior way of life. The catechist, who was also a *luluai* (i.e., a village chief appointed by the government), decided that the way to achieve these things was through emulation of the Christian Passion. His friend agreed, and the catechist arranged the erection of a platform surrounded by an enclosure and called a meeting there to which he invited the bishop and the village people. He addressed them, as well as the sun, the moon, and the stars. He then killed his friend with the latter's cooperation. Later he explained that the spirit of God had come to his friend and told him that he must die, as had Jesus Christ, to ensure a wonderful change in the lives of the people: prosperity and an end to fighting, stealing of pigs, and quarrels over women. This man's beliefs were not held in the same persistent way by his *wantoks* (kinsmen). Yet the friend's cooperation in his own death was consistent with a folie à deux.

A middle-aged epileptic man from the Morobe Province predicted the end of the world. While in a state of preictal irritability, he gave the day, month, and year when this would happen. A *guria* (earthquake), he said, would allow the ancestors to return from below bearing unlimited amounts of goods. For this reason work would be no longer necessary, and children would not have to go to school. Unfortunately, his followers destroyed their money and damaged their property in anticipation of the new era.

Potential Leaders: The Grandiose-Paranoid Reaction

The grandiose-paranoid reaction occurs in the young man generously furnished with cargo cult ideology. It is a reversible condition in which the person concerned usually asserts that he is Jesus Christ, or some other prominent figure, and in the course of so doing informs other people and so is referred for examination. One avowed he had a 20 million-dollar bank account and owned a ship and an airline, which were to assist in the reception of cargo. Another had been appointed by God, he said to lead the country as prime minister to ensure a more rapid cargo from the ancestors. This condition needs careful differentiation from the purely political aspirations of immature youth. Evidence of gross distortion of reality defined as such by the alien medical examiner and the patient's own kinsmen will usually clarify the issue. The reaction is short-lived and is analogous to the persecutory paranoid reaction common in technologically complex cultures. One danger with this class of patient is his recruitment of followers. Should he come in contact with some of the acephalous collective hysterias, two possibilities may ensue. His overdetermined ideas may well become reinforced and consolidated into more permanent delusions and/or he may precipitate a cult.

The Deputies

Deputies more commonly exhibit a personality consistent with sociopathic disorder.

The Followers

In the course of my work, I have examined many cult followers. As far as can be determined, the pattern of mental disorder among them appears to vary little from that of other people in rural areas. The psychological contagion to which they are subjected has, however, led to widespread destructive activities through the exploitation of allegedly rational institutions.

Although some people appear to be more readily susceptible to cult recruitment than others, it is impractical to examine each and every cult follower; the distribution of the beliefs is very widespread and their character is ever changing, often over short periods of time. An individual might go through a whole series of phases and at various times may be procult, anticult, noncult, or a fence-sitter. His viewpoint may be colored by his attitude to his rivals or competitors. If he is jealous of the cult leader in the next village, his response might color his beliefs and he might take an opposing stand. If he is in the same village, he might prefer to remain quiet concerning his own assessment of the facts, as vocalization might lead to sorcery retribution and in some cases to assassination. A man was jumped on and suffered fatal injuries when he cast doubt on and mocked the grandiose delusional beliefs of a village leader in the Southern Highlands in 1974.

VIOLENCE

There have been instances of human sacrifice in the cargo cults. One has been described in this chapter, when a serious attempt was made to speed up the arrival of cargo through the emulation of the Christian Passion. In another instance, a man took a child behind a village house and decapitated him. This made him God, he said, and he would ensure that plenty of cargo in the form of automobiles, houses, food, transistor radios, and other material goods would arrive by ship and aircraft. The evidence obtained from rural informants suggests that the sacrifice pattern might not be all that rare, particularly when we take into account the fact that information on deaths in many rural areas is inevitably secondhand, so that the true incidence of sacrifice is unknown.

Guiart (1951) considered cargo cults to be the forerunners of Melanesian Nationalism. This argument ignored the nonpolitical medicopsychological factors that make up cargo cults. But there are political components, and for this reason brief mention is made of certain cargo analogues associated with violence. Guillaime (1956) gave a detailed account of the Mahdi legend and how its power and vitality among certain groups in North Africa was the result of their feeling that they were members of a body deprived of its rights. He observed that messianism is a widespread phenomenon, and that the British army engaged in warfare against at least two abnormal Mahdis, the Mahdi of the Sudan and the Mad Mullah of Somaliland. The maumau in Kenya has now been explained as a cargo cult activity (Rosensteil, 1953; Nottingham and Rosberg, 1966). Carothers (1954) described the maumau leaders as egocentric psychopaths who used the people for their own ends. MacKenzie (1957) noted that the maumau leader Dedan Kimathi became prey to Caesarism and his grandiosity ended in delusional psychosis. If Guiart is correct in his assessment, and if the cults of Papua New Guinea and elsewhere evolve in the way he has described, then such development poses the threat of sick people occupying crucial roles in society. There have been quite a number of prominent instances of this sort in more recent times, which should alert us all to the danger. Early diagnosis and treatment may play their part in reducing the hazard.

CONCLUSION

Group paranoia signifies those delusional attitudes that are displayed by, or appear to be displayed by, the majority of a given group of people. The crucial factor appears to be the acceptance of paranoid leadership, but not necessarily the presence of paranoid membership in all instances. Hartmann and Stengel (1932) have shown how certain paranoiacs have a specific motivation to establish a following. Those compulsive characters with a high narcissistic need tend to settle conflicts by an appeal to exogenous sources rather than by self-imposed penalties.

Grandiose delusions, cargo thinking in a specifically cargo cult context, and other deficits of a medicopsychological nature characterize the expression of cargo cult syndromes. They could, of course, be classified in accord with generally accepted and standard nosologies. This would be a mistake, in my opinion, for it denies the significance of the cultural factor in diagnosis. To limit ourselves in this way and to ignore the inextricably interwoven character of cultural factors in illness is to restrict our knowledge of human behavior as well as our capacity to help the patient.

REFERENCES

Abel, C. W., 1902, "Savage Life in New Guinea," p. 104, London Missionary Society, London.
Ackerknecht, E. H., 1943, Psychopathology, primitive medicine, and primitive culture, Bull. Inst. Hist. Med. Johns Hopkins Hosp. 14:30.
Bodley, J. H., 1975, "Victims of Progress," Cummings, Menlo Park.
Brown, P., 1966, Social change and social movements, in "New Guinea on the Threshold" (E. K. Fisk, ed.), p. 155, Australian National University Press, Canberra.
Burridge, K. O. L., 1960, "Mambu, A Melanesian Millenium," Methuen, London.
Burton-Bradley, B. G., 1967, "Some Aspects of South Pacific Ethnopsychiatry. With Special Reference to Papua and New Guinea," South Pacific Commission, Noumea.
Burton-Bradley, B. G., 1973, The psychiatry of cargo cult, Med. J. Aust. 2:388.
Burton-Bradley, B. G., 1975, "Stone Age Crisis," Vanderbilt University Press, Nashville.
Carothers, J. C., 1954, "The Psychology of Maumau," Government Printer, Nairobi.
Carothers, J. C., 1972, "The Mind of Africa," Tom Stacey, London.
Chinnery, E. W. P., and Haddon, A. C., 1917, Five new religious cults in British New Guinea, Hibbert J. 15:458.
Christiansen, P., 1969, "The Melanesian Cargo Cult," Akademisk. Forlag, Copenhagen.

Cochrane, G., 1970, "Big Men and Cargo Cults," Clarendon Press, Oxford.

Cohn, N., 1957, "The Pursuit of the Millenium," Secker and Warburg, London.

De Bruyn, J. V., 1949, De mansren cultus de Biakkers, *T. Volkenk* 83:313.

Firth, R., 1951, "Elements of Social Organization," Beacon Press, Boston.

Guiart, J., 1951, Forerunners of Melanesian nationalism, *Oceania* 22:81.

Guillaime, A., 1956, "Islam," 2nd ed. (rev.), Penguin Books, Harmondsworth.

Hartmann, H., and Stengel, E., 1932, Studien zur Psychologie des induzierten Irreseins, *Jahrb. Psychiatr. Neurol.* 48:164

Inglis, J., 1957, Cargo cults: The problem of explanation, *Oceania* 27:149.

Jarvie, I. C., 1964, "The Revolution in Anthropology," Routledge and Kegan Paul, London.

Kennedy, R. J., 1893, *In* "Annual Report on British New Guinea," p. 71, Government Printing Office, Port Moresby.

Kenyatta, J., 1937, Kikuyu religion, ancestor-worship and sacrificial practice, *Africa* 10:308.

Kwekmarin, L., Jamenan, J., and Lea, D., 1971, Yangoru Cargo Cult, *J.P.N.G. Soc.* 5:3.

La Barre, W., 1972, "The Ghost Dance," George Allen and Unwin, London.

Lawrence, P., 1964, "Road Belong Cargo," Melbourne University Press, Melbourne.

Le Bon, G., 1879, "The Crowd: A Study of the Popular Mind," T. F. Unwin, London.

Leeson, I., 1952, "Bibliographie des 'Cargo Cults' et Autres Mouvements Autochthones du Pacifique Sud," South Pacific Commission, Noumea.

Lipowski, Z. J., 1977, Psychosomatic medicine in the seventies, *Am. J. Psychiatry* 134:233.

MacKay, C., 1932, "Memoirs of Extraordinary Popular Delusions," L. C. Page, Boston.

MacKenzie, N., 1957, "Secret Societies," Aldus Books, London.

Maher, R. F., 1961, "New Men of Papua: A Study of Culture Change," University of Wisconsin Press, Madison.

Mair, L. P., 1948, "Australia in New Guinea." Christophers, London.

Martin, E. D., 1920, "The Behavior of Crowds," W. W. Norton, New York.

Mihalic, F., 1971, "The Jacaranda Dictionary and Grammar of Melanesian Pidgin," Jacaranda Press, Brisbane.

Mooney, J., 1896, The ghost dance and the Sioux outbreak of 1890, Bureau of American Ethnology 14th Annual Report, Part 2:641.

Muhlmann, W. E., 1961, "Chialismus und Nativismus," Reimer, Berlin.

Nottingham, J., and Rosberg, C., 1966, "The Myth of the Maumau," Praeger, New York.

Pareto, V., 1935, "The Mind and Society," Harcourt, Brace, New York.

Rosensteil, A., 1953, The anthropological approach to Maumau, *Pol. Sci. Q.* 68:419.

Schwartz, T., 1962, "The Paliau Movement in the Admiralty Islands, 1946–1953," American Museum of Natural History Anthropological Papers, New York.

Smelser, N. J., 1962, "Theory of Collective Behavior," Free Press, New York.

Stanner, W. E. H., 1953, "The South Seas in Transition," Australasian Publishing, Sydney.

Steinbauer, F., 1971, "Melanesische Cargo-Cults," Delp, Munich.

Strecker, E. A., 1940, "Beyond the Clinical Frontiers," W. W. Norton, New York.

Thrupp, S. L., 1962, "Millenial Dreams in Action," Mouton, The Hague.

Toch, H., 1965, "The Social Psychology of Social Movements," Bobbs-Merrill, Indianapolis.

Virchow, R., 1849, "Die Einheitsbestrebungen in der wissenschaftlichen Medizin," Reimer, Berlin.

Wallace, A. F. C., 1956, Revitalisation movements, *Am. Anthropol.* 58:264.

Wallis, W. D., 1943, "Messiahs: Their Role in Civilization," American Council on Public Affairs, Washington, D.C.

Williams, F. E., 1923, "The Vailala Madness and the Destruction of Native Ceremonies," Anthropological Report No. 4, Government Printer, Port Moresby.

Williams, F. E., 1934, The Vailala madness in retrospect, *in* "Essays Presented to C. G. Seligman" (E. E. Evans-Pritchard, ed.), Kegan Paul, London.

Wilson, E. O., 1978, "On Human Nature," Harvard University Press, London.

Worsley, P. M., 1959, Cargo cults, *Sci. Am.* May:117.

Worsley, P. M., 1968, "The Trumpet Shall Sound: A Study of Cargo Cults in Melanesia," 2nd ed., Schocken Books, New York.

Yap, P. M., 1954, The mental illness of Hung Hsiu-chuan, leader of the Taiping Rebellion, *J. Asian Stud.* 13:287.

12

Possession States and Exorcism

E. MANSELL PATTISON

INTRODUCTION

Our Western views of health and illness, cause and effect, reality and fantasy are the products of a construction of reality that is largely determined by the empirical rationalism of experimental science. The Western mode of thought and its explanation of reality have often been the measure against which all other cultural constructions of reality were assessed, while so-called primitive cultures were considered to be irrational, simplistic, and naive.

Yet Western science and its vision of reality are terribly fragmented. The naturalistic system of the world of the West, rooted in the empirical rationalism of latter-day humanism, provides proximate and limited explanations of isolated fragments of human life. Without ontological grounding it may fail to provide a rationale, a purpose, or a meaning to life.

Sartre (1959) states the dilemma of modern Western man succinctly: "The existentialist ... thinks it very distressing that God does not exist, because all possibility of finding values in a heaven of ideas disappears along with him ... everything is permissible if God does not exist, and as a result man is forlorn, because neither within him nor without does he find anything to cling to ... we find no values or commands to turn to which legitimize our conduct. So, in the bright realm of values, we have no excuse behind us, nor justification before us. We are alone, with no excuses" (pp. 22–23).

The psychoanalyst Allen Wheelis (1971) similarly writes: "At the beginning of the modern age science did, indeed, promise certainty. It

---

E. MANSELL PATTISON • Department of Psychiatry, Medical College of Georgia, Augusta, Georgia.

does no longer. Where we now retain the conviction of certainty we do so on our own presumption, while the advancing edge of science warns that absolute truth is a fiction, is a longing of the heart, and not to be had by man . . . our designations of evil are as fallible now as they were ten thousand years ago; we simply are better armed now to act on our fallible vision" (p. 114).

In contrast, so-called primitive views of reality provide a much more coherent, cohesive, and comprehensive model of the world and of human behavior (Levi-Strauss, 1966). For example, in Foster's (1976) comparison of naturalistic versus supernaturalistic systems of thought about health and illness, he finds that Western naturalistic systems view misfortune and illness in atomistic terms. Disease is unrelated to other misfortune; religion and magic are unrelated to illness; and the principal curers lack supernatural or magical powers, for their function is solely technical task performance. On the other hand, supernaturalistic systems integrate the totality of all life events. Illness, religion, and magic are inseparable. The most powerful curers are astute diagnosticians who employ both technical and symbolic means of therapeusis.

Indeed, careful ethnological studies of folk healers reveal a complex and sophisticated description of reality in which there is indeed differentiation between accidents, distortions of natural process such as malformed fetuses, hazards such as snakebites, psychosomatic diseases, and existential disorders of impaired human relations. Similarly, within the supernaturalistic system there exists a range of interventions practiced by a variety of healers with skills suitable to the curing of the misfortune.

POSSESSION*

It is within this supernaturalistic belief system that possession is embedded. The concept of possession by "other forces" is both ancient and widespread. The level of abstraction, however, varies widely through time and culture. At the concrete end of the spectrum, there is a high degree of personification and specification. Thus, one may be possessed by a specific spirit of a specific person or animal, which produces specific behavior in the possessed person. In the middle, there is possession by generalized spirits, ghosts, or supernatural beings, which may in

*The literature on possession is enormous. Early history of religious possession is given by Russell (1979), medieval history by Knox (1950), renaissance history by Thomas (1971), and recent history by Podmore (1963). The classic early review of possession states was written by Oesterreich (1966), followed by extensive anthropological analyses (Mair, 1969; Douglas, 1970; Lewis, 1971; Bourguignon, 1973, 1976; Rush, 1974; Landy, 1977). Empirical field and case studies have been published from a social science perspective (Goodman et al., 1974; Lebra, 1976; Loudon, 1976; Crapanzano and Garrison, 1977; Tiryakian, 1977), while psychiatrically oriented volumes have also appeared (Kiev, 1964; Prince, 1968; Cox, 1973; Yap, 1974).

turn produce specific acts or generalized sets of behaviors. Finally, at the most abstract level, we have possession by thoughts, impulses, memories, or images. One may be possessed by either good objects or bad objects, and possession may produce either socially desirable or undesirable behavior (Lambert et al., 1959). For the most part, however, possession usually involves bad objects that produce undesirable behavior. The panoply of different possession concepts invoked in different cultures is shown in Figure 1.

While belief in demonic possession is widespread, the actual occurrence of possession is limited. The emergence of demonic possession and exorcism is seen in rather particular sociocultural milieux. The eruption of demonology is usually coincident with an oppressive social structure, a loss of trust in the efficacy of social institutions, and a seeming inability to cope with the evils of the social structure. The personification of the social evil is seen in evil demons, and displaced social protest is evidenced in accusations of witchcraft and personal experiences of possession. Being possessed of social evil is personified, while accused, accuser, and exorcist symbolically act out the social dilemma in safely displaced form, avoiding active social protest and attempt at reform. Bourguignon (1973) thus finds that the distribution of demonic possession in folk societies is correlated with conditions of social oppression and stagnation. Wijesinghe et al. (1976) report a high incidence of possession in a low-status subcommunity of Sri Lanka, and Carstairs and Kapur (1976) describe possession in the most oppressed persons of an Indian community.

Sociocultural studies have emphasized the social dynamics that produce demonology (Wilson, 1967; Douglas, 1970; Thomas, 1971). Yet individual psychology must also be taken into account. Freud (1922) states the classic psychological formulation as follows: "The states of possession correspond to our neuroses . . . the demons are bad and reprehensible wishes" (p. 72).

This interpretation, however, reduces demonology solely to individual psychopathology. In contrast, Rosen (1968), a medieval historian, observes: "Witch hunting expresses a dis-ease of society, and is related to a social context. . . . To be sure, some individuals involved in witch trials were mentally and emotionally disordered. Most of those involved were not. In part, their reactions were learned, in part, they conformed because of fear-producing pressures" (pp. 7–8).

The historian Russell (1972) states: "But it will not do to assume that the witches were on the whole mentally ill. They were responding to human needs more universal than those of individual fantasy; universal enough to be described in terms of myth. . . . The phenomenon of witchcraft, whether we are talking about the persecutors or the witches, was the result of fear, expressed in supernatural terms in a society that

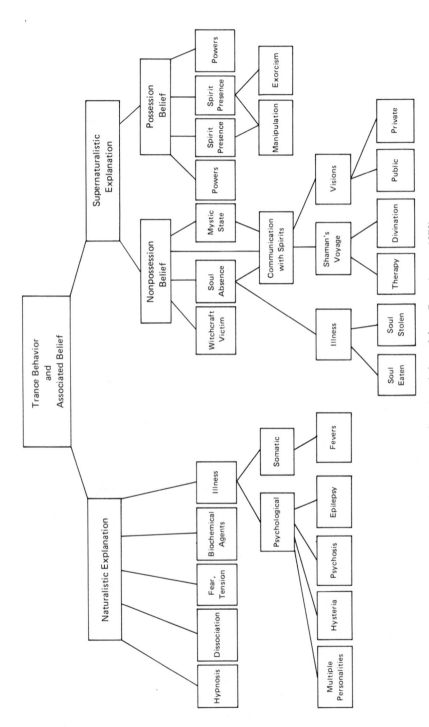

FIGURE 1. Possession explanations (adapted from Bourgignon, 1973).

thought in supernatural terms, and repressed by a society that was intolerant of spiritual dissent. In most respects a variety, or at least an outgrowth, of heresy, witchcraft was one manifestation of alienation . . ." (pp. 273–274). And the anthropologist DeVos (1976) concludes: "We must maintain a clear distinction between the internal structuring of personality related to a concept of adjustment and social-behavioral responses, which can be seen as adaptive or maladaptive for the individual within his social nexus. . . . To understand the interrelationships of social structure, possession behavior, and personality, one must use a dual level of analysis with a structural-functional distinction to delimit and interrelate the concept of adjustment to psychological structure on the one hand, and adaptation to social functioning on the other" (pp. 280–281).

Finally, LeVine (1973) stresses a *psychosocial* interpretation of demonology. He notes that within a culture there will be degrees of potential, for some individuals, to act out demonic possession. When belief in demonic possession is no longer culturally modal, only those with specific psychological propensities are likely to use such beliefs as ego defense.

A CLINICAL CASE STUDY

The foregoing ideas are highlighted in this case, which is an example of possession and exorcism in the changing culture of the Yakima Indians of North America. This case demonstrates the psychosocial nature of demonic possession and therapeusis through a synthesis of Western naturalistic and non-Western supernaturalistic belief systems.

The Yakima are located on several thousand acres of farming and lumbering land in central Washington state, in the rich agricultural Yakima Valley. As on many Indian reservations, these people live in close proximity to white Western culture, but life on the reservation is isolated from the world in which it is located. The reservation culture is in the midst of decay. The "long-hair" Indians cling to the traditional Yakima mores, while their middle-aged children flounder in bewilderment, part of neither the white culture nor the Indian. Meanwhile, the grandchildren attend the local white schools and watch television in the homes of their grandparents.

Mary, an adolescent girl, was brought to the attention of her physician by her family. She was crying, incoherent, and running around the house in a state of panic. The physician reported to me that he found the girl in an agitated state, babbling incoherently about ghosts and her fear of death. He gave her an intramuscular injection of chlorpromazine and this calmed her down and put her to sleep. He made a diagnosis of acute schizophrenic psychosis and requested that the family bring the girl to the U.S. Public Health Clinic for further evaluation and treatment.

When I saw mother and daughter, they were both sullen, guarded, and withdrawn. The girl was a pretty, well-developed 13-year old; she was dressed like a typical high school girl, but she was hunched over, her eyes were downcast, and she spoke in barely audible tones. She stated that her problems had begun the prior August, when she had gone off to a week-long summer camp for Indian girls. One night, after lights were out and the counselors were in bed, Mary and several of her girl friends crept out of their cabin to frolic in the moonlight among the tall fir trees. As they ran about in the moonlight they looked up in the trees and saw human figures. These ghostlike figures drifted down from the trees, and the girls recognized them as their tribal ancestors. The girls talked to the ghosts and the ghosts talked to the girls. After a few minutes, however, the girls became frightened, ran back to their cabin, jumped into their beds, and hid under the covers.

Yet a ghost followed Mary into the cabin. He jumped on her as she lay in bed, and tried to choke her. She fought and struggled against the ghost, gasped for breath, and screamed for help. The counselors came running into the cabin, but they could not calm her. Sobbing and screaming, Mary was sure the ghost would kill her. Finally, the counselors bundled her into a car and drove her to the local hospital, where she was given an intramuscular tranquilizer before being taken home to her parents.

The stage was set, and a routine pattern became established. Mary would go off to high school every day without a care in the world. She would participate in her daily high school activities like any teenager. She was an honor student, a cheerleader, and a student body officer. When she came home, though, a different Mary appeared. She combed her hair into long Indian braids. She put on long-skirted traditional Indian clothes and wandered about the house as if in a daze. She would see ghosts at the window and cry out in fright. She would walk in the fields and often saw blood on the ground. She would think that the ghosts would attack and kill her younger brothers and sisters. Often she could not be calmed down and would be taken to the hospital for an injection. The next morning she would always get up and go to school like a normal adolescent girl.

Mary and her mother had no explanation for this behavior. The mother turned to me and asked what I, as a psychiatrist, thought of this behavior. Was her daughter crazy? I stated that I did not yet know what this all meant, but I encouraged her to share any ideas she might have with me.

The mother said she had heard that psychiatrists did not believe in religion. Did I believe in religion? I told her that I thought religion was very important in the lives of people.

"Look at my face! Do you see any scars?"

"No, I don't."

"Well, my father healed me. Do you believe that?"

"Yes, I do."

"Well, he was a witch doctor; he used to care for the whole tribe. And when I was a girl, I fell in a fire and burned my face. And he made a pack of mud with his spittle, and anointed my face and said his prayers. And said I would be healed and have no scars. He said I would have a beautiful face. Do you think he was right? Is my face beautiful?"

"Yes, I think it is."

"Doctor?"

"Yes?"

"Should I say this? Maybe I shouldn't. I've never talked about this before. My daughter doesn't know about this. I've never told her. Well, you see, my father, the witch doctor, he told me that his powers would be passed on when he died. But not to his children, not to me. His powers would be passed on to his grandchildren. And the oldest, this daughter, this girl, would have his powers."

"Do you think that Mary's experience has something to do with your father?"

"Oh, yes," she answered. "But we don't talk about those things anymore, because, you know, we're Presbyterians now, and people don't believe in witchcraft anymore."

"But what if they did?" I asked. "How would you handle something like this?"

The mother was now animated, and the daughter was listening intently.

"Well, we knew what to do. You see, in the old times, when someone was going to be given the powers of the spirits, was to be given the gifts of the witch doctor, you had to struggle with the spirits. You had to prove you could rule them."

"Well, what would you do?" I asked.

"Oh, there's nothing we can do. If this were the old times, we would just open the door and let Mary wander out of the house at night. And she would go out and meet the spirits. And she would have to fight with them. And then she would come back with the powers . . . or maybe we would just find her out there after a few days, but that's the way it happens. . . ."

"I see. Well, what do you think about this now? Since this is not the old days, what do you think might be the best way to help Mary now?"

"Well, you know, doctor, I've been thinking about that. You can't really practice much as a witch doctor these days. It might be better if Mary were a Presbyterian and didn't accept the gift her grandfather left her."

"Well, how would you work that out?"

"You see, doctor, we have to get rid of the spirits. We have to tell them that Mary doesn't want to fight with them. And then they'll go away and leave her alone. And she'll be okay."

"H'm. Well, what do you have to do?"

"Oh, I don't know how to do that."

"Who does?"

"Oh, Grandma does. She and some of the other old women know the ceremony. We all have to get together, and we have to dress Mary up in the ceremonial dress and we have to say prayers, and offerings, and we have to anoint her, and say the prayers. . . ."

After some time, Mary, her mother, and I reached an agreement that it was not appropriate for Mary to attempt to achieve the mantle of power her grandfather had bequeathed her. That would be looking backward. We agreed, rather, that Mary should renounce the legacy and look forward to becoming part of the modern world. The mother stated that she would call the grandmother and see if she and the other tribal women could conduct a ritual of exorcism that night. I would return in 1 month.

I returned in January. With some trepidation I awaited their arrival. They came early! They were delighted to see me. I was a great doctor. The ceremony of exorcism had been conducted and it had been successful. Mary was healed. Indeed, since that night of exorcism, the strange behavior had disappeared.

I had the opportunity to follow this family for many months thereafter. Mary remained healthy and happy. In contrast to her mien that first cold, snowy December morning, she was thereafter bright and bouncy, talkative and enthusiastic, like any other energetic adolescent girl beginning to become a woman.*

---

*I am reminded of the Old Testament story in which Jacob wrestles with the angel of the Lord, in order to obtain power over the spirits: "And Jacob was left alone; and there wrestled a man with him until the breaking of the day. And when he saw that he prevailed not against him he touched the hollow of his thigh; and the hollow of Jacob's thigh was out of joint, as he wrestled with him. And he said, Let me go, for the day breaketh. And he said, I will not let thee go, except thou bless me. And he said unto him, What is thy name? And he said, Jacob. And he said, Thy name shall be called no more Jacob, but Israel: for as a prince hast thou power with God and men, and hast prevailed. . . . And Jacob called the name of the place Peniel: for I have seen God face to face, and my life is preserved . . . and he halted upon his thigh" (Gen. 32:24–310). What is remarkable is that over a span of perhaps 6,000 years and over many continents, this story resembles Mary's: One gains power over spirits by fighting with them, and if he or she wins, the person then has special powers and can command the spirits. The person is a shaman, a healer, a witch doctor. It is dangerous, though, for to acquire special powers requires potentially mortal combat.

DISCUSSION

Although we have limited clinical material, we may speculate on some of the psychodynamics of this family. Mary's mother presented herself as the favored daughter of her father. Father had healed her, she said, using his spittle (semen?). Mother framed her acceptability as a person around her external appearance, her beauty and sexuality. She asked for acceptance as a desirable woman from the therapist (father). Mary, a maturing adolescent, was viewed as a threat and a competitor. Mary, intuiting her mother's feelings, projected the disapproving mother into the hallucinatory ghost object who would kill her. However, the projected and forbidden object was also the father figure who lay upon her in bed—the incestuous father. Mary wandered in the field and found blood on the ground (menstrual blood?). The competitive rivalry between mother and daughter was projected into Mary's fear that her siblings would be killed by the spirits.

The conflict was resolved when the therapist reaffirmed mother's attractiveness. She, in turn, in concert with her own mother, participated in a symbolic ritual that gave Mary the sanction and approval to mature, grow, and become a sexually mature woman.

These speculations, although they may be appropriate and accurate, do not, however, completely account for the conflict that Mary and her mother experienced. We should look at this possession state not only from a Western psychodynamic perspective but also from a psychosocial point of view. Mary's family, I believe, was caught in a cultural bind. If the family had been living within the traditional Indian culture, it would have followed a prescribed pattern of response, and it is likely that her deviant behavior would have been speedily resolved. The family, though, was torn between two cultures and belief systems and was consequently immobilized. Mary's behavior was congruent with the belief system of an old culture, which was in conflict with the new belief system represented by doctors and hospitals.

Mary's dilemma was not just one of growing up but also one of growing up with a competing belief system. I think that I was able to help her resolve her conflict by assisting in finding a bridge between the Western and non-Western belief systems. I accepted the traditional Indian values in which the family was embedded and of which they were not entirely aware. I did not attempt to translate the problem from one belief system to another. Rather, I supported an intervention within the system, and ensured that the healing would take place through the symbolic modes of the indigenous culture.

In summary, demonic possession is highly correlated with social oppression or stagnation; it expresses both individual and social unrest.

Belief in demonic possession is embedded in a rich and cohesive super-naturalistic belief system, and treating a case of demonic possession requires an understanding of the specific cultural construction of reality.

REFERENCES

Bourguignon, E. (ed.), 1973, "Religion, Altered States of Consciousness, and Social Change," Ohio State University Press, Columbus.

Bourguignon, E., 1976, "Possession," Chandler & Sharp, San Francisco.

Carstairs, G. M., and Kapur, R. L., 1976, "The Great Universe of Kota. Stress, Change and Mental Disorder in an Indian Village," University of California Press, Berkeley.

Cox, R. H. (ed.), 1973, "Religious Systems and Psychotherapy," Charles C Thomas, Springfield, Ill.

Crapanzano, V., and Garrison, V., 1977, "Case Studies in Spirit Possession," Wiley, New York.

DeVos, G. A., 1976, The interrelationship of social and psychological structure in transcultural psychiatry, in "Culture-Bound Syndromes, Ethnopsychiatry, and Alternate Therapies" (W. P. Lebra, ed.), pp. 278–298, University of Hawaii Press, Honolulu.

Douglas, M. (ed.), 1970, "Witchcraft Confessions and Accusations," Tavistock, London.

Foster, G. M., 1976, Disease etiologies in non-western medical systems, Am. Anthropologist 78:773.

Freud, S., 1922, A seventeenth-century demonological neurosis, in "Collected Works" (1961), Hogarth Press, London.

Goodman, F., Henney, J. H., and Pressel, E., 1974, "Trance, Healing, and Hallucination: Three Field Studies in Religious Experience," Wiley, New York.

Kiev, A. (ed.), 1964, "Magic, Faith and Healing," Free Press, New York.

Knox, R. A., 1950, "Enthusiasm: A Chapter in the History of Religion," Oxford University Press, London.

Lambert, W., Triandes, L., and Wolf, M., 1959, Some correlates of beliefs in the malevolence and benevolence of supernatural beings: A cross-cultural study, J. Abnorm. and Soc. Psychol. 58:162.

Landy, D., 1977, "Culture, Disease, and Healing: Studies in Medical Anthropology," Macmillan, New York.

Lebra, W. P. (ed.), 1976, "Culture-Bound Syndromes, Ethnopsychiatry, and Alternate Therapies," University of Hawaii Press, Honolulu.

LeVine, R. A., 1973, "Culture, Behavior, and Personality," Aldine, Chicago.

Levi-Strauss, C., 1966, "The Savage Mind," University of Chicago Press, Chicago.

Lewis, I. M., 1971, "Ecstatic Religion: An Anthropological Study of Spirit Possession and Shamanism," Penguin Books, New York.

Loudon, J. B. (ed.), 1976, "Social Anthropology and Medicine," Academic Press, New York.

Mair, L., 1969, "Witchcraft," McGraw-Hill, New York.

Oesterreich, T. K., 1966, "Possession: Demoniacal and Other Among Primitive Races in Antiquity, the Middle Ages, and Modern Times," New York University Press, New York.

Podmore, F., 1963, "From Mesmer to Christian Science," University Books, Hyde Park, N.Y.

Prince, R. (ed.), 1968, "Trance and Possession States," R. M. Bucke Society, Montreal.

Rosen, G., 1968, "Madness in Society. Chapters in the Historical Sociology of Mental Illness," University of Chicago Press, Chicago.

Rush, J. A., 1974, "Witchcraft and Sorcery: An Anthropological Perspective on the Occult," Charles C Thomas, Springfield, Ill.

Russell, J. B., 1972, "Witchcraft in the Middle Ages," Cornell University Press, Ithaca.

Russell, J. B., 1979, "The Devil: Perceptions of Evil from Antiquity to Primitive Christianity," Meridian Press, Bergenfield, N.J.

Sartre, J. P., 1959, "Existentialism and Human Emotions," Philosophical Library, New York.

Thomas, K., 1971, "Religion and the Decline of Magic: Studies in Popular Beliefs in Sixteenth and Seventeenth Century England," Weidenfield & Nicolson, London.

Tiryakian, E. A. (ed.), 1977, "On the Margin of the Visible: Sociology, the Esoteric, and the Occult," Wiley, New York.

Wheelis, A., 1971, "The End of the Modern Age," Basic Books, New York.

Wijesinghe, C. P., Dissanayake, S. A. W., and Mendis, N., 1976, Possession in a semi-urban community in Sri Lanka, Aust. N.Z. J. Psychiatry 10:135.

Wilson, P. J., 1967, Status ambiguity and spirit possession, Man 2:366.

Yap, P. M., 1974, "Comparative Psychiatry," University of Toronto Press, Toronto.

13

The So-Called Hystero-Psychoses

Latah, Windigo, and Pibloktoq

CLAUDE T. H. FRIEDMANN

INTRODUCTION

In this chapter, three unusual syndromes are discussed—latah, windigo and pibloktoq, plus a number of others believed to be related to them. These intriguing syndromes have a number of things in common. First, of course, they have curious and strange names, made even more exciting by the addition of such exotic appellations as "the Jumping Frenchmen of Maine," "miryachit," "olonism," "imu," "misala," and "Arctic hysteria." Second, they are found in diverse and interesting regions: Our discussion will take us from the steaming jungles of Malaysia to the coldest reaches of the Arctic Circle, and include other locales such as New England, Nyasaland, Japan, and Siberia. These travels will bring us into contact with an unusual array of peoples, including such groups as the Ojibwa Indian, the Eskimo, the Malay, and the Tungu. Third, the syndromes are all dying out, and their literature is becoming old. Many of the writers are gone, several were renowned scholars, many were great adventurers. Through their eyes, cross-cultural psychiatry, anthropology, and exploration were merged.

Many fascinating questions are raised and explanations offered as to the nature and meaning of these syndromes. Are the syndromes linked? Do they represent "primitive" psychoses? Are they really "hysterias," as is the common consensus, and, if so, do they represent different manifestations of the same illness? To what extent are they culturally deter-

---

CLAUDE T. H. FRIEDMANN • Department of Psychiatry, University of California at Irvine College of Medicine, Orange, California.

mined? Or are they a product of geography, race, or religion? Are there genetic roots? Psychodynamic roots? Experiential roots? And why are they, after all, no longer so prevalent on the world map? These and many other questions come to mind as one delves into the so-called hystero-psychoses.

WINDIGO (WIHTIGO, WHITICO, WIHTIKO)

Description and Setting

The winter in the sub-Arctic of North America is cold, white, and long. The Ojibwa male hunted alone. His territory was large, but game was always in short supply. He would see no one, save perhaps his wife and children, for months on end. His entire life had been a rigorous training for individuality, self-reliance, and survival (Landes, 1938). He practiced starvation, communed with spirits, and eschewed affection. Only in the brief summertime would he mingle with other families, there to confront rivals, compete with the other men, and become suspicious. Indeed, hostility and paranoia were said to be culturally bred into the Ojibwa male, along with grandiosity and competition. If one did well in the hunt, one was by definition in touch with powerful spirits. If one did poorly, one's rival had hexed the hunt. The more powerful one was, the more the community feared and distrusted him. The man who was too powerful was eventually killed. It was a paradox—and a cultural trap. Unless one refused to hunt, compete, commune with spirits, etc., one's success automatically became one's undoing.

It is against this bleak, frozen background that the phantom of the windigo arose like a giant iceberg, cannibalizing all in sight. The windigo was the embodiment of all who starved to death (Meth, 1974). A giant snowman, a skeleton of ice, it was an insatiable monster. The man possessed by the windigo could only obey its orders. Possession by the spirit was complete. Murder and death were the results—unless the possessed man were a shaman who himself had supernatural strength and powers. Then the result might be less bloody, but generally more prolonged.

The windigo became manifest when the Ojibwa had bad hunting (Landes, 1938; Parker, 1960). He assumed that a shaman with whom he quarreled during the summer was the cause of his bad luck. He became acutely depressed (Landes, 1938); manifestations included sleeplessness, withdrawal, and anorexia. When lucid, he felt sad, but in the main he was out of touch with reality. He had the delusion that his wife and children were game animals, juicy and tender. After a while he ceased to brood and became violent, murdering and cannibalizing. The idea was fixed and obsessional. He must kill, eat, and kill again. He was a danger to all and eventually he would be killed. Since all windigos die or become weak over the summer when ice and snow melt, the possessed man was most likely to perish then—if he had not been killed sooner. In rare cases, the community might try to cure the person over the summer, rather than execute him. If lucky, the windigo was aborted during the melancholic early phase by an alert wife or child. Death could also occur by suicide.

More atypical windigo occurred without the classic depressed phase, and with less acute violence. The outcome, eventually, was the same, however. When the windigo attacked a shaman, though, the situation was remarkably different, because shamans had the power to fight back. If he could defeat his enemy, usually another shaman, he might survive. Generally, the result, as with a "commoner," was terminal, but the illness was much less acute and might last for years and years. The onset was the same: poor hunting leading to melancholia. However, cannibalism did not ensue. Rather, it was aggression against his rival—or, where possible, direct combat with the spirit itself.

Occasionally, women contracted windigo (Hallowell, 1934; Landes, 1938). Those who did were generally raised in the traditions of male children, or in other ways were forced into male roles. Clearly this was an affliction mainly of men.

In addition to the Ojibwa, windigo occurred among the eastern Cree (Saindon, 1933; Cooper, 1933), located in northern Ontario, and the Berens River Salteaux of Ontario and Manitoba (Hallowell, 1934; Lehmann, 1975).

Cooper (1934) stated that windigo psychosis was rare among the eastern Cree. When it occurred, it was, he felt, the result of a conflict between the strict tribal taboo against cannibalism and the need to eat human flesh during periods of extreme starvation. The cases among the Salteaux described by Hallowell were generally mild. He postulated an extreme "anxiety state" as the cause. Psychophysiologic manifestations (nausea, vomiting, and anorexia) were generally present, and crying and weeping were also reported. The Salteaux, like the Ojibwa, had a cultural fear of cannibalism. When the physical symptoms did not abate, the victim fancied himself/herself a "windigo." The entire village became aware and watched the victim day and night. If not cured, the person was put to death. Actual homicide, then, among the Salteaux was rare.

Etiology and Classification

Regardless of the tribe, those who became windigos were believers in a mythology and folklore of ancient peoples. They believed in magic, ghosts, spirits, and witchcraft. Prior to onset, they suffered from severe sensory deprivation, privation, starvation, and isolation. They became severely depressed. Then they became psychotic, delusional, murderous, and cannibalistic, or, in the case of the shaman, obsessed with a war against one's enemies. Yap (1952) believes windigo to be a form of hysteria—hysteric possession and dissociation—in a peculiar cultural setting. However, unlike most hysteria, men—not women—were the victims. As the tribes involved have become Westernized, acculturated, and "civilized," the affliction has all but vanished (Lehmann, 1975). Futhermore, neighboring tribes and groups (i.e., Eskimos) never manifested windigo. These facts reinforce Landes's and Parker's notion that culture must play a major etiologic role in this affliction. The severe environment, of course, is also a crucial etiologic factor.

We must conclude that the windigo psychosis is a rare, culturebound syndrome that, although it shares features of hysteria, psychotic depression, and sensory deprivation syndrome, cannot be easily classified in Western psychiatric terms.

PIBLOKTOQ (PIBLOKTO)

Description and Setting

We now look further north, to Greenland, and the Eskimo. Like their more southern counterparts, the Eskimo live in a harsh land, frozen and bleak. But there are several differences between the Eskimo and the Ojibwa. Geographically, the Eskimo live by the ocean, and their life is dominated by the sea. It is not the friendliest of oceans, but game is more plentiful. Land and territoriality are less obviously "staked out" for hunting; the domain is instead largely sea and ice. In addition, the Eskimo culture is quite social and communal, not competitive and isolative, as is the Ojibwa's. Nature, in a sense as much the Eskimo's enemy as the Ojibwa's, seems nonetheless somewhat tempered by the ocean. According to Freuchen (1965), the Eskimo love company, are at home with friends and relatives, and do not quest for power and status in any real sense of the word. Eskimo society, prior to European enculturation, was very communal, with a strict division of labor between the men and the women. Communication with spirits and the use of *angakoks* (faith healers) were part of the culture. The *angakok* would use trance states in healing; communal ceremonies incorporated them, and individuals might go into a trance at any time, become hysterical, then emerge with a "revelation." The belief was that the trance state was sacred and brought one in touch with spirits (Freuchen, 1965). Those in the trance were "respected," not ill. The long, dark polar nights of winter were full of evil spirits, apparently, whereas the summers were more benign. (Note: The windigo also died in the summer.)

Perhaps no single point about the Polar Eskimo better illustrates the combination of the spiritual and communal as the act of naming a child. The Eskimo believe in a type of reincarnation, and children are named for deceased ancestors in such a way as to continue a long chain of historical and genetic linkage (Freuchen, 1965).

In short, whereas the Ojibwa and Eskimo share much in common (harsh climate, long winter nights, constant fight for survival, animism, etc.), the culture, especially as it affects the males, is very different. The Ojibwa male meets his spirits alone, the Eskimo usually in the company of many. The Ojibwa learns to be a loner, to compete, and to be suspicious of others. The Eskimo shares most everything—including sexual partners. Perhaps for that reason, windigo does not exist among the Eskimo.

Pibloktoq, however, has been described among the Eskimo by several authors (Lehmann, 1975; Brill, 1913; Achranecht, 1948). Considered by Brill as "primitive hysteria," it is not unique to the Eskimo but, apparently, more prevalent in that society than most others. In any event, it is thought by some to have much in common with such states as latah. Most commonly occurring in the long Arctic night of fall or winter, and thought by Brill to be precipitated by a loss of a loved one, lack of love, or some sexual difficulties, pibloktoq is an acute reaction resembling a dissociative state. The Eskimo consider it to be caused by spirits and thus do not interfere with its course. Virtually all cases are said to occur in females, last 1 to 2 hours, and end in a crying spell and/or sleep. During the attacks, the patient appears to be in an altered state of consciousness and usually does not recall the episode. Brill, however, discussed one patient who appeared at least partially aware during an attack when a photographer was present, and who chided the person after she recovered. In any event, recovery is usually very quick and complete.

Classically, a woman will start to sing or sway rhythmically, then tear her clothes off and run into the snow. She may imitate birds or animals, beat her breasts, clap her hands, throw objects, jump into the icy water, or scream. Finally, she will collapse, weep profoundly, and fall asleep. She will awaken with a clear mind and resume her normal activities. One case described to Brill by MacMillan was suggestive of epilepsy: The woman foamed at the mouth, struck people, and became bloodshot and congested. This does not seem to be the general rule, however.

Freuchen, in a case not previously described in the medical literature, presented pibloktoq in an entirely different sense: a case of a male suicide. Since Freuchen married an Eskimo and lived among them for a long time, his use of the word casts some doubt upon our supposed understanding of the syndrome. Indeed, much of what has been described so far seems to be seen by the Eskimo as benign, normal, and a representation of spirit activity—not as psychopathology. Indeed, the Eskimo in no way cast out the possessed person or considered him insane. Rather, the Eskimo avoided the possessed person until the spirit left.

Freuchen's case (1965, p. 182) is as follows: "Miuk . . . suddenly got the feeling the pibloktoq was to come over him. . . . He began to chant louder and louder, and nobody dared to come near him . . . it would be dangerous to touch Miuk. For the spirits who want revenge do not consider whom they punish. . . . But in a short time he became quite violent and began to shout. . . . Then he struck [a] knife into his wrist so that the blood sprayed out. But Miuk laughed and carried the knife up along his arm, ripping up the skin . . . up to the shoulder and across the chest . . . down the right arm . . . to the wrist. . . . He collapsed on the floor. . . . Soon he got back his thoughts, [and] said that he didn't know what moved him to use the knife. . . . When he had said this, his voice left him, and in another moment he was dead."

Freuchen made no attempt to ascribe psychodynamic or medical meaning to the behavior, nor did he give us any clue as to any antecedent event. He treated this case rather casually, as though it were one of many and as though the spirits were the cause. Unfortunately, he described only this one case in his book. Nonetheless, it is clear that the word *pibloktoq* to the Eskimo is a state brought on by spirits acting at times indiscriminately ("it came upon him"), and clearly not always benign. The result can be death. The victim can be male. The victim need not strip or run in the snow. The reaction is acute, and the mind clears quickly.

Etiology and Classification

Brill saw the cause of pibloktoq, in general, as sexual (love) difficulties resulting in acute hysterical reactions. Whitney, as stated by Czaplicka (1914), ascribed the etiology to the dark, gloomy, silent Arctic night. Yap (1952) preferred to think of pibloktoq as one of several "instinctive" responses to acute fright or stress that "primitive" peoples manifest. He felt that trancelike states of immobility (Van Loon, 1927), a pibloktoq-like fright reaction of the Cree Indians (Cooper, 1934), and an amok-like syndrome among the Samoyedes and Yakutz (Czaplicka, 1914) were similar to pibloktoq and may represent a biological reaction to fear or upset. Although Brill finally concluded that pibloktoq was truly hysteria, because it occurs mainly in women and involves relationship prob-

lems with sexual overtones, Yap (1952) seemed to prefer a simpler explanation—primitive dissociation secondary to fright or upset, but not true
"hysteria." It seems that pibloktoq is truly an acute psychotic reaction of
some sort, probably with multiple causes such as epilepsy, fear, anxiety,
depression, and anger. In that sense, then, it is similar to windigo, and
to latah and other unusual phenomena. It is also similar to these other
syndromes in that it is dying out. Lehmann reports seeing only one case.
There are no recent cases in the literature.

LATAH

Description and Setting

A number of afflictions that seem to be the same as—or similar to—
latah, exist in Siberia and carry the appellation "Arctic hysteria" (Novakovsky, 1924). More specifically, some of the many names used are "amu-
rakh" among the Yakuts, "olan" among the Tungus, "irkunii" among the
Yakughirs, "menkeiti" among the Koryaks, and "ikoto" among the
Samoyedes. The Russian word for this syndrome, encompassing the
above tribal variants, is *miryachit* (Hammond, 1824). Shirokogoroff (1935)
and Czaplicka (1914), however, used the term *olonism* to describe the
latah-like phenomena among Siberian tribes. They felt that *Arctic hysteria*
was too global a term, which covered more than the "imitative mania"
that they wished to encompass. As Yap has pointed out, *olonism* is
derived from a Tungus word. It means "to be suddenly frightened," and
it also means "doing something stupid and useless because of sudden
fear."

In addition to Siberia, latah has been reported in Japan, Maine, Lap-
land, the Philippines, Mongolia, and Thailand. Moreover, cases of similar syndromes have been reported from India, Africa (Repond, 1940;
O'Brien, 1883a; Aberle, 1952), and Tierra del Fuego (Meth, 1974), and
some Eurasian and non-Siberian Russian (Ellis, 1897; Czaplicka, 1914)
cases have also been noted. Although latah is indeed extraordinary,
unusual, and rare, its distribution is quite wide. The Mongols call it
"belenci" (Aberle, 1952), and among the Ainus of northern Japan it is
known as "imu" (Uchimura, 1935; Winiarz & Wielawski, 1936). Some of
the other names include "mali-mali" (Philippines), "yaun" (Burma), and
"bah-tsi" (Thailand) (Yap, 1952; Chapel, 1970).

In addition, a latah-like syndrome was reported from Maine. The so-
called Jumping Frenchmen of Maine, although not French at all and not
just from Maine, were 18th- and 19th-century Shakers who lived in New
England, Appalachia, and Canada (Beard, 1880; Yandell, 1881; Yap, 1952).
A religious sect, they used a collective hysteria as part of their religious

ceremonies. Also known as Holy Rollers, they would on command, at times even by the thousands, jump, roll, jerk, run, and/or bark like dogs on all fours, until exhausted (Yandell, 1881). Occasionally, members developed a latah-like syndrome whereby, as Beard described, a sudden noise, a laugh, or a command would cause an individual to laugh uncontrollably or roll on the ground or mumble religious phrases. A pointed finger might be enough to start the rolling. Beard noted that a door slamming or an animal howling would result in such a reaction. If ordered, they would jump in the air (hence the term *Jumping Frenchmen of Maine*) or strike one another or jump into water or fire. If startled while carrying a weapon, they were apparently quite dangerous. Young children could be affected and men were more often affected than women. Tickling and ceremonial trances were thought to be preludes to the syndrome.

Among the symptoms of Arctic hysteria, Novakovsky (1924) noted: "(1) Fit, (2) Unconscious state, (3) Impressionableness, (4) Unintentional visual suggestion, (5) Mania of imitation by an inclination to repeat all visual and auditory impressions, all gestures, and words and sometimes even those of an unknown language, (6) Susceptibility to hypnotic suggestion, (7) Clairvoyance, (8) Susceptibility to fight, (9) Feeling fright and timidity, (10) Monotonous, mournful improvisation, (11) Singing while asleep, (12) Spasms, (13) Epileptoid seizures, (14) Melancholy, (15) Inclination to suicide, (16) Sometimes, cramps of the vagina, (17) Often, utterances of erotic expression." Many of these will be noted in the descriptions below of latah itself.

Aberle (1952), in his study of Mongolians, discussed several cases of latah. One was that of a Khalkha who, it was said, became "belenci" because of being constantly tickled. If startled, he could be induced to imitate a person writing by writing on his skin with a lighted cigarette. If someone pretended to drink, he would imbibe until he vomited. Once he imitated a jumping horse until the horse had to be held by friends. When alarmed, he would recite obscenities about male genitals.

Another case was that of a Chakar woman who, when startled once by a frog, fainted, and from then on was phobic about frogs. If she saw one, or if a person croaked like a frog in her presence, she might be induced to disrobe, or be echopraxic or echolalic. Another woman became belenci secondary to falling on her husband's dead body. In all these cases, the people seemed normal between episodes but were constantly susceptible to a new reaction. In addition, some Mongols' response to being startled was coprolalia, but without any echolalia or echopraxia. One such was a Chakar woman who shouted "cunt" whenever alarmed. Occasionally, a victim would be dangerous, for there were some who, when startled by a phobic object, would attack it (or its would-be surrogate), i.e., attack a piece of yarn said to be a mouse. In

Mongolia—indeed, in all latah-prone groups but the Manchus and Shakers—affected women outnumber affected men. The onset is from late
adolescence onward. Among the Mongols, belenci is a source of amusement and not considered an illness to be cured. Among the Mongols, it
is not considered spirit possession, but among Siberian tribes it may be
considered as such.

Imu (Winiarz and Wielawski, 1936; Uchimura, 1935; Yap, 1952)
mainly affects older women, as does latah. It occurs among the Ainus, a
tribe that was an early inhabitant of Japan. Occasionally, Japanese raised
in Ainu homes might be affected, too. The Ainus have a cultural fear of
snakes, and imu is often an apparent result of a frightening experience
with a serpent. Imu literally means "possessed" (Yap, 1952). Once imu
starts, it is irreversible and may become worse over time. The person
becomes timid, may at times be aggressive or run when startled, and may
show echoing and automatic obedience (Yap, 1952). Like belenci, it
becomes monotonized and stereotyped, may result in a fit, and may have
accompanying loss of consciousness.

As for latah proper, Yap (1952) provides several classic examples
from among the Malay. Like imu, it may also occur in other Malaysian
ethnic groups with close proximity to a Malay household, and like imu
its incidence is much higher in the primary groups. It occurs predominantly in females—usually in middle to old age. It is often a community
entertainment. It is not considered by the Malay to be mental illness.
Those affected tend to be of limited intelligence and education and are
often of lower social caste and possess a passive disposition. Here are two
of Yap's illustrative cases.

"A *nonya*, aged 60. . . . Her symptoms had been noticeable 15 years
previously; during the Japanese occupation two of her four children had
died within a few days of each other and her illness was said to have
taken a more severe turn then. For the previous two years she had ceased
to go out (because of) fear of cars. . . . When asked her age, she . . . made
a play of figures—'50, 60, 70 . . .'—giggling all the while. When touched
unawares, she would . . . accelerate and raise the pitch of whatever she
[was] saying . . . or (show) definite echolalia. . . . Her word play normally
turned round a word or phrase . . . meaningful to the situation; e.g.,
when suddenly touched on the arm, she exclaimed ' . . . I'm done for,
done for, eh, done for, so indeed.'. . ."

"A Malay woman, aged 50. . . . She had been latah for more than 20
years, but the onset was not related to any special occurrence. . . . She was
. . . dull and stupid. . . . She was incapable of sustaining conversation and
showed no spontaneous speech. The remarkable feature was that she

needed no stimulation to show the symptoms. It was a case of being per-
manently in the latah state. All that was necessary was in an ordinary
way to engage her attention. . . . When asked in English, 'Do you speak
English?' She at first said 'No' and then echoed . . . the question, which
she could not have fully understood. . . . When I thrust a cigarette at her,
she said 'Kotek, Nonok' [male and female organs]. . . . When I handed
her my hat she put it on, made a half-salute, spoke . . . in imitation of
English [and] took it off. . . . Sometimes negativism would appear as, e.g.,
when asked to allow her pulse to be felt, she would at once hold out her
wrist and then withdraw it again. Echopraxia she showed perfectly. . . .
She would [throw a match-box] back at once. . . . When I put out my
tongue, she did the same, but shot it in and out, as though to tease and
insult. . . . Her husband [said] if the session were prolonged, she would
. . . use a knife on someone [if ordered] . . . and become very exhausted
and faint. . . . [Once she was frightened by a pedicab] and had to be carried home in a coma."

   Other illustrative cases include those of Murphy (1973) and O'Brien
(1883a, 1883b): Murphy paraphrases Clifford (1898): A cook saw a pot fall
over and a boy made a try to save it. The cook, being latah, imitated the
boy and went into the fire, grasping the scalding metal. The boy, being
a brat, continued to pretend to grab the pot, and the cook kept putting
his hand into the fire. The result was a very severe burn. The case of
O'Brien is even more chilling: A latah seaman, holding a baby, is induced
by others, through mimicry, to toss the child up into the air. His tormen-
tor eventually lets a stick of wood fall on the ground and the latah lets
the baby fall to its death.
   The literature is replete with other cases. They range from mild
coprolalia without mimicry to mimicry without coprolalia to both
together; from being induced to dance to being prompted to disrobe or
fight or attack; from the "village clown" to the tragedies discussed above.
But, in all cases, according to Malay tradition, the latah is thought to be
"possessed," but not insane; eccentric and enjoyable, but not mad. (For
classical descriptions, see Yap, 1952; Clifford, 1898; O'Brien, 1883a, 1883b;
Ellis, 1897; Logan, 1849; Swettenham, 1896; Abraham, 1911, 1912.)
   In summary, the symptoms of latah and the latah-like syndromes
include (1) usually sudden onset after an acute fright, but sometimes
insidious onset with no apparent cause; (2) variability of symptoms,
depending on the culture and the individual; (3) several common features: echopraxia, echolalia, and coprolalia, which may occur simultaneously or separately in the same individual, or in part only in some
individuals; (4) episodic nature; (5) episodes induced by teasing, tickling,
or startling the victim; (6) episodes generally accepted by the culture as

a "state" rather than a disease; (7) episodes generally entertaining to the community; (8) episodes generally occurring in poorly educated and lower-class people within a given culture; (9) episodes occasionally, but not usually, resulting in violent behavior; and (10) episodes of variable course, but often tending to chronicity and worsening with age. In addition, the patient, though unable to resist the latah phenomenon, is aware of it and may protest being forced to do things, while simultaneously performing the action. Memory for the episode is variable, but usually present.

Etiology and Classification

In Malay, *latah* means "ticklish" or "love madness" (Chiu *et al.*, 1972). Being tickled in the woods was thought to be causal to the "Jumping Frenchmen" and belenci. Other folk beliefs as to causes include possession, dreams, and severe fright. Western writers have ranged in their conclusions regarding the nosology of this entity. Some, like Pfeiffer (1968) and Ullman and Krasner (1969), consider latah to be a unique culture-bound phenomenon. Opler (1967) and Rosenthal (1970) propose that it is a manifestation of schizophrenia. Kline (1963), Uchimura (1935), Kraepelin (1909), Bleuler (1936), Van Loon (1927), and others have considered latah as a "primitive hysteria." Indeed, the term *Arctic hysteria* used by so many authors supports this appellation even further—albeit informally. Other support for hysteria as the proper diagnostic classification comes from the prevalence of spirit-possession as a considered cause by many of the natives involved, as well as the apparent altered state of consciousness common to many of its victims; the episodic nature of the disease; the fact that an entire army once had mass latah among the Mongols (Yap, 1951) (i.e., mass hysteria); and the fact that women predominate as victims and sexual acts (i.e., disrobing) and coprolalia are so prevalent. Other possibilities include epilepsy (Novakovsky, 1924), genetics (Ellis, 1897), climate and sensory deprivation (Novakovsky, 1924), European encroachment with subsequent cultural and personal conflicts and stress (Murphy, 1973), the prevalence of the trance in ceremony, ritual, and child play in many of the latah-prone cultures (Murphy, 1973; Lehmann, 1975), and social reenforcement (Chapel, 1970).

Yap (1952), after reviewing the above possibilities, concluded that none was valid. He felt that hysteria required secondary gain and latah had none. (I suspect he did not consider the attention brought to the victim by teasing villagers as secondary gain.) He also felt that latah differed in many other ways from Western hysteria. Clearly, in this, he is correct. His conclusion was that latah was a "fright neurosis," i.e., "traumatic neurosis," akin to combat neurosis and compensation neurosis. He concluded, "A theory of automatic obedience and the echoreactions is given: this states that fright provokes inhibitory processes which bring about 'suppression' . . . of perceptual activities; [which] leads to a dissolution of the boundaries of the ego . . . so that the behavior becomes more directly determined by the total behavioral [Gestalt] field; this manifests itself in echo-phenomena and automatic obedience. Coprolalia is interpreted as a symbolic [verbal] defensive act. . . ." Aberle supported Yap's view with his theory that latah "is a defense against being overwhelmed." He felt that imitative behavior is an "identification with the aggressor" and that coprolalia is a compromise both to drive back unconscious material and to allow simultaneous partial expression of anger or sexuality. He pointed out, as we did earlier in this section, that most latah patients are of a low station. The possibility that mimicry and coprolalia in a semidissociated state represent an acceptable solution to the problems of emotional expression (especially negative ones and sexual ones) in an otherwise passive, subservient, uneducated person has not been overlooked (Murphy, 1973; Meth, 1974).

It is thus obvious that even at the elementary level of classification and nomenclature ("hysteria," "schizophrenia," "culture-bound," etc.) the latah syndrome is still far from clearly defined. What is clear is that its incidence and prevalence are diminishing dramatically (Murphy, 1973). As with windigo and pibloktoq, the coming of "civilization" seems to be coupled with a sharp diminution of the syndrome.

Chiu et al. (1972) studied a sample of over 12,000 Malaysians, half Malay and half Iban. A total of 50 cases of latah were found. Seven "firm" diagnoses were made: depressive neurosis (3), hysterical neurosis (2), schizophrenia (1), and adjustment reaction (1). In addition, 14 patients were less firmly diagnosed: hysterical personality (2), hysterical neurosis (1), depressive neurosis (4), manic depression (3), psychotic depression (2), paranoid personality (1), and psychophysiologic disorder (1). Sexual conflicts seemed to play a role in many of these cases; all were female. As in the previously discussed literature, most were of middle and older age. The main points from their study are the incidence in the early 70s of latah was low (less than 2% of females); bona fide mental illness among the victims was low (7/50 and, even when diagnoses were unsettled, less than 50%); depression at the time of onset was very often the prevailing affect.

We can only conclude that latah and the myriad latah-like syndromes described here represent a final common pathway for a wide spectrum of disorders, ranging from mild acute adjustment reactions to schizophrenia and organic brain syndrome. In addition, much of latah is not readily classifiable in Western psychiatric terms. Clearly, cultural patterns that support the latah state (i.e., trance-states, teasing, mythology) must also be present, as well as poor education and low social status. As European civilization encroached, many of the old native belief-systems crumbled. Latah apparently increased in incidence initially on the boundaries of Western influence ("acute adjustment reaction"?) but now is apparently waning as new cultural norms take hold. The reduction of classical "conversion hysteria" among literate and acculturated Western populations might be an appropriate analogy. Windigo and pibloktoq are undoubtedly victims of the same changes. It becomes clear, as one studies such diverse and intriguing rare syndromes, that the mythology, tolerances, and beliefs of a society and culture are crucially important to the concept of mental illness of each society.

SUMMARY

Latah, windigo, and pibloktoq are three unusual psychiatric syndromes that have been generally grouped under the heading "hysteropsychoses." Although each contains many hysterical elements, a close look at the literature makes such easy classification suspect. More than likely, many types of illness, from acute reactions to schizophrenia and organic brain syndrome, can be expressed via one or another of these syndrome complexes. The key variable seems to be culture, in all of its social, mythological, and geopolitical aspects. Latah, a syndrome of echolalia, echopraxia, coprolalia, and mimicry, is the most widely distributed of the three, occurring on virtually every continent and among a wide variety of peoples. Pibloktoq is almost completely the domain of the Eskimo, and windigo occurs among a few American Indian tribes. Pibloktoq is classically thought of as a dissociative episode involving screaming, disrobing, and running in the snow, but our review has cast doubt upon such a narrow spectrum of behavior as regards the Eskimo's concept of the term. Windigo involves witchcraft, depression, delusions, cannibalism, and isolation during the winter hunt. With the encroachment of Western civilization, all three syndromes are becoming less common, if not downright rare, and, in some cases, perhaps, extinct.

REFERENCES

Aberle, D. F., 1952, "Arctic hysteria" and latah in Mongolia, Trans. N.Y. Acad. Sci. 14:291.
Abraham, J. J., 1911, "The Surgeon's Log; Being Impressions of the Far East," E. P. Dutton, New York.
Abraham, J. J., 1912, Latah and amok, Br. Med. J. 1:438.
Achranecht, B. H., 1948, Medicine and disease among Eskimos, Ciba Symp. 10:916.
Beard, G. M., 1880, The jumping Frenchmen of Maine, J. Nerv. Ment. Dis. 7:487.
Bleuler, E., 1936, 1951, "Text-book of Psychiatry," Dover, New York.
Brill, A. A., 1913, Piblokto or hysteria among Peary's Eskimos, J. Nerv. Ment. Dis. 40:514.

Chapel, J. L., 1970, Latah, myriachit, and jumpers revisited, *N.Y. State J. Med.* 70:2201.

Chiu, T. L., Tong, J. E., and Schmidt, K. E., 1972, A clinical and survey study of latah in Sarawak, Malaysia, *Psychol. Med.* 2:155.

Clifford, H., 1898, "Studies in Brown Humanity: Being Scrawls and Smudges in Sepia, White and Yellow," G. Richards, London.

Cooper, J. M., 1933, The Cree whitico psychosis, *Primitive Man* 6:20.

Cooper, J. M., 1934, Mental disease situations in certain cultures—A new field for research, *J. Abnorm. Soc. Psychol.* 29:10.

Czaplicka, M. A., 1914, "Aboriginal Siberia," Clarendon Press, Oxford.

Ellis, W. G., 1897, Latah: A mental malady of Malays, *J. Ment. Sci.* 43:33.

Freuchen, P., 1965, "The Book of the Eskimos," Fawcett, New York.

Hallowell, I., 1934, Culture and mental disorder, *J. Abnorm. Soc. Psychol.* 29:1.

Hammond, W. A., 1824, Myriachit, a newly described disease of the nervous system and its analogues, *N.Y. Med. J.* 39:191.

Kline, N., 1963, Psychiatry in Indonesia, *Am. J. Psychiatry* 119:809.

Kraepelin, E., 1909, "Lehrbuch der Psychiatrie," Barth, Leipzig.

Landes, R., 1938, The abnormal among the Ojibwa Indians, *J. Abnorm. Soc. Psychol.* 33:14.

Lehmann, H. E., 1975, Unusual psychiatric disorders and syndromes, *in* "Comprehensive Textbook of Psychiatry" (A. M. Freedman, H. I. Kaplan, and B. J. Sadock, eds.), pp. 1724–1736, Williams and Wilkins, Baltimore.

Logan, J. R., 1849, Five days in Naning, *J. Indian Archipelago East. Asia* 3:24.

Meth, J. M., 1974, Exotic psychiatric syndromes, *in* "American Handbook of Psychiatry" (S. Arieti, ed.), pp. 724–729, Basic Books, New York.

Murphy, H. B. M., 1973, History and the evolution of syndromes: A striking case of latah and amok, *in* "Psychopathology: Contributions from the Social, Behavioral and Biological Sciences" (M. Hammer, K. Salzinger, and S. Sutton, eds.), pp. 33–55, Wiley, New York.

Novakovsky, S., 1924, Arctic or Siberian hysteria as a reflex of the geographic environment, *Ecology* 5:113.

O'Brien, H. O., 1883a, Latah, *J. Straits Branch R. Asiat. Soc.* 11:143.

O'Brien, H. O., 1883b, Latah, *J. Straits Branch R. Asiat. Soc.* 12:283.

Opler, M. K., 1967, The dimensions of culture and human values, *in* "Culture and Social Psychiatry" (M. K. Opler, ed.), pp. 64–166, Atherton Press, New York.

Parker, S., 1960, The windigo psychosis in the context of Ojibwa personality and culture. *Am. Anthropol.* 62:603.

Pfeiffer, W., 1968, New research findings regarding latah, *Transcult. Psychiatr. Res.* 5:34.

Repond, A., 1940, Le lattah: Une psychonerveuse exotique, *Ann. Méd.-Psychol.* 98:311.

Rosenthal, D., 1970, "Genetic Theory and Abnormal Behavior," McGraw-Hill, New York.

Saindon, J. E., 1933, Mental disorders among the James Bay Cree, *Primitive Man* 6:1.

Shirokogoroff, S. M., 1935, "Psychomental Complex of the Tungus," Trubner, London.

Swettenham, F. A., 1896, "Malay Sketches," John Lane, London.

Uchimura, Y., 1935, Imu, a malady of the Ainu, *Lancet* 228:1272.

Ullman, L. P., and Krasner, L., 1969, "A Psychological Approach to Abnormal Behavior," Prentice-Hall, Englewood Cliffs, N.J.

Van Loon, F. G. H., 1927, Amok and latah. *J. Abnorm. Soc. Psychol.* 21:434.

Winiarz, W., and Wielawski, J., 1936, Imu: A psychoneurosis occurring among Ainus, *Psychoanal. Rev.* 23:181.

Yandell, D. W., 1881, Epidemic convulsions, *Brain* 4:339.

Yap, P. M., 1951, Mental disease peculiar to certain cultures: A survey of comparative psychiatry, *J. Ment. Sci.* 97:313.

Yap, P. M., 1952, The latah reaction: Its pathodynamics and nosological position, *J. Nerv. Ment. Sci.* 98:33.

14

Psychological Disorders Among the Australian Aboriginals

HARRY D. EASTWELL

The Australian Aboriginals were nomadic hunter-gatherers who built no permanent dwellings, made no pottery, and used spears rather than bows and arrows. They shared the honor of last place in the race toward cultural complexity with the Bushmen of the Kalahari (Waterman and Waterman, 1970). This failure to advance technologically is explained by the unsuitability of the native animals for domestication and the native plants for growth as crops.

In the 1950s about 1000 Aboriginals remained in the bush, living a life relatively untouched by the Western world until the Australian government accelerated its program to settle all Aboriginals in towns. The ostensible motive for this policy was the prevalence of disease and malnutrition among the bush dwellers. By 1960 only a few families remained in the bush and they usually had access to Western foods to supplement their own. Today the life of the tribesmen is centered around 11 mission-towns and 6 government towns (Figure 1). They are the population centers for 10,500 persons of homogenous Australoid descent.

In the towns, home gardening is still not practiced because it is considered un-Aboriginal and without ancestral precedent. Almost all foodstuffs are imported. A cash economy was introduced only in the 1960s, making the skills of hunting and foraging redundant. Polygamy is still common in the eastern towns, with one-third of the men having plural wives. Christianity has made little headway and ancestral beings still dominate religious thought; ceremonies commemorating them are reg-

HARRY D. EASTWELL • Department of Psychiatry, University of Queensland, Brisbane, Queensland, Australia.

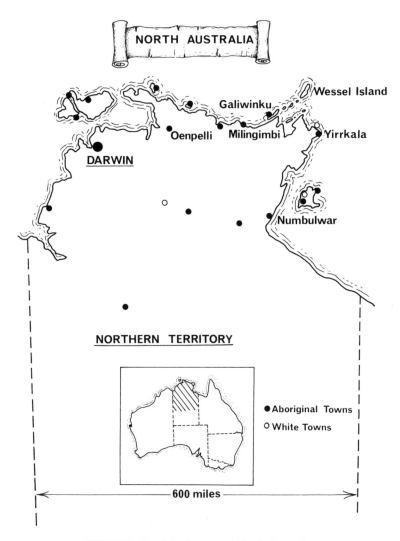

FIGURE 1. Aboriginal towns of North Australia.

ularly reenacted. Young men are formally initiated into tribal life, usually by circumcision, but in some areas by the much more radical operation of subincision, whereby the penile urethra is slit. There is a
personal adherence to a philosophy of the timelessness of life, entirely
alien to Westerners, and an acceptance of magical explanations for
events. Concepts of the individual's control over his own life and destiny
are poorly developed. The complex kinship system survives, with fami-

lies grouped by dialects into clans or lineages of 50 to 100 members. Sickness, both physical and psychological, is commonly attributed to the
malevolence of rival clans, through acts of sorcery. The Aboriginal *lex
talionis* is still not completely supplanted by white Australian law in the
more isolated districts, with accounts of revenge killings occurring fairly
regularly in Australian newspapers. Schooling is available but is
regarded ambivalently because it is thought to subvert Aboriginality,
and fewer than 70% of eligible pupils actually attend. No Aboriginals
have proceeded to tertiary education and only a handful have completed
secondary school. The standard of English is low, with the original dialects still used as first languages. In all dialects Aboriginals refer to themselves as "the real people." The population adjusts confusedly to town
life because clanship erodes the sense of community. In reaction to the
essentially roleless life, a movement back to small settlements in the bush
has gained momentum. This is known as the Homelands movement.
Enthusiastic support for it is shown by the fact that about one-quarter of
the population now live in small settlements up to 100 miles from the
nearest town. At these places the precepts of Aboriginal life continue in
a neotraditional way, but without foodstuffs brought in from the town
this emulation of the old life-style could not continue. Overall, the goods
and services of Western society have been slow to penetrate this part of
the world, which has been described as a "backwater within a backwater" (Cawte, 1972). The whole of North Australia contains only three
other towns, almost exclusively white, and one small city, Darwin.

THE FIVE-YEAR EPIDEMIOLOGIC SURVEY

Psychiatric clinics were established in this area in 1966 under the
aegis of the Flying Doctor Service. These became regular in 1971, with a
survey to assess the epidemiology of psychological disorders. A field
team was sent to each of the small towns, along the lines used by Cawte
(1972) in another northern part of Australia, North Queensland. The
field teams monitored psychiatric illness between the trimonthly visits
of the psychiatrist, the present writer. They consisted of a white nurse at
the town and one or two Aboriginal aides. In addition, nonmedical white
staff who knew many townspeople were also enlisted. Aboriginals living
on the Homelands were visited during the survey. The field teams were
supported for 5 years, 1971 through 1975, and a case register was com-
piled. Only patients who corresponded to the World Health Organization definition of mental illness (1960) were included. This definition
states that the symptoms of psychiatric illness should be severe enough
to debar the patient from ordinary social life and work and that the ill-

ness should resemble some established psychiatric entity. Thus, many mild symptoms were excluded.

Over the 5 years, 435 patients were encountered (211 males, 224 females) among the population of 10,500, a prevalence rate very roughly equivalent to that of illnesses of the same degree in the Western world. Of the 435 patients, some were known prior to the creation of field teams in 1971; they were 123 patients with chronic disability, 63 males and 60 females. The field teams identified a further 312 "new" patients (148 males, 164 females) during the survey period. It should be noted that there are almost equal numbers of males and females in the series, a finding at variance with the Western world, where females predominate. It should also be mentioned that alcoholism among males is very frequent but that this condition was difficult for whites to assess due to lack of cooperation. This same difficulty was encountered by Morice (1976) in his survey of towns in Central Australia. Thus, for reasons of rapport, alcoholism was not included.

The results of the survey are given in Table I, using the diagnostic framework of the International Classification of Disease, 8th Revision (1967). This is recommended by Yap (1974) as providing sufficient leeway for transcultural diagnosis. Classification and diagnosis in any remote culture is always problematic and the field teams encountered practical difficulties. For example, extreme reactions of shame resembled reactive depressions but, because of the lack of indigenous labeling of such states of illnesses, many tended to be overlooked by Aboriginal field team members and none were recorded at some towns. As another example of the difficulties, whites readily labeled repeatedly aggressive persons as personality disorders. But there was a surprising lack of agreement by Aboriginals, who often refused to label them as ill, even though they may have suffered at their hands or been inconvenienced by them. White and Aboriginal investigators differed in their perception of what is an illness. The advantages of the International Classification for cross-cultural comparability are certainly reduced by such anomalies. Similar difficulties with classification are noted in Papua New Guinea by Burton-Bradley (1978), who contributes to this volume.

The clinical aspects of the most common diagnoses encountered by the field teams appears to be unique and culture-related. These are found in illnesses wherever Aboriginal culture still exists in recognizable form. Nevertheless, it is too extreme to claim that they are "culture-bound" because the illnesses resemble those of developing peoples in other parts of the world. Examples of the most common diagnoses are now given for the consideration of the reader and will introduce the psychiatric illnesses of North Australia.

TABLE I. Five-Year Survey of Northern Aboriginal Reserves (Population
11,000)
Diagnoses Using the International Classification of Disease

	Males	Females	Total
Reactive psychosis (a fear-of-sorcery syndrome)	53	4	57
Depressive neurosis (shame as dominant dynamic)	25	74	99
Hysterical neurosis—dissociation	11	43	54
Hysterical neurosis—conversion[a]	1	3	4
Hypochondriacal neurosis	14	33	47
Anxiety neurosis	7	3	10
Schizophrenia	10	17	27
Manic depressive psychosis and reactive depressive psychosis (often reactive to "rolelessness")	13	14	27
Acute brain syndrome (all causes, usually alcohol)	15	—	15
Chronic brain syndrome (all causes)	12	5	17
Moderate and severe mental retardation	10	4	14
Mild mental retardation (difficult to diagnose)	6	1	7
Major epilepsy ("idiopathic")	1	5	6
Transient situational disorder[b]	13	8	21
Personality disorders	12	8	20
Other diagnoses	3	2	5
Insufficient detail for diagnosis (in persons living remote from towns)	5	—	5
Total	211	224	435

[a]Many patients with minor conversion symptoms were included under their major diagnoses—depressive neurosis.
[b]Includes episodes of self-injury.

UNIQUE SYNDROMES

The Fear-of-Sorcery Syndrome

The first illness common to the Aboriginals, and the most dramatic, is an anxiety state with paranoid features magnified to psychotic proportions. The patient fears imminent death from sorcery, and the severity of concurrent autonomic signs is a noteworthy feature. Sorcery is part of the psychological reality of the people.

One such case was a 19-year-old youth who lived in a remote part of a reserve that received food supplies from a nearby cattle ranch. His tribal country was isolated for months at a time by monsoon. He was escorted to the hospital in an agitated, tremulous state, perspiring freely. He had the firm conviction that he was soon to die as the result of sorcery from a tribal elder. Noises outside the ward were misinterpreted as evidence of the sorcerer waiting to kill him; he was vigilant and pacing through the night. A classificatory "brother" who traveled with the patient was puzzled by his reaction. He recounted how the patient had suddenly broken off relations with a young woman who was forbidden to him by tribal law, being convinced that tribal elders knew about his affair and that punishment would ensue. As far as the brother knew, his affair was a well-kept secret. The patient suspected that sorcery emanated from the tribal elder whose duty it was to properly bestow the girl. Despite the severity of the presenting symptoms, the patient recovered in 2 weeks with the use of chlorpromazine. Thereafter, he was discharged to the care of relatives who lived some distance from his usual home.

    Such reactions are referred to in the International Classification of Disease as "reactive psychosis." There was distortion of reality in that no elder had, in fact, detected his sexual offense and no one was clearly intent on punishing him. A paranoid flavor is common to many types of illness among these people (Eastwell, 1978), but it is not considered dominant enough to label this psychosis as paranoid schizophrenia. Such states resemble *bouffée délirante*, which occurs commonly among Africans. In Australia there is a selective distribution for this condition; it is almost wholly restricted to men of middle age or younger; old men are apparently immune and women are rarely affected. The aspect of social labeling is important in the causation of these reactions, along the lines laid down by Waxler (1974). The society defines young and middle-aged men as vulnerable to sorcery because their loss caused the greatest disruption to life in precontact times. Also, the old are not vulnerable because they achieve that status only by their immunity to sorcery, which is thought to be almost omnipresent. This defines them as not able to suffer such conditions. The patient is not rejected by his clan, who close ranks in indignation against the putative sorcerers. Fifty-seven of the total of 435 cases were of this kind. A paradox was noted confirming the cultural causation of this syndrome: Although sorcery is feared as potentially affecting everyone in the culture, actual evidence for the performance of any sorcery ritual is very difficult to obtain. Clear-cut rituals were recorded on only five occasions, three of these by one clan leader with a personality disorder. Apparently the sorcery fears do not need reinforcement by the present day enactment of the appropriate ritual. The anthropologists R. M. and C. H. Berndt (1951) also failed to find evidence for sorcery ritual. They state: "It is extremely doubtful whether the forms of sorcery alleged to exist in this region are practiced at all. They are real, however, in the sense that they are firmly believed to exist."

Hysterical Trance States

A second common reaction is the local variant of a dissociative state. It is seen especially in young women and reflects the ideologies of soul loss or possession by an alien spirit. These dissociative states are recurring episodes at times of personal stress. Unlike many tribal cultures, there are no occasions when trance states or other forms of dissociation are normal among the Aboriginals.

Living in a coastal town, Motiti was an 18-year-old girl who had so far produced no children although married for 4 years. She repeatedly collapsed outside her hut in an immobile, unresponsive, and mute state. Each time she was carried totally rigid to the local clinic. She confided that she was possessed by the spirit of a recently dead man to whom the sea tide was of special totemic significance, and her "turns" occurred only at times when the tide was high. She claimed that the dead man had been in a "joking" relationship to her, since there had been bantering quasi-sexual remarks between them. Later it became known that the patient's husband was negotiating for a second wife on the grounds of her childlessness and this new wife would become the senior if she produced a child first. After some months, the patient became pregnant and her husband relinquished his claim on the second wife; the patient's "turns" ceased.

Such conditions are indistinguishable from acute catatonic schizophrenia—unresponsiveness, immobility, catalepsy, mutism, negativism, and automatic obedience can all be seen. But the rapidity of their resolution is pathognomonic; most of these dissociative states resolve in hours or a few days. Two autonomic accompaniments deserve recording: low systolic blood pressure and urinary retention for the duration of the trance.

One aspect of Aboriginal life-style is of importance in promoting these reactions. Aboriginals exist in a remarkably nonprivate world. They live, eat, and often sleep outside their huts in the company of their extended family. This open-air existence means that dissociative states create the maximum visible disturbance, in the nature of secondary gain. Of the 435 cases, 54 were of this general type; dissociation plays a much more prominent part in the illnesses of this culture than in those of the urban West.

Depression Mediated by Shame

The third and most common illness (99 of the 435 cases) is a depressive state marked particularly by apathy and restriction of social relationships (although the patient might still be regarded as gregarious by Western standards of withdrawal). The patient lies on a blanket in a shady place for days on end, in full public view. Statements by the patients actually reflecting a downturn in mood are not common. Instead, appetite is severely curtailed and emaciation quickly ensues. Irritability is common, especially in men: They are quick to take offense and brandish their spears. Sleep disturbance, on the other hand, is surprisingly difficult to detect; such a history, even with optimal interpreting, is difficult to elicit. Indeed, many patients show an apparent hypersomnia. The cultural surrounds of the concept of sleep are vastly different from those of the West. Aboriginals believe that the soul vacates the body in sleep, as evidenced by dreams, and also that dreams are experienced concurrently by close clan relatives.

These depressions are mediated by shame as the dominant dynamic, and the public display of shame in the form of apathy and unhappiness often conveys passive reproach to others. Thus, a young woman forced into an unwanted marriage may develop these symptoms to reproach both her own relatives who arranged the marriage and her husband; an older man may be shamed by the refusal of a young woman to marry him and may seek to reproach the woman and her relatives. The public aspect of shame in the patient or of seeking to shame others is important in these reactions. Internalized guilt is not a feature of these illnesses (Cawte, 1964; Jones, 1972) and this absence has been noted in African tribal peoples (Carothers, 1953). In cases where guilt might be expected, it is rationalized and projected into others.

The field team called attention to a middle-aged widow who began sitting apart, taking little part in communal life. She was apathetic about her appearance and took no interest in food preparation. Weight loss was obvious, but sleep disturbance was denied. Questioning soon elicited her concern about the sexual behavior of an unmarried daughter, who she planned to rightfully bestow to an older man. To add to the difficulties, she had accepted the requisite bride-price (about $400). Shame at the daughter's conduct and an inability to return any of the bride-price money was the key feature of this reaction.

Mimetic Illnesses

A fourth type of illness is a folie communiquée among members of a clan group. This illness was quite common in the 5-year survey, with 49 patients identified. For statistical purposes, these individuals were classified separately, as there is no suitable category in the International Classification of Disease. The fear-of-sorcery syndrome, dissociative states, and depressive reactions were all noted to be shared by members of the one clan group. On the other hand, instances of epidemic hysteria, the commonest shared reaction in the developing world, were not found. The term *associative*, following Gralnick (1942), is appropriate for these shared illnesses. They resemble folie à deux, or à trois, except that there is no primary dominant patient and no secondary submissive patient. The dominant psychodynamic is identification, often cross-identification, between clan members. Cultural dictates facilitate this circulation of illness, especially the common fear-of-sorcery syndrome. These dictates are that sorcery affects the whole clan and not just one of its members. If the first clansman to become ill recovers, then others expect to become ill because the sorcery is still operative. When a clansman recovers, he is seen to be "too strong" for the sorcery and there is no recurrence in his case. This tends to suggest that social labeling is effective in the causation of this sorcery-fear syndrome, as already noted. Such mimetic illnesses were probably underrepresented; there was a tendency for the field team to focus on the one identified patient, thus restricting observation of close relatives. The mediating dynamic for these shared illnesses, identification, is thought to have been useful as an adaptation to clan life in small bands in the bush. At the present time, it is maladaptive because it limits independence, autonomy, and the need to achieve as an individual.

Shared Depressive Illness

The paradox with depressive illness is that it too is often shared by mimesis, or identification, with other close relatives. This is in contrast to experience among Westerners where the illness affects only the individual. There were nine patients encountered who were symptomatically depressed in identification with a preexisting patient with the same condition. The primary patient in these pairs had offended against the traditional mores. In clan society, relatives share the same stigma of blame for any offense committed by the individual. They too react with shame. On this topic, the first missionary in the east of North Australia had this to say: "Every member of it [the clan] shares in the honour or disgrace of any of its number. An offence by one member is regarded as an offence by the whole of the offender's [clan], all are held equally guilty" (Webb, 1934).

One young woman repeatedly postponed her marriage to an old man who had already had three wives. He had paid the requisite bride-price to her parents and all her clan were shamed by her vascillating attitude. When interviewed, she was downcast in mood and notably inactive, spending most of the day lying on her blanket. Weight loss was obvious. Her sister, only a year younger, also became conspicuously apathetic and gave up her job. She failed to join the circles of people on the sand playing cards, previously her major interest. She was preoccupied with her sister's dilemma but improved when the old man relinquished his claim on the primary patient. Hypersomnia rather than insomnia appeared to be a major symptom in both, with weight loss. Although they were obviously ill from an outsider's point of view, they were not considered ill by relatives who understood the cause of the reaction. This cultural blindness to depressive reactions probably led to many being overlooked in the course of the survey.

An Explanatory Framework

As the survey proceeded, it became obvious that most of the psychopathology encountered could usefully be viewed as an exaggeration or a caricature of behavior commonly seen in subclinical degrees. This is a concept recently discussed by Draguns (1973). Thus, the fear of sorcery is present in any Aboriginal group; dissociation is a caricature of the withdrawal behavior seen, say, in any Aboriginal who wishes to isolate himself from an unwanted situation in which he may be called to fight; depressive reactions in subclinical proportions represent the psychological pain felt by many young people where conflict occurred between the old system of arranged marriages and the new ethic of assortative mating, as actively promoted by missionaries. In this view of psychopathology as a caricature of common behavior, one of the more striking paradoxes of Aboriginal psychiatry emerged.

PARADOXICAL OMISSIONS FROM THE NEUROTIC REPERTOIRE

Anxiety neurosis, obsessive-compulsive neurosis, and phobic neurosis form a subject of singular interest among those studying Aboriginals. The very existence of these three types of neurosis has become a topic of debate. Eight surveys of psychiatric illness among Aboriginals of homogeneous Australoid descent have failed to identify anxiety neurosis in anticipated numbers, and phobic states and obsessive-compulsive neurosis have not been identified at all. Yet transcultural psychiatrists have previously commented on the worldwide distribution of these symptom neuroses (Kiev, 1972; Yap, 1974). Their relative or complete omission from the neurotic repertoire of Australian Aboriginals is examined here in the light of the paradoxical finding that anxiety is very common in the form of sorcery fears. It is free-floating anxiety that is so rare. Similarly, phobiclike and obsessive-compulsivelike ideation are common in the culture. How is it possible that anxious, obsessive, and phobic behavior is commonly recognized, yet the corresponding neuroses are rarely described?

The stage for this debate was set by Kidson and Jones (1968), who commented: "No syndromes clearly resembling Western classical neurosis—anxiety states, phobic states or obsessive-compulsive states, were detected. No special factors were found which would explain why they should not come to notice. It therefore seems likely that these disorders do not occur."

This provocative claim stimulated Yap's response (1974) on the worldwide incidence of neurosis: "The standard forms of neurosis are everywhere encountered. As far as I know only one study, that of Kidson and Jones, claims categorically that in the Aborigines of Western Australia the standard textbook forms are not to be found, but in their place more 'exotic' conditions like the spirit-possession syndrome. We are inclined to dispute this and would query whether it is not artlessly easy altogether to overlook anxiety and obsessional states because of cultural barriers to communication. Obviously further studies are called for."

But, the Kidson and Jones finding was not an isolated one. Indeed, with the exception of a few anxiety states, these neuroses have not been diagnosed in any Aboriginal town where tribal organization persists. The findings of all surveys are listed in Table II. Wittkower and Dubreuil (1968) quoted the Kidson and Jones findings and also commented that obsessive-compulsive neurosis is rare in rural Africa and rural India. It should be noted, of course, that obsessive-compulsive states are not very common in the psychiatry of developed countries, either. But the situation is very different with free-floating anxiety. A standard psychiatric text by Freedman, et al. (1975) mentions a prevalence rate of 5%. Likewise, phobias are common in Western nations, sometimes seen in the context of other illnesses.

Anxiety Neurosis Encountered in This Survey

The field team survey supports the previous findings in respect to free-floating anxiety: They found only ten patients with symptoms of anxiety, and five of these were suffering from a life-threatening or disabling disease (carcinoma, leprosy, motor neuron disease, obstructive airways disease, and congestive cardiac failure). The other five with free-floating anxiety were all from the small number of acculturated (or "sophisticated") Aboriginals. These five patients without physical disease account for only 1.2% of the total series of 435. This low prevalence of free-floating anxiety is in marked contrast to the number of patients

TABLE II. Conclusions and Key Statements on Anxiety Neurosis, Phobic
Neurosis, and Obsessive-Compulsive Neurosis in All Surveys of Aboriginal
Townships

Cawte, J., 1964: Kalumburu, Western Australia; population 300.
  No cases specifically identified as anxiety neurosis, phobic neurosis, or obsessive-
  compulsive neurosis.
Kidson, M. A., 1967: Yuendumu, Central Australia; population 650.
  The symptom neuroses, anxiety states, phobias, obsessive-compulsive states, and the
  rest are conspicuously absent.
Nurcombe, G., and Cawte, J., 1967: Mornington Island, North Queensland; population
  280 children.
  Most striking of all is the scarcity of disorder with overt psychoneurotic
  symptomatology. There were no individuals with well-evolved obsessive-
  compulsive, phobic, or dissociative syndromes or with free-floating anxiety states.
Kidson, M. A., and Jones, I. H., 1968: Warburton Range, Western Desert; population 441.
  No syndromes clearly resembling Western classical neurosis-anxiety states, phobic
  states, or obsessive-compulsive states were detected.
Cawte, J., 1972: Mornington Island, North Queensland; population 190 adults.
  No cases specifically diagnosed as anxiety neurosis, phobic neurosis, or obsessive-
  compulsive neurosis, but the common Malgri syndrome and preoccupation was
  recognized to have anxiety, phobic, and obsessive-compulsive features—hand
  washing and mouth washing removed the spirit contamination incurred by
  poaching on the estate of a rival clan.
Jones, I. H., 1972: Jigalong and Fitzroy Crossing, Western Australia; population 118.
  Obsessive neurosis has yet to be seen and free-floating anxiety was only present in
  one of the most sophisticated members of the most sophisticated mission.
Morice, R. D., 1976: Neotraditional desert outstation, Central Australia; population 90.
  (Investigation into this isolated group's "language of psychiatry")
  There was an apparent absence of true free-floating anxiety. No terms suggestive of
  anankastic personality disorder or of obsessive-compulsive neurosis were elicited.
This survey: Five-year survey of Aboriginal townships of North Australia; population
  10,500.
  No single case of phobic or obsessive-compulsive neurosis, as Westerners
  understand it, was encountered. Anxiety neurosis was found in only ten
  acculturated or physically ill patients.

(13%) who exhibited a fear state in which anxiety was displaced or projected to culturally defined dangers, as already described, in the fear of
sorcery. In traditional times, anxiety was always projected, displaced, or
otherwise attributed to the world outside, as in sorcery fears.

  None of the five patients suffered severe or totally disabling symptoms, but all fulfilled the criteria of psychiatric illnesses as prescribed by
the World Health Organization. The stresses that precipitated their
symptoms were clear-cut and the symptoms were of a few weeks' duration only. Four of the five were young adults under 30 years of age. The
diagnosis was made on their description of the physiological accompan-

iments of anxiety. (This is the approach used by Beiser *et al.*, 1972, in his assessment of anxiety states among the Serer of Senegal.) Because of the language barrier, even in these acculturated persons, it was not possible to obtain descriptions of the psychological concomitants of anxiety such as tenseness or feelings of impending doom. One of the few cases of free-floating anxiety is described.

Bargaru, aged 28 years, was from a northern township, but he worked on a mission in Central Australia a thousand miles away. On his way home to obtain permission for his marriage to a Central Australian girl, he became anxious and presented to the Darwin base hospital for treatment. He knew that his relatives had been paying off the install-ments on the bride-price for another young woman at his home town-ship. The money paid by his relatives would be lost if he did not marry this woman. In the hospital he refused to believe that his symptoms were the result of sorcery. Later, when he was interview in his hometown in the bush, he mentioned that his relatives suggested that he had really been ensorcelled by the clan who were expecting to provide him with a wife, and for whom payments had now ceased. One year later, with his marriage negotiations completed, he again returned home, this time with his Central Australian bride.

The main factor reducing the incidence of anxiety neurosis is the ease with which anxiety is projected to become a fear of sorcery. This is essentially a cognitive explanation. However, personality factors must also be considered and child-rearing patterns must be explored. The warmth and extreme permissiveness of Aboriginal mothering reduces the formation of infantile anxiety, which is generally seen to be the fore-runner of adult anxiety states, on the principle of antecedent conflict. The close physical contact of infancy sets the pattern for a gregarious life in which the individual is rarely alone. The Aboriginal is surrounded by kinsmen who are auxiliary egos (and ids and superegos), who share his conflicts, and who enter disputes with him or alternatively restrain him. In the words of one of the first missionaries in North Australia, T. T. Webb (1934): "[R]arely does a man act on his own initiative or assume and maintain an individual attitude in regard to any matter." It is note-worthy that three of the five patients with primary anxiety were sepa-rated from kinsfolk by geographical or social factors.

Another Aboriginal characteristic that possibly reduces anxiety is low motivation for achievement, coupled with little sense of penalty for failure. Their limited aspirations are clearly realizable and there is little incentive to adopt a problem-solving approach to life. As evidence for this factor, it has been mentioned that schools are poorly attended. On any one school day only 50–80% of the enrolled pupils attend.

Phobic Neurosis: The Absence of Clinically Identifiable Cases

No patients with a phobic illness were encountered in any of the surveys, yet phobic ideation is common in the culture. Whole communities feared "danger place," usually nearby tracts of rain forest thought to be inhabited by malevolent spirits. If patients intruded unwittingly into a "danger place," the resultant illness was clinically a fear state—fear of possession by the local malevolent spirit. By far the commonest subclinical phobia was fear of the dark, more specifically a fear of nocturnal spirits. Some of the most acculturated men were affected by this phobiclike ideation, which was not considered by Aboriginals to be pathological. Cawte (1964) comments on the phobiclike fear of the gremlin Tjimi in the Kimberley district: "Fear of Tjimi presumably fulfills a social function by preventing children from wandering off and becoming lost, or women being available for trysts."

The Absence of Obsessive-Compulsive Neurosis

No patients with this condition were reported in any of the surveys. Of course, Aboriginals are not involved in counting or ritual handwashing: There is no concern with bacterial contamination or sanitary obsessions. In an Aboriginal language studied carefully there was no term suggestive of anankastic disorder (Morice, 1976). However, Murphy (1976) reminds us: "The absence of a single label for some of the phenomena we call mental illness, such as neurosis, does not mean that the manifestations of such phenomena are absent." But a paradox is again encountered since obsessive-compulsive behavior is carried out with obsessive observance of detail. Mistakes are feared in the depiction of sacred emblems (bark and body paintings and sand designs), with the artists working with obsessive concern supervised by clansmen. Members of a hunting party are carefully anointed with a clan leader's protective sweat before hunting or traveling on his territory. There is also an obsessive fear of contaminated people—brothers and sisters must avoid each other. Brothers cannot even be handed a pill by sisters who are nursing assistants. A man must carefully avoid his mother-in-law, who in North Australia is often not much older than he is. Although these avoidances are culturewide, there is considerable variation among individuals as to their observances. But none of this individual variation is elaborated to "illness" proportions. The question may be best phrased: When does a taboo become a phobia? Aboriginals are ridden by taboos (of place, ritual, relationships); why are they not reported as phobic and viewed as a psychiatric problem, as occurs in the common phobias of the West (heights, crowds, confined spaces)?

Explaining This Low or Absent State of Risk

The simplest explanation focuses on the problem of negative information in the relatively small numbers of Aboriginals surveyed. It assumes that cross-cultural surveys employ too coarse a filter to identify patients with neurosis. A close, accurate, and empathic communication is the *sine qua non* of the understanding of psychoneurosis to many psychiatrists, and this is difficult to achieve because of linguistic barriers to a culture as "remote" as that of Australian ex-hunter-gatherers. None of the previous surveys was made by psychiatrists who had more than a smattering of the local languages, and Aboriginals fluent in English are quite rare. This is the interpretation for the deficient or sparsely filled categories of psychoneurosis made by Cawte. In his surveys (1964, 1972) he did not identify clinical cases, and he refrained from commenting that they were not present, because of the difficulty in labeling them. It seems that the taboo system, as anthropologists would describe it, is poorly related semantically to the anxiety-phobic system, as psychiatrists would describe it. If this interpretation is correct, it has important implications for transcultural psychiatry; a finer filter is necessary to avoid overlooking large segments of psychopathology, especially among peoples culturally removed like the Aboriginals. It is here suggested that this is the most likely explanation for the failure to identify and label these neuroses.

An Alternative Explanation: Do Taboos Act to Replace Phobias?

Given the widespread prevalence of ideation resembling both phobic and obsessive-compulsive states, are there cultural factors that prevent its assuming the dimensions of clinical neurosis? As outlined, psychiatric illness reflects an extreme of psychopathology that is common subclinically. Thus, subclinical anxieties about sorcery are the ground swell from which arises the common psychotic fear state. In addition, an important finding is that the breaking of taboos that are maintained by phobiclike or obsessional ideation also results in fear states. Thus, inadvertent foraging in a "danger place" (always likely in the desert, where such places are less well defined) leads to fear of possession by a malevolent spirit. Too casual a performance of sacred dances or perfunctory rendering of sacred art results in fear of ancestral revenge. Walking alone at night results in fear of attack, supernatural or physical. In each case something external to the transgressor is feared, so that there is less internalized conflict, which is necessary for the clinical appearance of phobic and obsessive states. Cawte (1964) and Jones (1972) have remarked on the apparent absence of internalized guilt in depressive neurosis, whereas shame, which is much less internalized, is commonly seen. Morice (1976) reached a similar conclusion from his "language of psychiatry" investigation in a remote desert dwelling community. He stated: "As there appears to be only one word to cover both [guilt and shame], it can be assumed that guilt is not differentiated from shame and therefore as a distinct entity it is not experienced."

Childbearing practices of Aboriginals explain to a great extent this decreased internalization—all observers unanimously describe these as extremely permissive (Hipler, 1978). In this explanation it is this reduced internalization of conflict among Aboriginals that protects against the appearance of these symptom complexes called psychoneuroses and that channels individual decompensation into other avenues.

THE PARADOX SURROUNDING PERSONALITY DISORDERS

A major difficulty besets the investigation of aggressive or antisocial personality disorders among Aboriginals. There is the lack of congruence between those designated as abnormal by whites and those so designated by Aboriginals. Two surveys found aggressive and antisocial personality disorders to be common. The first of these was reported by Australia's first transcultural psychiatrist, Dr. J. Cawte (1972). He found personality disorders to be the most frequent psychiatric illness at a North Queensland mission. But he has since made an important retraction (1976, personal communication): "If I had my work to do over again, I suspect I should be less impressed by Aboriginal personality traits, and more impressed by the environmental situations to which such behaviours are a predictable response. In other words, I tend now to attribute the behaviours in question more to a response to the demand characteristics of the environment, the boredom, oppression or institutionalization, than to fixed dispositions, the subjects' personalities. All the same, 'Rosenthalism,' or the emphasis on the demand characteristics of the environment, is unsatisfying by itself. One still has to explain why some individuals are more adversely affected by the environmental deprivations than others."

Similarly, Jones (1972) used information gathered from white nurses and found personality disorders to be very common. The criteria he used in diagnosis were the frequency of aggressive acts and the length of time they had been in evidence.

However, in this survey carried out by the field teams, a high estimate of aggressive personality disorders as defined by the white members was counterbalanced by the reluctance of Aboriginal members to label aggressive behavior as abnormal, whatever their private opinion might have been. This was also noted by Berndt and Berndt (1951) at Oenpelli, in North Australia.

Similarly, the field team's careful survey at Numbulwar, a remote township, revealed that Aboriginal informants did not consider that three patients whose history featured grossly aggressive behavior were in fact abnormal. Aboriginal informants' opinions persuaded the field team to remove one case from the cohort. It is rewarding to scrutinize these individually.

A 43-year-old clan leader had a history of intimidating others with spears or clubs, for many years. On at least three occasions he brought the life of the township to a halt by public performance of sorcery rituals. In the first of these, he rendered drinking water taboo; in the second, all firewood was made "sacred" and was unable to be used for cooking; in the third, he pronounced the local store as ensorcelled. On these occasions no adults went to work and children stayed home from school. Clearly, by Western standards he could be considered an aggressive personality. He was listed as such in the survey.

Another male patient, aged about 60 years, suffered from a frontal lobe syndrome. He had a fist-sized depression on his frontal bone—a result of an old injury. His history included murdering one of his wives and seriously wounding another, before he was certified insane. Thereafter he spent 5 years in a Southern Australian Mental Hospital. Lesser degrees of aggressive behavior continued on his return. Informants were reluctant to label him abnormal in any way, because they felt his ability to live in the bush with his remaining wives, away from the township, was evidence to the contrary.

A middle-aged man was frequently involved in serious spear fights. He had a history of killing two wives in the bush before he came to live in the township. These were passed off as due to measles, which was epidemic at the time. Informants and all his peer group treated him with high respect and refused to consider him abnormal. He was therefore not included in the survey.

There was thus good evidence that the Berndts' observation of the acceptance of aggressive acts applies in this remote, unacculturated township of Numbulwar. At the more acculturated township of Galiwinku, informants were more ready to label troublemakers abnormal, but once again, certain patients, who were clearly aggressive personalities in Western eyes, were not spoken of as abnormal. These included young men with repeated offenses against white property, such as break-ing into the school or the store. If, however, these patients were involved in sexual misdemeanors that transgressed the kinship code, they were considered abnormal.

The reluctance to consider aggressive individuals as abnormal is probably accounted for by the Aboriginal group cohesiveness. It is the whole clan, rather than just the individual miscreant, that must take the responsibility for aggressive acts. Webb (1934) is again a clear commen-tator: "Though the tribe as a whole may strongly disapprove of the action of one of their members by whose action hostility has been created between them and another tribe, they, knowing they are all involved, must nevertheless stand behind this particular individual. In serious offenses as occasion the shedding of blood, the members of the injured tribe or division make no special attempt to avenge themselves upon the individual who has actually committed the offense, but are well satisfied if they succeed in punishing any member of the party to which he belongs."

With these attitudes prevailing, only the most recalcitrant aggressive Aboriginals were listed in the survey as aggressive or antisocial person-alities. Influences from traditional culture and influences from the pres-ent-day environment are conceived as explaining much aggressive behavior, without too confidently attributing the behaviors to fixed dis-positions in the subjects' personalities. Thus, the cultural relativity of the diagnosis is clear. Yet a purely cultural interpretation of aggressive behavior is not satisfying. The question remains: Who is a bully? For bul-lies are recognized by all societies and certainly by Aboriginal society. We may not always understand what makes a bully, but we know what keeps him in check: a working system of law and order. The age-old sys-tem of kin control is still the mechanism for this in North Australia.

HOMOSEXUALITY ABSENT IN ADULTS?

No investigator has found evidence of an exclusively homosexual orientation in any adult male from an Aboriginal society that is orga-nized along traditional lines. J. Money and his co-workers (1970) carried out a careful investigation in the large township of Galiwinku (Elcho Island), in eastern North Australia, and remarked to "the virtual com-plete freedom from homosexuality and related disorders of gender iden-tity." Jones's surveys (1972) of more than 2000 Aboriginals in the Central Australian Desert also revealed no adult of homosexual orientation. In addition, this present field team's survey failed to disclose any adult male homosexual despite extensive questioning of Aboriginal informants and of whites living in close contact with Aboriginals. The question was tackled from a different direction by Morice (1976). He made an exhaustive study of the "language of psychiatry" among the most remote desert dwellers—the Pintupi. He found that they had a word for anal intercourse between a man and a woman, but his informants denied any knowledge of the existence of male homosexuality and even seemed ignorant of the concept.

This is not to deny that homosexual acts occur, especially between teenage youths. For example, one group of three boys aged 13–15 years cross-infected each other with gonorrhoea while boarding at high school. Later, another group of three teenage males was treated who suffered from secondary syphilis with anal condylomata. Homosexual practices are also known among youths disinhibited after inhalation of gasoline vapor. The anthropologist Meggitt (1962) mentions homosexual practices between teenage youths who were segregated prior to their initiation. These are apparently the only references to homosexuality in the literature. Morice (1976) reports that there are no words in the Central Australian dialect he studied for "womanlike man" or "manlike woman." Such terms occur among the Eskimos (Murphy and Leighton, 1965).

The absence of homosexuality invites our conjecture for possible explanations. Once again, there is the problem of negative information in a remote culture. Was the filter fine enough to detect cases? In his classic work among New Guineans, Malinowski (1922) commented on the absence of homosexuality and attributed it to the general permissiveness of heterosexuality. Aboriginal men have been described as notably uxorious (Meggitt, 1962), and the same leniency of heterosexuality might here be proffered as a partial explanation.

More specific factors are listed by Money et al. (1970) as facilitating a heterosexual orientation and suppressing homosexuality. The first factor they considered is the normalcy of nudity up to the age of 5 or 6 in both sexes. Next, they observed the sexual play of children up to the age of 7 or 8, with boys and girls of this age imitating the sex acts of their elders. Adults do not restrain the children if they belong to kin categories that can rightfully engage in sexual activity. Finally, Money comments on the extreme polarization of male–female roles and the rigid division of labor in hunter-gatherer society. This is developed to a degree that is quite at variance with present Western attitudes. Women provide certain foods, men others—men were never gatherers because this was considered "women's work." Women provide all the firewood and carry the water. This rigid division of roles extends to apparently minor detail—the style of cooking fire used by women is constructed differently from fires made by men. Evidence of this division of labor is still an obvious facet of town life. For example, the most numerous clan at

Galiwinku is the tradition-oriented Galpu. Since the men of this clan no longer engage in the traditional male activities, hunting and fighting with other clans, they refuse to do any other work at all. All the Galpu men are supported by the wages of working wives—often multiple, since they are notably polygamous.

Ambivalence Between the Sexes

Another feature of the Aboriginal social order that reinforces the polarization of roles and is of importance in the gender orientation of the individual is the ambivalence and antipathy between the sexes. The basic cause of ambivalence and the personal dilemmas that flow from it are a result of the clan system and the need for exogamy, or marrying outside the clan. Oversimplifying the situation, Aboriginal men reason thus: "We give our sisters in marriage to another clan and she provides them with sons. Soon they outnumber us and become stronger than we are." This reasoning might continue: "Besides, we suspect the clan into which our sister will marry is responsible for the death [by sorcery] of our esteemed kinsman So-and-So." (Men not uncommonly make accusations of sorcery against their sister's husband or his clan. To compensate for this there is a cultural injunction that is just the opposite, that a man should be friendly with his brother-in-law.) The public display of affection between husband and wife is not condoned in this culture. Also, Aboriginal mythology is replete with references to antipathy between sexes. Native societies in New Guinea are also organized along clan lines and are similarly divided by male–female ambivalence or antipathy (Williamson, 1979). Homosexuality is also rare in New Guinea, with the exception of a few circumscribed areas where specific forms of it are culturally prescribed.

Avoidance of Certain Female Relatives

Ambivalence and antipathy between the sexes is most conspicuous in the avoidance relationships. The mutual avoidance of a man and his sisters is the most important of these, although women in other kin categories are also avoided. Males of all ages are prohibited from talking freely with their sisters, but often the avoidance is expressed more forcibly. For example, many female nursing assistants will not even dispense a pill to their brothers. (The central feature of the avoidance relationship is a prohibition of looking directly at a sister, face to face. Eye contact is a prelude to seduction, since it is believed that one person looks directly into the other's soul.) Among town dwellers, brother–sister avoidance presents many practical difficulties. For example, a man must not be in a position to see his sister walk into the toilet. In the towns, as the female expression of this ambivalence, women readily voice their dissatisfaction with their domestic work load or, if they are employed, with the demands made on their pay packet by their menfolk.

The conclusion to be drawn is that two groups of social forces act to suppress homosexuality. First, there is the acceptance of sexuality in childhood, and second, the ambivalence and antipathy between the sexes reinforce a rigid definition of roles. These forces are apparently strong enough to keep repressed the homosexual behavior found in any society.

THE LOW INCIDENCE OF SUICIDE: THE PARADOXICALLY HIGH INCIDENCE OF UNCONSCIOUS SELF-DESTRUCTION

In his survey of over 2000 Aboriginals in the Western Desert, Jones (1972) found no cases of suicide and no history of it in the recent past. He concluded that the Aboriginals were protected by their tendency to act out and to project hostile impulses. The field teams' findings are similar to those of Jones, but with important qualifications. It is necessary to raise the issue of self-destruction consummated without fully conscious intent. People die from the effects of their own actions, though it is open to question whether they have, in the legal sense, *mens rea*.

The field teams found only one case of overt suicide among the 10,500 people of the northern reserves over the period 1971–1975. Because any death commonly gave rise to psychiatric sequelae among clansmen, the field teams systematically inquired into recent deaths during the survey. It is unlikely that any cases of suicide were missed. The rate of explicit suicide can then be expressed as under 2 per 100,000 per year. The rate for Australia as a whole is 12 or 13 per 100,000 per year, as quoted by Burton-Bradley (1975), a representative figure for most Western nations. The one overt suicide is described.

W., from Milingimbi, was married, 31 years of age, and known as a very heavy drinker. In 1971 he returned to his home after drinking for several months in Darwin. When he stepped off the mail plane he mentioned to clansmen that he was ensorceled and that he was intent on shooting himself. This he did within an hour of his return. It is noteworthy that his action took place on his home territory, where he was a member of the dominant clan. Aboriginals wish to die in their own country so that their souls can be recycled to animate future clansmen. The association of this suicide with alcoholism should be noted. It is likely that he was recovering from an acute brain syndrome due to alcohol, the symptoms of which he misinterpreted as ensorcellment. Alcoholic complications interpreted as ensorcellment commonly occurred in other patients. W.'s suicide perplexed his clansmen, who sought to justify it by accusing his widow of infidelity, thereby throwing the blame onto her. (Burton-Bradley, 1975, records the same response among clansmen of New Guinea suicides.) This accusation heightened the widow's grief reaction, which now became one of frank depression. She responded to this situation realistically, by moving with her sister to another township. The sister was also noted to have depression symptoms in sympathy with her. The sister shared the insult made against the widow and other members of their clan.

Collective Suicides Among Aboriginals

Dispite the rarity of individual suicide, there were collective suicides among at least two groups in the recent past. Two generations ago the Wessel Island clans (in the eastern part of North Australia) were locked in internecine warfare, and members of the clans jumped from cliffs in collective suicide rather than fall into the hands of their enemies. There was only one survivor. In 1947, the Kaiadilt of Bentinck Island, off the North Queensland coast, were almost exterminated by a series of ecological disasters. Shortages of resources then sparked off warfare between rival clans. In the face of these multiple privations, a number of the survivors suicided (Cawte, 1972).

Cross-Cultural Comparisons

The low rate of explicit suicide conforms to the Durkheimian hypothesis relating social structure to suicide (Durkheim, 1893/1952). Thus, societies that have rigid social structures have a low incidence of suicide. Where substantial parts of the original culture are lost, the suicide rate rises. This phenomenon is clearly demonstrated by native American Indians, whose current suicide rate is very high. Among Eskimos, suicide was a positively sanctioned act for the middle-aged and elderly and these suicides were often of an altruistic kind, intended magically to protect sick infants. Nowadays, the suicide pattern has changed to include young Eskimos (Kraus, 1971). In rural Africa, where the original social structure has been preserved, the suicide rate is low, as reported for the Tallensi (Fortes and Meyer, 1967) and for rural Uganda (Orley, 1970). Suicide is not recorded among present-day hunter-gatherers in Africa, the Bushmen, according to Truswell and Hansen (1976).

Unconscious Self-Destruction

Subintentional self-destruction is present among Aboriginals. Self-destruction is a likely factor in drinking, since drunkenness is widely known among Aboriginals to be a risky condition, especially while visiting white towns on drinking holidays. Some men seem indifferent as to whether they live or die, and they drink so excessively that death is likely. It is common for Aboriginals to be admitted to hospitals comatose from alcohol. For example, one man was found comatose in a drinking camp on the outskirts of the town. He died soon after admission with a high level of blood alcohol. One day later his tribal "brother" and drinking companion was admitted from the same camp in the same condition. He died some days later. Another alarmingly common form of risk-taking ends in the death of pedestrians while drunk at night. In white towns this risk is also well recognized and much feared, yet such deaths are a common occurrence; realistic precautions are rejected. Young men often recount with amusement how a motorist had to brake at the last moment to avoid them.

Explanations for this behavior are difficult to formulate. Risk-taking by young men is strongly inculcated in this culture. In precontact days they were the warriors, and a high proportion were killed in skirmishes (Warner, 1937). In those times this behavior facilitated polygamy.

Explaining the Low Risk of Overt Suicide

From his work in Brazil, Stainbrook (1954) listed four factors to account for a low incidence of suicide among preliterate peoples. These are an extended family pattern, elaborate mourning rituals, culturally patterned outlets for hostility, and esteem-sustaining roles for all age groups. The first three of these factors certainly operate among Aboriginals. The family is extended, with the clan as the basis of social organization; mourning rituals are the most complex rites regularly performed; culturally patterned outlets for hostility are found in the belief in sorcery and in the "payback" principle to avenge clan deaths. The belief system also protects against overt suicide. The death of an adult is regarded as diminishing the strength of the clan as a whole, and it must be avenged. Aboriginals still expect revenge to be exacted from a traditionally hostile clan after their death; this will be a just retribution for their own. An act of overt self-destruction will run counter to this belief and counter to the talion principle of "a life for a life."

The generalized conception of the locus of control as external to the self is fundamental to these beliefs. An orientation of externality, as opposed to internality (Rotter, 1975), attributes the cause of death always to others, never to the person himself. This orientation helps to explain why Aboriginals readily participate in activities that they themselves regard as dangerous, and that expose them to increased risk of accidental death. To them, causes of danger are entirely external and the individual can do little to influence them—his own actions do not count. Perhaps the certainty that their soul will return to clan territory, whence it can animate successive generations of clansmen, contributes.

Sardonic Death, A Quasi-Suicidal Act

A middle-aged man of traditional orientation suffered from chronic obstructive airways disease. When pneumonia supervened, he was hospitalized in Darwin. He insisted on taking his discharge, against medical advice, saying he wished to visit relatives at another township. There he disregarded his strict and clear instructions to take antibiotics. When he returned home he claimed that he was dead, that his soul had already returned to its traditional territory (the clan's hunting range), that he was animated only by ancestral spirits. Death followed in 2 weeks. Although there was certainly a nihilistic, resigned flavor to his statements, there were no other depressive symptoms.

This case calls attention again to the possibility of less explicit forms of suicide, much influenced by cultural suppositions. It was found that customs were still extant that hastened the deaths of certain elderly people and with which the victims were in tacit agreement. These have been commented on among other native peoples as well (Murphy, 1976). These deaths fall outside the Western classification of deaths as either natural, accidental, suicidal, or homicidal. In fact, they have elements of both suicide and homicide. These are referred to here as sardonic death.

The term *sardonic* derives from the Roman accounts of the Sards, who pushed their elderly over the cliffs of Sardinia. They then laughed, according to these accounts, "sardonically." The Aboriginals may not laugh after hastening the death of one of their elderly or enfeebled, but they do enjoy the funeral ceremonies, particularly the festival of dancing. More importantly, the funeral ceremonies are seen as a revitalization of the corporate clan spirit, the life force for all the surviving members. They respond with a mild euphoria, reversing the apathy of the institutionalized town life. The morale of the clan is greatly enhanced and the psychological importance of the practice lies in this aspect.

Warner (1937) noted a process of "mortification" prior to deaths in North Australia and attributed it to the person becoming "socially dead." The withdrawal of social support is the most obvious feature of these deaths. Relatives who previously sat close to the elderly person move back to a distance of 10 or 20 yards and commence funeral rites while the person is still conscious and alert. No one approaches the mortified person, who accepts his fate without protest, even cooperating with it (Warner, 1937). The water container is taken away and physical death occurs rapidly, presumably from dehydration in this region of high ambient temperatures. Jones (1972) mentioned similar deaths in the

Western Desert and implicated dehydration as the cause. Death occurs in 36 to 48 hours, about the time necessary for dehydration and electrolyte imbalance to take effect.

On the other hand, the psychological isolation and the suggestion implicit in the commencement of the funeral rites is perhaps equally lethal. This effect should not be underestimated. The quasi-suicidal aspect of the practice is illustrated by the finding that four of the mortified persons observed by the field teams were physically capable of walking for water when their funeral rites began. Another died without protest in a room possessing a water tap. In these deaths where the person accepts his fate, one can again discern the powerful influence of the externally perceived locus of control. Death is the decision of others and the individual must accept it—it is totally beyond his control.

This practice is also noted when a patient is dying from a physical illness. Water and food are withheld when the person is judged to be near death, health workers about to administer injections are turned away, and the singers and dancers begin before actual death. Very occasionally, the patient's compliance is misjudged. Mourners were foregathered around one old man, who sat up and dismissed them. One patient described below (case 6) was saved on one occasion by the use of phenothiazine medication. He succumbed to "singing" a year later.

Maku was an elderly widow of indeterminate age. She was hospitalized at Yirrkala clinic with a chronic disease, probably tuberculosis. The following report was given by the white nurse: "One morning an old woman appeared at the clinic and said she dreamed she was going to die. She brought singers and dancers who began outside. From that time she was not given food or water, and we were asked not to help her. But this meant that everything I learned as a nurse had to be put aside. We spoke sharply to the Aboriginal nurses to make them attend her. Larrinyin [the senior Aboriginal nursing assistant] agreed with me about helping her—she knew what to do to make people comfortable. But once our backs were turned she did what the old men ordered. She did not turn up for work the next day. The old woman's tongue was misshapen from dehydration and she died the next day. Her body lay in the camp for four days while they sang and danced. Then all her belongings were put on the bed and everything was burnt, and all the relatives left for the bush."

Cases of Sardonic Death, 1971–1975, North Australia (Eastern Area)

The following is a list from field team records of six old or infirm persons who died under similar circumstances.

1. Y.—Female, about 70 years old, widow; town: Galiwinku; physical illness: mild intermittent diarrhea.
2. M.—Female, about 75 years old, widow; town: Galiwinku; physical illness: mild diarrhea.
3. W.—Female, about 60 years old, widow; town: Galiwinku; no
   physical illness: relatives said, "Time for her to die."
4. Me.—Female, about 60 years old, widow; town: Galiwinku; blind.
5. B.—Male, about 85 years old, widower; town: Galiwinku; senile.
6. Ma.—Male, 35 years old, single; town: Yirrkala; physical illness:
   brain stem hemorrhage.

The Relevant Beliefs

In terms of the Aboriginal mores, all these individuals were without
value to society; they were dependent consumers of the products of the
food quest and their presence disrupted daily foraging. With the advent
of the white economy, this reasoning no longer applies; at the time of
their deaths all were recipients of some form of social welfare payment,
which was shared among relatives. The explanation for their being
"sung to death" must therefore be sought in the adherence to traditional
practices. The belief system dictates that "social death" may precede
actual physiological death, once the spirit or vital essence is displaced
from the body. In sardonic death, the spirit that is held weakly in place
by an enfeebled body is dislodged by the power of the mortuary rites
and is dispatched to its ancestral home. The spirit of a clansman that has
properly returned to the clan territory is not lost but will be reincarnated
through future generations; it is important to ensure its proper return for
future use.

A relevant insight into Aboriginal attitudes to death comes from the
Dance of the Lone Crow, which is regularly a feature of funeral rites.
This was formerly construed as an invocation to the crow's scavenging
capabilities, because bodies were left exposed on platforms in the bush.
Hiatt (1976) interprets the festive dance as expressing "What's all this
fuss about?"—a message that death is part of the natural order.

Cross-Cultural Parallels

Murphy (1976) quoted W. H. Rivers (1926), who described a very
similar set of attitudes and practices in parts of Melanesia. Senile elders
were regarded "as if dead" and deprived of their rights and were then
buried while still alive. The Eskimos also practiced senilicide (Balikci,
1968). Balikci (1968) concluded that "the unproductive members of society were eliminated and the size of the family adjusted to the capacity of

the provider, and the survival of future hunters is maximized." Similar demographic controls were evidently necessary in the harsh North Australian environment. Yet J. Woodburn (1968) specifically warns of the danger of explaining the abandonment of the old and the lame in hunting societies as solely the result of ecological pressures. Adherence to cultural attitudes is also important since these old people nowadays contribute usefully to the family income through their welfare checks.

CONCLUSION

Cultural definitions of reality vary. Psychological illnesses, which are intimately related to a culture's perception of reality, also differ from group to group. In any study, we must use our Western classificology scheme cautiously and never forget that our own theoretical persuasions are also relative. The results of the study that has been reported here gain their validity, it is hoped, from the care with which these precepts were followed.

REFERENCES

Balikci, A., 1968, The Netsilik Eskimo. Adaptive processes, in "Man the Hunter" (R. B. Lee and I. de Vore, eds.), Aldine, Chicago.
Beiser, M., Ravel, J. M., Collomb, H., and Egelhoff, B. A., 1972, Assessing psychiatric disorder among the Serer of Senegal, *J. Nerv. Ment. Dis.* 154:142.
Berndt, R. M., and Berndt, C. H., 1951, The concept of abnormality in an Australian society, in "Psychoanalysis and Culture" (G. B. Wilbur and W. Muensterberger, eds.), International Universities Press, New York.
Burton-Bradley, B. G., 1975, "Stone Age Crisis: A Psychiatric Appraisal," Vanderbilt University Press, Nashville.
Burton-Bradley, B. G., 1978, Correspondence, *Br. J. Psychiatry* 133:282.
Carothers, J. C., 1953, "The African Mind in Health and Disease: A Study in Ethnopsychiatry," W.H.O. Monograph Series, Geneva.
Cawte, J. E., 1964, Australian ethnopsychiatry in the field: A sampling from North Kemberley, *Med. J. Aust.* 1:467.
Cawte, J. E., 1972, "Poor, Cruel and Brutal Nations," University of Hawaii Press, Honolulu.
Draguns, J., 1973, Comparisons of psychopathology across cultures, *J. Cross-Cultural Psychol.* 4:9.
Durkheim, E., 1893, "Le Suicide," Routledge and Kegan Paul, London. (Translated, 1952.)
Eastwell, H. D., 1976, Associative illness among Aboriginals, *Aust. N.Z. J. Psychiatry* 10:89.
Eastwell, H. D., 1978, Projective and identificatory illnesses, among ex-hunter gatherers, *Psychiatry* 40:330.
Fortes, M., and Meyer, D. G., 1967, Psychoses and social change among the Tallensi of Northern Ghana, *Transcult. Psychiatr. Res.* 3:19.
Freedman, A. M., Kaplan, H. I., and Saddock, B. J. (eds.), 1975, "Comprehensive Textbook of Psychiatry," Williams and Wilkins, Baltimore.
Gralnick, A., 1942, Folie á deux. The psychosis of association, *Psychiatr. Q.* 16:230.

Hiatt, L. R., 1976, Burara obsequies, Presented at the Biennial Conference of the Australian Institute of Aboriginal Studies, Canberra, May 1976.

Hipler, A., 1974, The North Alaska Eskimos: A culture and personality perspective, *Am. Ethnologist* 1:449.

Hipler, A., 1978, A culture and personality perspective of the Yolngu in East Central Arnhemland, *J. Psychol. Anthropol.* 1:221.

Jones, I. H., 1972, Psychiatric disorders among Aborigines of the Australian Western Desert, *Soc. Sci. Med.* 6:263.

Jones, I. H., 1978, Severe illnesses with anxiety following a reported magical act on an Australian, *Med. J. Aust.* 2:93.

Kidson, M. A., 1967, Psychiatric disorders in the Walbiri, Central Australia, *Aust. N.Z. J. Psychiatry* 1:14.

Kidson, M. A., and Jones, I. H., 1968, Psychiatric disorders among the Aborigines of the Australian Western Desert, *Arch. Gen. Psychiatry* 19:413.

Kiev, A., 1972, "Transcultural Psychiatry," Penguin Books, Middlesex.

Kraus, R., 1971, Suicide among Bavadian Eskimos, *Transcult. Psychiatr. Res.* 8:24.

Malinowski, B., 1922, Argonauts of the Western Pacific," Routledge, London.

Meggitt, M. J., 1962, "Desert People," Angus and Robertson, Sydney.

Money, J., Cawte, J., Bianchi, G., and Nurcombe, B., 1970, Sex training and traditions in Arnhem Land, *Br. J. Med. Psychol.* 43:383.

Morice, R. D., 1976, The language of psychiatry in a preliterate speech community. Unpublished M.D. thesis, University of New South Wales, Sydney.

Morice, R. D., 1978, Psychiatric diagnosis in a transcultural setting, *Br. J. Psychiatry* 132:87.

Murphy, J. M., 1976, Psychiatric labelling and cross-cultural perspective. *Science* 191:109.

Murphy, J. M., and Leighton, A. H., 1965, Native conceptions of psychiatric disorders, *in* "Approaches to Cross-Cultural Psychiatry" (J. M. Murphy and A. H. Leighton, eds.), Cornell University Press, Ithaca.

Nurcombe, G., and Cawte, J., 1967, Patterns of behaviour disorder amongst the children of an Aboriginal population, *Aust. N.J. J. Psychiatry* 1:119.

Orley, J. H., 1970, "Culture and Mental Illness: A Study from Uganda," East African Publishing House, Nairobi.

Rotter, J. B., 1975, Some problems and misconceptions related to the construct of reinforcement, *J. Consult. Clin. Psychol.* 43:56.

Stainbrook, E., 1954, A cross-cultural evaluation of depressive reactions, *in* "Depression" (P. Hock and J. Zubin, eds.), Grune and Stratten, New York.

Truswell, A. S., and Hansen, J. D., 1976, Medical research among the Kung, *in* "Kalahari Hunter-Gatherers" (R. B. Lee and I. DeVore, eds.), Harvard University Press, Cambridge.

Warner, W. L., 1937, "A Black Civilization," Harper, New York.

Waterman, R. A., and Waterman, P. P., 1970, Directors of cultural change in Aboriginal Arnhem Land, *in* "Diprotodont to Detribalization" (A. R. Pilling and R. A. Waterman, eds.), Michigan State University Press, East Lansing.

Waxler, N., 1974, Culture and mental illness: A social labelling perspective, *J. Nerv. Ment. Dis.* 159:379.

Webb, T. T., 1934, The Aborigines of East Arnhem Land, "Ninth Methodist Laymens' Memorial Lecture," The Methodist Laymen's Missionary Movement, Melbourne.

Williamson, M. H., 1979, Who does what to Sago? *Oceania* 49:210.

Wittkower, E. D., and Dubreuil, G., 1968, Cultural factors in mental illness, *in* "The Study of Personality" (E. Norbeck, D. Price-Williams, and W. McCard, eds.), Holt, Rinehart & Winston, New York.

Woodburn, J., 1968, Discussion Part 2, in "Man the Hunter" (R. B. Lee and I. de Vore, eds.), Aldine, Chicago.
World Health Organization, 1960, Epidemiology of Mental Disorder. Technical Report Series No. 185, Geneva.
World Health Organization, 1967, Manual of the International Statistical Classification of Diseases, Injuries and Causes of Death, Geneva.
Yap, P. M., 1974, "Comparative Psychiatry," University of Toronto Press, Toronto.

15

Atypical Cycloid Psychoses

KAY REDFIELD JAMISON

Summer and winter, and pleasure and pain
And everything everywhere in God's reign,
They end, and anon they begin again:
Wane and wax, wax and wane:
Over and over and over amain
End, ever end, and begin again—
End, ever end, and forever and ever begin again!

Herman Melville

OVERVIEW

Atypical cycloid psychoses are fascinating to clinical scientists for a number of reasons: They reflect the extremes in human moods, they tend to recur, and they almost always remit. As we shall see in discussing the nature and treatment of these atypical psychotic mood disorders, recent advances in psychobiological research make difficult the notion of "typical" or "atypical." Are syndromes atypical because their clinical presentations are unusual, because their response to treatment varies significantly from the normal, or because their patterns of recurrence are either abnormally predictable or singularly unpredictable? In any event, most of the phenomena classified by earlier clinicians as atypical cycloid psychoses now would be regarded as variants of bipolar manic-depressive illness. Thus, rapid progression in the study of affective disorders has profoundly altered earlier conceptions of the extreme mood disorders. Important among these advances, and particularly relevant here, are (1) increasingly sophisticated diagnostic systems (Akiskal and Webb, eds., 1978; Spitzer *et al.*, 1978); (2) natural history studies that overwhelmingly

KAY REDFIELD JAMISON • University of California at Los Angeles, Affective Disorders Clinic, Department of Psychiatry, UCLA School of Medicine, Los Angeles, California.

support the recurrent nature of the affective disorders (Angst and Grof, 1976; Zis and Goodwin, 1979); (3) the use of lithium for diagnostic and taxonomic purposes, and as a therapeutic agent (Dunner and Fieve, 1978); and (4) studies of the relationship between biological rhythms and affective illness (Wehr and Goodwin, 1978).

For the purposes of this chapter, we will limit our discussion of atypical cycloid psychoses to those falling within the affective range; atypical schizophrenias and schizoaffective disorders are covered in Chapter 16. We shall assume that, in many respects, we are not talking about atypical or extraordinary symptoms so much as we are about extraordinary phasing, patterning, or periodicities of a group of mood disorders.

HISTORICAL PERSPECTIVES

Severe, cyclic disorders of mood were observed and described by ancient poets and physicians such as Homer, Plutarch, and Hippocrates. Although these writers discussed both depression ("melancholia") and mania in great detail, the occurrence of mania and depression in the same person was not systematically investigated until 1684, when Bonet described *folie mania-comélancolique*. In the 19th century Falret and Baillarger both described periodic disorders in affect, activity, and cognition, which they termed *folie circulaire*. Then, in the 1890s, Kraepelin published a monograph on manic-depressive illness in which he described patients in different stages of their illness and presented his view that these stages of mania and depression "represent manifestations of a single morbid process." Although the advances in the study of mood disorders have been remarkable since Kraepelin's time, his writings on psychotic disorders of mood remain unparalleled in the literature. He described, in great detail, the natural history and phenomenology of psychotic disturbances of mood. Likewise, he observed that "attacks of manic-depressive insanity may be to an astonishing degree independent of external influences." He and his contemporaries hypothesized several possible causes of the disorder (many of them based on arguments of periodicity) including "periodic disturbances of vasomotor innervation," metabolic changes, insufficiency of thyroid activity, autointoxication by "glandular" or "internal poisons," and abnormal behavior of the nerve tissue itself. Kraepelin, in addressing the issue of periodicity within the cycloid psychoses, also discussed the problem of taxonomy and, tangentially, the subject of typicality:

> The morbid form of manic-depressive insanity, as it has here been delimited and described, is composed of a great number of clinical component parts, which otherwise frequently receive a different interpretation. The starting point of this conception of the disease is formed by the doctrine of the peri-

odic, or, as Magnan named them, intermittent psychic disorders. This doc-
trine was elaborated principally by the French alienists. The attention of
these investigators was then directed to one of the most striking characteristics of our morbid group, to its tendency to multiple repetition in life. At
the same time it could not escape their notice that the return of the attacks
takes place sometimes in the same, sometimes in changing form. This experience led next to the separation of periodic mania and melancholia; then,
as already mentioned, the compound forms were again divided according to
their changing course into a series of varieties till they were collected later
under the name of circular insanity, which originally was valid only for the
continuous alternation of mania and depression.

Further experience, as it could not permit of the individual kinds of
circular insanity being regarded as separate diseases, has also taught that the
separation of the simple periodic forms from the compound cannot be carried through. (Kraepelin, 1921)

More recently, Kleist introduced the concept of *cylcoid psychoses,*
which he felt were neither schizophrenic nor manic-depressive in
nature; he did believe, however, that such psychoses were closely related
to manic-depressive insanity. Leonhard, whose diagnostic system and
clinical descriptions are presented below, developed Kleist's conceptual
work; his writing forms a natural bridge to recent research studies of
these disorders.

CLINICAL DESCRIPTION

Leonhard (1961) described a group of acute recoverable psychoses
that he, like Kleist before him, thought to be neither schizophrenic nor
manic-depressive. He divided these cycloid psychoses into three
subgroups: (1) *motility psychoses,* (2) *confusion psychoses,* and (3) *anxiety-
elation psychoses.* As we shall see later when we discuss modern diagnostic
systems for the affective disorders, there is striking overlap between
Leonhard's cycloid psychoses and the bipolar affective disorders. Here
we briefly present the nosological work of Leonhard with short clinical
vignettes from his case studies.

The motility psychosis, according to Leonhard, has a "hyperkinetic
pole" and an "akinetic pole," and, "whereas manic-depressive illness
affects thinking, affectivity and psychomotor activity in the same way,
motility psychosis is a pure psychomotor illness" (Leonhard, 1961).
Although Leonhard conceptualized the motility psychosis as an excess or
absence of activity, it is clear that many other features of bipolar illness—
including marked changes in cognition and mood—are present in his
case histories. He cites the lack of certain "classic" manic symptoms (e.g.,
pressure of speech), but modern diagnostic systems allow such absences
of symptoms as long as a sufficient number and type of other symptoms
are present; i.e., the Research Diagnostic Criteria and DSM-III, discussed

later, allow for considerable individual variance. Below are excerpts from Leonhard's (1961) case descriptions of the hyperkinetic and akinetic poles of the motility psychosis; interestingly, when presenting the akinetic pole, Leonhard notes that the major differential diagnosis would be the catatonias, many types of which would be now subsumed within the affective disorders.

"(Helga K.) . . . Her behavior was free and easy, and although she laughed she was also somewhat irritable. Later she expressed ideas of reference of an erotic kind and reported dreamlike experiences. She also claimed to have given birth to twins. She became even more disturbed, she took her bed to pieces, tore her underclothes, danced, sang and sometimes beat her head against the wall. A diagnosis of hebephrenia was made. On 27 February, 1960 she was transferred to our clinic at the request of her mother. . . .

On 15 March, 1960 I presented this patient at a lecture. At this time she showed the following clinical picture. She was smiling when she came into the lecture theatre and behaved as an equal of the nurse. Then she broke free from the nurse who wished to take her to a chair and ran past the benches with mincing steps, saying 'very many here.' When requested she sat down on the chair, not in the quickest way but made gestures to the lecturer and the audience. Scarcely had she sat down when she jumped up again, walked a few steps, turned back and then sat down for a few minutes. However, her hands continued to move and expressive movements of the face went on in a lively way. These movements partly consisted of laughing but partly were made up of other exaggerated expressions. Thus, she showed movements expressing attentiveness or astonishment in relation to some event in the environment or coquettish behaviour, or feigned indignation or some other psychic content. Although this play of expression for the most part appeared to be completely unfounded, it took place in a natural way so that there was no suggestion of grimacing. The gestures and the play facial expression fitted neatly together. After a while, the patient began to play with her legs and threw them about, so that one of her shoes came off and fell in front of a student. She ran to pick up the shoe but she did not put it on straight away. Instead she swung it around in a circle so that everyone expected she was going to throw it at someone. She was unable to put the shoe on because other movements interrupted her attempts. Finally the nurse was obliged to help her with it. Then she began to skip about, turned round in a circle and with a pathetic gesture said 'Shall I sing?' She was encouraged to do so and began to sing a popular song, but stopped almost immediately. She turned towards a student and shouted something to him but it was so poorly articulated that one could not understand what she had said. Then she turned away with almost a jumping movement, ..."

"(Irmgard D.) ... she again became quiet and withdrawn. She stopped eating and again began to talk about her morbid fears. She ran into the cellar and crept into a corner. On 24 December, 1959 she was readmitted to our clinic. At this time she hardly spoke at all but sometimes she shook her head almost imperceptibly. On one occasion she said 'yes' very softly but apart from this she said nothing. At the same time she produced no movements but sat motionless with a rigid facial expression. She did not look after herself so that she had to be fed and taken to the toilet. She was treated with cardiazol shock therapy but she only improved for one day after each treatment and then relapsed. At the beginning of February, 1960 I presented this patient in the lecture theatre. She sat stiffly on the chair and did not look up when questioned. She did not look round but only stared straight ahead. When she was asked to walk she did so slowly and held her body stiffly. On insistent questioning I obtained a few completely monosyllabic replies. When questioned her facial expression did not change and she did not move.

During February the inhibition gradually declined. D. began to speak and her posture and expressive movements became more lively. Finally her psychomotor activity was completely free and normal and her attitude was friendly and sensible. She was discharged cured on 14 March, 1960. When seen fourteen days later she was quite normal. She was back at work."

Leonhard characterized his second type of cycloid psychosis, the confusion psychosis, as affecting thinking but not psychomotor activity and affectivity. He differentiated excited confusional thinking from manic thinking by less distractiblity and more disorientation; pressured speech is shared in common by the two disorders (again, we shall later notice the striking overlap between current concepts of bipolar illness and the confusion psychosis). The other end of the pole, inhibited confusion psychosis, is characterized by a poverty or a complete absence of speech. In the clinical excerpts from Leonhard we again see the many mood and behavior changes, understated by him, which also accompany these disorders and parallel the affective illnesses.

"*Confusion psychosis:* Liselotte E., a commercial clerk, was born in 1920. She had always been sociable, cheerful, and well-balanced. She was also very musical. There was no known family history of nervous or mental illness. Her school record at the ordinary school and high school was good. She took up a commercial course and married at the age of twenty. During the war she was a bookkeeper, telephonist and interpreter."

(Leonhard then goes on to describe in this patient a recurrent, alternating course following the general pattern described above.)

"In 1947 she suddenly became very quiet. She was perplexed, anxious, taciturn and was scarcely able to produce a coherent sentence. She was, however, able to express the idea that other people had changed in their attitude towards her and said, 'It is all so comical.' She expressed the fear that she would be cremated in the fireplace. On 16 June, 1947, she was admitted to Clinic B. At this time her thinking, speech and motor behaviour were all retarded. The case notes mention the searching and questioning element in her mimic expression. After admission she lay in bed apathetically, her mood was depressed and she wept occasionally, but would later smile in a perplexed uncertain way. Only when she was spoken to in an insistent manner would she reply in monosyllables, saying that there was something going on against her and that the nurses behaved strangely. Two weeks after admission she suddenly began to speak confusedly and produced an incoherent pressure of talk. She was quiet and perplexed again on the following day and her verbal expressions were inhibited. After two days the inhibition of speech became more marked and led to mutism. She began to speak again ten days later but always in a hesitating manner. 'Everything is so comical, so many names, which are so well known to me, I do not see through it at all any more. They run about so much in black and make comical indications. . . . I must think about my relatives a lot. If I think of one someone sits straight up in bed; if I think of another, someone coughs; I do not see through it.' The psychosis died away with electro-shock therapy. Three months after admission her thought and speech had become normal. She had acquired insight into her abnormal fears and ideas of reference. She was discharged on 15 September, 1947."

In the anxiety-elation psychosis only the affectivity is involved; one pole is represented by anxiety, the other by ecstasy. Leonhard differentiates this from manic-depressive illness by stating that in the latter disorder patient affect is "cheerful or sad," and ideas of reference, extreme grandiosity, religious ecstasy are not present. However, much that Leonhard describes is quite typical of what would now be known as euphoric, expansive mania or paranoid, irritable, and dysphoric mania.

"*Anxiety-elation psychosis:* Wolfgang Sch. . . . was treated as an inpatient for the first time from 30, October, 1953, to 4 December, 1953. While on holiday, he became restless, anxious and later excited for no apparent reason. He was admitted to Clinic C. where he claimed he was a writer and that he had discovered the gift of hypnotism. He had also discovered the philosophers' stone. He made up many theories about Marxism and explained that he was stronger than Marx, Engels, Lenin and Stalin since they were frightened of dying and he was not. He wrote very much during his stay in the Clinic and made many political suggestions. He also wanted to help the other patients in the Clinic to get better and believed he had the ability to do this. He improved following cardiazol shock therapy but still showed some anxiety. On 4 December, 1953, he was discharged at his brother's request. The diagnosis at this time was schizophrenia.

After his discharge in 1953 his mood changed into one of anxiety which was associated with the feeling that he was being watched. This led him to the conclusion that he should renounce his intellectual work. He then became a forestry worker. After nine months, he felt well again and wanted to take up intellectual work. He took a position as a director of a home and shortly after this he married. . . . He was subject to mood swings at this time."

In summarizing his classification system, Leonhard noted that the three cycloid psychoses were characterized by being acute, recurrent, recoverable, neither manic-depressive nor schizophrenic, and bipolar (in that two contrasting clinical states could occur at different times). He also commented that these disorders were associated with good prognosis, and that the three subgroups were not "sharply delimited from each other, so that overlapping clinical pictures occur."

We have discussed Leonhard's taxonomy of cycloid psychoses and later will see how these illness systems were the precursors of modern thinking about bipolar affective disorders. Let us now briefly turn to an interesting subgroup of cycloid psychoses that are manic-depressive in nature but atypical in their periodicity. This is a group of patients with 48-hour manic-depressive cycles; other patterns of cycling are, of course, well known (e.g., mania in October, depression in May; 6-month cyclers; annual cyclers; 14-day cyclers) and will be mentioned later in the discussion of biological rhythms and affective disorders. For those patients with 48-hour cycles, the regularity and predictability of their mood cycles is so strikingly consistent that from both a phenomenological and a statistical point of view they are truly atypical cycloid psychoses. Bunney and Hartmann (1965) reviewed the literature on patients who had 48-hour mood cycles and found ten such cases in French, German, and Italian literature. The first patient was reported by Dömling in 1804; this patient had virtually uninterrupted 2-day cycles for 15 years and was described tersely as follows: "On the manic day the patient was gay and on the depressed day he was very depressed and had dull eyes" (Dömling, 1804).

For 10 months in a hospital research ward, Bunney and Hartmann

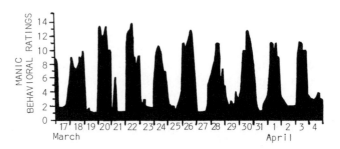

FIGURE 1. Study of a patient with 48-hour manic-depressive
cycles (from Bunney and Hartmann, 1965, p. 613).

(1965) observed a 43-year-old woman with a 2-year history of rapid, 48-hour mood cycles. Every 2 hours a nursing research team rated, on a 15-point rating scale, the patient's mania level during the preceding observation period. Figure 1 shows a randomly selected 19-day period during the patient's hospitalization. The authors describe below a typical 48-hour manic-depressive cycle, general behavior on a manic day, and general behavior on a depressed day.

"Description of a typical 48-hour manic-depressive cycle: A typical high day starts rather abruptly at 3:30 A.M. The patient awakens full of energy, ideas, and ambitions for the day. She gets up, starts to rearrange the furniture, and may start to type a short story. The manic behavior remains elevated during the day, decreasing somewhat in the evening. The patient usually falls asleep about 12:30 A.M., sleeps for an average of about five hours, awakens at 5:45 A.M., depressed, sad, and feeling guilty about the previous day's activity. She remains depressed throughout the day with an almost complete absence of manic behavior. She may nap periodically. Aspects of the manic behavior break through periodically in a muted form and account for the low-manic rating and the fact that the ratings are not at the 0 point. Also, manic ratings from 0 to 2 are within normal limits. The patient goes to sleep about 12:45 A.M., sleeps for three hours, and wakes again at 3:30 A.M. in a manic state."

DIAGNOSTIC ISSUES

Current diagnostic systems for recurrent, psychotic mood disorders rely upon a constellation of relatively clear signs and symptoms obtainable from a patient's history and mental status. Thus, the Research Diagnostic Criteria (and the DSM-III, which is largely derived from the Research Diagnostic Criteria) systematize many of the affective, cognitive, and behavioral symptoms we saw in the case histories presented by Leonhard (1961) and Bunney and Hartmann (1965). Specifically, these criteria require the *presence* of (1) a given *mood*, (2) a certain number or type of *behavior changes*, or *symptoms*, (3) a given *duration* for the episode (varying from a minimum of 1 to 4 weeks, depending on the researcher or clinician), (4) a *severity of disturbance criterion*, and (5) the *absence* or exclusion of other *preexisting psychiatric* and *medical problems* that occurred within a year prior to the onset of the affective episode. Table I lists the specific diagnostic criteria for mania and major depressive disorders.

One of the more recent, and the most empirically supported, classification schemes in the development of the taxonomy of the affective disorders is the unipolar–bipolar distinction (interestingly, first described by Leonhard *et al.*, 1962). *Unipolar* depression refers to a mood disorder characterized by depressions only; unipolar mania, where a patient has no history of depressions, exists but is a very rare disorder. *Bipolar* depression requires the occurrence of both depression and a hypomanic or manic episode. A large research literature exists that demonstrates significant genetic, biochemical, psychosocial, and biological differences between these two types of depression. Table II lists a few of these differences.

Diagnostic criteria for cyclic and other affective disorders are assessed during a structured clinical interview, which also inquires into family history of affective disorders, suicide, psychiatric hospitalizations, and alcoholism; current and past medical problems that might account for the same symptoms (e.g., thyroid disorders or illnesses treated with mood-altering medications such as steroids, antihypertensive agents, etc.); substance-abuse patterns; suicidal ideation and attempts; and many other variables of importance in a comprehensive evaluation.

The importance of taking a thorough affective and family history was well demonstrated by Carlson and Goodwin (1973), who studied acute, untreated manic episodes in 20 patients. They delineated three basic stages during the accelerating course of mania. Table III summarizes the affective, cognitive, and behavioral features of these stages. All 20 patients progressed through Stages I and II; 70% went through Stage III as well. Figure 2 shows the course of a single manic episode for one patient who experienced all three stages.

The acceleration period started with a mild hypomanic phase, progressed through a clearly disorganized and psychotic stage, and finally returned to normal behavior; it lasted about 3 weeks. In the course of their longitudinal behavior analysis, Carlson and Goodwin also found that the behavior of patients in Stage III mania was frequently indistinguishable from that of paranoid schizophrenics, although a positive history of affective disorder, good premorbid functioning, and a good

TABLE I. DSM-III Criteria for Manic-Depressive Illness[a]

Diagnostic criteria for a manic episode

A. One or more distinct periods with a predominantly elevated, expansive, or irritable mood. The elevated or irritable mood must be a prominent part of the illness and relatively persistent, although it may alternate or intermingle with depressive mood.

B. Duration of at least 1 week (or any duration if hospitalization is necessary), during which, for most of the time, at least three of the following symptoms have persisted (four if the mood is only irritable) and have been present to a significant degree.
  1. increase in activity (either socially, at work, or sexually) or physical restlessness
  2. more talkative than usual or pressure to keep talking
  3. flight of ideas or subjective experience that thoughts are racing
  4. inflated self-esteem (grandiosity, which may be delusional)
  5. decreased need for sleep
  6. distractibility, i.e., attention is too easily drawn to unimportant or irrelevant external stimuli
  7. excessive involvement in activities that have a high potential for painful consequences that is not recognized, e.g., buying sprees, sexual indiscretions, foolish business investments, reckless driving

C. Neither of the following dominates the clinical picture when an affective syndrome is absent (i.e., symptoms in criteria A and B above).
  1. preoccupation with a mood-incongruent delusion or hallucination
  2. bizarre behavior

D. Not superimposed on either schizophrenia, schizophreniform disorder, or a paranoid disorder.

E. Not due to any organic mental disorder, such as substance intoxication.
  Note: A hypomanic episode is a pathological disturbance similar to, but not as severe as, a manic episode.

Diagnostic criteria for major depressive episode

A. Dysphoric mood or loss of interest or pleasure in all or almost all usual activities and pastimes. The dysphoric mood is characterized by symptoms such as the following: depressed, sad, blue, hopeless, low, down in the dumps, irritable. The mood disturbance must be prominent and relatively persistent, but not necessarily the most dominant symptom, and does not include momentary shifts from one dysphoric mood to another dysphoric mood, e.g., anxiety to depression to anger, such as are seen in states of acute psychotic turmoil. (For children under 6, dysphoric mood may have to be inferred from a persistently sad facial expression.)

B. At least four of the following symptoms have each been present nearly every day for a period of at least 2 weeks (in children under 6, at least three of the first four).
  1. poor appetite or significant weight loss (when not dieting) or increased appetite or significant weight gain (in children under 6, consider failure to make expected weight gains)
  2. insomnia or hypersomnia
  3. psychomotor agitation or retardation (but not merely subjective feelings of restlessness or being slowed down) (in children under 6, hypoactivity)
  4. loss of interest or pleasure in usual activities, or decrease in sexual drive not limited to a period when delusional or hallucinating (in children under 6, signs of apathy)
  5. loss of energy, fatigue

TABLE I. (*continued*)

6. feelings of worthlessness, self-reproach, or excessive or inappropriate guilt (either may be delusional)
7. complaints or evidence of diminished ability to think or concentrate, such as slowed thinking, or indecisiveness not associated with marked loosening of associations or incoherence
8. recurrent thoughts of death, suicidal ideation, wishes to be dead, or suicide attempt
C. Neither of the following dominates the clinical picture when an affective syndrome is absent (i.e., symptoms in criteria A and B above):
   1. preoccupation with a mood-incongruent delusion or hallucination
   2. bizarre behavior
D. Not superimposed on either schizophrenia, schizophreniform disorder, or a paranoid disorder.
E. Not due to any organic mental disorder or uncomplicated bereavement.

*a*Source: American Psychiatric Association, *Diagnostic and Statistical Manual, 3rd ed.*, 1980.

response to lithium therapy did distinguish between the two disorders. Interestingly, no relationship was found between the level of psychotic disorganization during the acute manic episode and the level of functioning at follow-up.

Increasingly, good response to lithium has raised diagnostic questions about types of affective illness and their relationship to one another, and about other periodic psychoses, schizoaffective disorders, and the so-called affective equivalents (e.g., alcoholism, premenstrual depression). Dunner and Fieve (1978) discussed at length the impact of lithium on diagnostic practice and state that "lithium, more than any other psychoactive drug, has forced us to reconsider our diagnostic criteria. Lithium has already effected a revolution in American psychiatric diagnostic practice." Although it is beyond the scope of this chapter to deal with lithium's impact on diagnosis, it is interesting that many of the nonaffective illnesses for which lithium has been prescribed share in common a recurrent, cyclical, or episodic basis (e.g., epilepsy, recurring aggression, periodic catatonias, premenstrual tension). More directly related to our current discussion is the fact that the disorders once described as cycloid psychoses—typical or atypical—respond well to lithium (see Treatment section below). Thus, not only are signs and symptoms important in the determination of cyclic affective disorders, so too is medication response.

THEORETICAL PERSPECTIVES

Psychological and biological formulations constitute the overwhelmingly majority of theoretical work on cycloid mood psychoses;

TABLE II. Characteristics of Bipolar and Unipolar Patients[a]

	Bipolar	Unipolar
Clinical features	Retarded in psychomotor activity; postpartum episodes; lower ratings of anxiety and physical complaints	Agitated (sometimes retarded) in psychomotor activity; higher ratings of anxiety and physical complaints
Family history	+ Mania, + depression, + suicide + alcoholism, + 2 generations affective illness; mania in primary relative 4–10%	Mania, + depression, alcoholism + sociopathy; mania in primary relative. 29–.35%
Proportion female	50%	64–68%
onset	Average age *younger*, mean age of onset 28.7	Average age *older*, mean age of onset 37.3
Follow-up	Average number of episodes *more* (>3 episodes per lifetime); episodes last 3–6 months	Average number of episodes *fewer* (usually 1–2 episodes in lifetime); episodes last 6–9 months
Suicide	*Higher* rate	*Lower* rate
Socioeconomic status	Significantly higher educational and occupational achievements compared to matched unipolars	Significantly lower socioeconomic status
Divorce rate	Higher	Lower
Premorbid personality	(Perris): Active and sociable (Rowe and Doggett): Intelligent, shy, active, good judgment; *not* insecure, ambitious, thrifty, or promiscuous	(Perris): Insecure, obsessional, sensitive (Rowe and Doggett): Shy, conscientious, sensitive with good judgment; *not* insecure, intelligent, egocentric, or promiscuous
Biochemistry	Subnormal steroid output; low platelet MAO activity	Above normal steroid output; normal platelet MAO activity
Neurophysiology	"Augmenter" on evoked potentials; lower threshold for response to flicker stimuli; lower sedation threshold	"Reducer" on evoked potentials; higher threshold for response to flicker stimuli; higher sedation threshold
Pharmacology	Lithium carbonate-responsive; may switch to hypomania if on tricyclic antidepressant; lithium useful as antidepressant	Less likely to respond to lithium; more likely to respond to tricyclic antidepressant

[a]Based on Akiskal and McKinney (1975), Grof, Angst, and Haines (1974), and Winokur (1978).

TABLE III. Stages of Mania[a]

	Stage I	Stage II	Stage III
Mood	Lability of affect; euphoria predominates; irritability if demands not satisfied	Increased dysphoria and depression; open hostility and anger	Clearly dysphoric; panic-stricken; hopeless
Cognition	Expansivity, grandiosity, overconfidence; thoughts coherent but occasionally tangential; sexual and religious preoccupation; racing thoughts	Flight of ideas; disorganization of cognitive state; delusions	Incoherent, definite loosening of associations; bizarre and idiosyncratic delusions; hallucinations in one-third of patients; disorientation to time and place, occasional ideas of reference
Behavior	Increased psychomotor activity; increased initiation and rate of speech; increased spending, smoking, telephone use	Continued increased psychomotor acceleration; increased pressured speech; occasional assaultive behavior	Frenzied and frequently bizarre psychomotor activity

[a]Adopted from Carlson and Goodwin (1973).

often, of course, the two overlap and, in many instances, complement one another. Biological theories have been postulated for both depressive and manic phases of the cycloid process; however, within the psychological theories (other than psychoanalytic), few have addressed hypomania and mania—only depression has been discussed. Abraham (1942) was one of the first psychoanalytic thinkers to address theoretical aspects of manic-depressive illness. He contended that both manic and depressive episodes represented domination by the same pathological complexes and that only the patient's attitude during depression (concern) differed from that which occurred during mania (indifference). Abraham felt that the "circular insanities" derived from many sources: constitutional factors, fixation of the libido at the oral level, and injuries to infantile narcissism through disappointments in love. Freud (1917) thought mania a defense against depression and a desire to regress to an earlier state. Lewin (1950, 1965) also stressed the importance of denial in the promulgation of mania, and he, like Abraham, saw mania as a way "out," not as a way "up." He set forth the "oral triad of mania": the wish to eat, the wish to be devoured, and the wish to sleep ("The manic state proper,

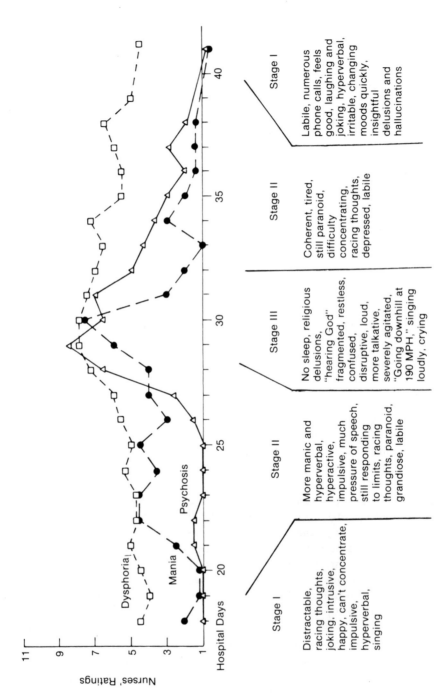

FIGURE 2. Relationship between stages of a manic episode and daily behavior ratings. Nurses on the hospital ward rated the patient's behavior twice a day on a global measure of mania. Additionally, they wrote down general observations of the patient's behavior during the day (from Carlson and Goodwin, 1973, p. 225).

with its overactivity and denials, is an attempted compromise between the wish to sleep and the wish to stay awake, i.e., to die and to live. The paradox of the manic's wakeful sleep is not in the formulation but in the conflict.").

Psychoanalytic theory has, as ever, an interesting, if somewhat idiosyncratic, view on the cycloid mood disorders. And although it is fair to say that these views do not represent psychoanalysis's finest hour (perhaps better reserved, in general, for the neuroses rather than the psychoses), it is noteworthy that many excellent biological researchers—including Bunney, Fieve, and Goodwin—were originally trained in, or strongly influenced by, psychoanalytic work. Many problems have arisen from psychoanalytic theories of mood psychoses: The most obvious one is scientific parsimony. There are now biological explanations (genetic and biochemical) that account for far more of the variance, more accurately and economically, and they are more readily testable. Other problems—for example, the psychoanalysts have generally equated mania with elation, ignoring the pronounced paranoia and irritability that often accompany manic states; too, they have not incorporated into their theories recent studies that demonstrate normal personality functioning in manic-depressive patients during euthymic periods (Hirschfeld and Klerman, 1979)—are important but not as compelling reasons for more recent emphasis on other theories of cycloid psychosis.

The psychological theories of mood disorders, briefly presented next, are useful and important as theoretical and heuristic contributions to the field, but they are highly limited in their explanations of manic behavior, the periodicity of these disorders, and the psychotic severity of the attacks when they do occur.

Personality theories suggest that individuals prone to develop clinical depression share certain maladaptive personality characteristics. The most frequently cited attribute in the psychological literature on depression is that of excessive emotional dependency (Chodoff, 1974). Predepressive personalities are thought to have a greater than normal need for love and approval from others. Secondary qualities believed to derive from excessive dependency are excessive envy, fear of competition, low self-esteem, and a lack of interest in or ability to deal with interpersonal nuances. This hypothesis has arisen primarily from intensive psychoanalytic studies of clinical patients, but it has not been validated by systematic studies using a large number of patients or control groups. Clearly, such a hypothesis relates well in a theoretical sense to the psychoanalytic separation hypothesis of depression, because intense emotional dependency can be a major consequence of early separation experiences.

In the case of bipolar manic-depressives, the literature suggests that between illness periods these patients have relatively normal and somewhat extroverted personality patterns. Psychodynamic theorists have questioned this judgment (Chodoff, 1974), however, and suggest that while these patients may appear normal on the surface, deeply seated problems of emotional dependency, derived from earliest parent–child experiences, still persist and are covered up until the next episode occurs. This is an interesting hypothesis, but difficult to test in the absence of prospective studies in which early life experiences are studied prior to the onset of depression; one would need to do "high-risk" prospective studies of depressive and manic-depressive individuals along the lines of current research with preschizophrenics.

Behavioral theories of depression conceptualize depression as the result of a substantial loss of positive reinforcement. Skinner (1953) explained depression as an extinction phenomenon in which established patterns of behavior, previously positively reinforced by the social environment, were, for some reason, interrupted. Relatedly, Ferster (1966) described depressed persons as people who evidenced fewer behaviors likely to generate positive reinforcement. He also saw depressed individuals as basically passive in their activities, that is, unable to act directly on their environments. Lewinsohn (1974) believes also that depressed behaviors elicit positive reinforcement in the form of concern, interest, and kindness shown by others, although several studies (Coyne, 1976; Hammen and Peter, 1978) indicate that, in fact, depressed people elicit many negative responses from those with whom they interact. Lewinsohn and his colleagues also postulate that a lack of social skills is crucially important in the development of depressive behaviors. Although they may be important in certain kinds of depression, the role of social skills in the more severe depressive disorders is unclear, and research indicates that the inability to socialize appears to be a state-dependent phenomenon. In other words, appropriate social behaviors appear to reemerge as the depression clears; likewise, studies of bipolar and unipolar patients that are conducted when the patients are not depressed do not show significant differences in social skills between normal persons and these groups. However, research does indicate that when depressed, individuals do elicit fewer positive reinforcements from others, show less social ease, and engage in fewer behaviors likely to result in positive experiences (Lewinsohn, 1974). Again, it is unclear whether these changes in behavior and reinforcement schedules cause depression or merely reflect it.

One very important aspect of depression is a sense of helplessness, the belief that no one can, or will, do anything to alleviate the fundamental problem. This sense of helplessness can be a reaction to an experience of loss in someone who has previously experienced the same sense of helplessness and who consequently has expended considerable energy to avoid a recurrence of that feeling (Schmale, 1973). The current loss may, in effect, challenge these defensive mechanisms and the individual may then experience the sense of helplessness once again. If he has never learned to effectively cope with this emotional state, it can precipitate a depressive reaction. Seligman (1974) has called this reaction "learned helplessness" and postulates that it grows out of experiences in which the individual does not have control over traumatic occurrences.

Beck (1967, 1970) has emphasized the role of a negative cognitive set, or negative way of thinking, as the core feature in depression. He postulates that a disturbance in thinking leads to a disturbance in mood (specifically, depression) rather than a disturbance in moods leading to problematic thinking. Individuals prone to depression, according to Beck, tend to have a deprecatory and pessimistic attitude toward themselves and, subsequently, toward other people and events. During times of stress these cognitive sets become distorted and lead to many of the typical thinking patterns associated with depression—for example, an unrealistic sense of duty and responsibility, suicidal ideation, severe self-blame, and indecision. Several types of cognitive distortion have been formulated by Beck and other cognitive theorists. Chief among them are overgeneralization, selective abstraction, and inexact labeling. Many studies have demonstrated that inexact labeling and other cognitive changes occur in depression; however, the theoretical issue of whether depressed moods precede or follow such alterations remains unresolved.

During the past three decades remarkable progress has been made in understanding the role of biological factors in depression and mania. In the early 1950s clinicians using reserpine to treat hypertension noticed that a significant percentage of patients receiving the drug developed moderate to severe depressions. Animal studies conducted during the same period found that reserpine depleted nerve endings of several of the important neurochemical transmitter substances, e.g., serotonin, dopamine, and norepinephrine. From a theoretical point of view, several criteria had to be met before assuming a biological substrate for disorders with such complex psychomotor, mood, cognitive, and behavioral manifestations (Goodwin 1977): (1) The biological substrate must have a complex, wide distribution in the brain; (2) it must be essentially integrative in nature; and, (3) it must be affected by drugs, which are known to produce changes in mood. Schildkraut's catecholamine hypothesis met most of these criteria in many important ways. In 1965 Schildkraut suggested that clinical depression is associated with a functional deficit of one or more monoamines in the central nervous system, and that mania is associated with a functional excess. He focused on the pivotal role of the catecholamines, although subsequent research has implicated serotonin (an indoleamine) as also important in depression and mania. Recently

Bunney *et al.* (1979) and others have stressed the probable role of a functional excess of dopamine, and a supersensitivity of the dopamine receptors in the CNS, in the manic process.

The amine hypothesis is supported by several kinds of clinical and scientific data. Mood-elevating drugs increase brain amines; for example, stimulant drugs, such as cocaine and amphetamines, increase amine function at the synapse. In the 1950s scientists noticed that pronounced mood elevation occurred in a significant percentage of patients treated with iproniazid for tuberculosis; iproniazid elevated brain amine levels by inhibiting the metabolizing enzyme, monoamine oxidase (MAO) (Kline, 1958). These monoamine oxidase inhibitor drugs have been used, of course, as antidepressant medications in the subsequent treatment of certain kinds of depression. The other major class of antidepressant medications, the tricyclic drugs, inhibit the uptake process by which the amines in the synaptic cleft are taken back into the neuron. This, then, increases the amount of amine available to interact with the receptor (Glowinski and Axelrod 1964; Mendels *et al.*, 1976).

Drugs that decrease the functional availability of certain amines (e.g., norepinephrine) can either cause depression (reserpine) or have an antimanic effect (lithium). A few of the pharmacological arguments for this amine theory of depression, specifically the norepinephrine theory, are summarized in Table IV.

There are several difficulties with the amine hypothesis. Drugs that act as stimulants in normal individuals are not generally therapeutic in patients with major depressive disorders; conversely, drugs that are therapeutic in depressed people do not have stimulant effects in normals. It is quite possible that a qualitative rather than a quantitative difference exists in the biological substrates between normal and clinical groups of individuals (Goodwin, 1977). Yet another problem with the amine theory is that it is difficult to understand how lithium exerts both an antimanic

TABLE IV. Pharmacological Evidence in the Norepinephrine Theory of Depression[a]

	Mechanism	Therapeutic
Tricyclic antidepressant	Potentiate norepinephrine (NE) by inhibiting uptake pump	Benefit depression
MAO inhibitors	Potentiate NE by inhibiting its destruction	Benefit depression
ECT	Increase NE synthesis	Benefit depression
Reserpine	Lower brain NE by decreased storage	Cause depression

[a]Adapted from Davis (1977).

and an antidepressant effect if it is acting largely on the availability of norepinephrine, although Bunney et al. (1979) present recent behavioral, receptor binding, and electrophysiological evidence that lithium can prevent the development of supersensitivity of dopamine receptors in the central nervous system. Of course, it is possible that many different mechanisms of action can cause similar effects in the central nervous system, and the amine hypothesis is a valid, useful (in terms of conceptualizing research findings and generating new hypotheses), but ultimately incomplete explanation.

Other biological theories of etiology have been proposed. The permissive theory states that an abnormality in two transmitter substances may be involved in depression (Prange, 1970; Kety, 1971). Like the norepinephrine theory, the permissive theory postulates that low norepinephrine is associated with depression and high norepinephrine is associated with mania. Additionally, however, serotonin levels must be low in both depression and mania. The two-disease theory of affective disorders postulates that there are basically two types of depressive illness, one based on functional deficits of serotonin, the other on functional deficits of norepinephrine. Some evidence supporting such a differentiation comes from clinical studies that have found that some patients respond better to those drugs exerting their primary effect on norepinephrine levels while others respond better to those drugs that affect serotonin levels (Maas, 1978; Asberg et al., 1976). Other biological theories have emphasized the role of membrane electrolyte balance and neuroendocrine function (Baldessarini, 1978). The hypothesized roles of neurotransmitters in the major biological theories of affective disorders are summarized in Table V.

Kramer and McKinney (1979), using a primate model, recently have suggested an interesting interaction involving neurotransmitter substances, psychosocial stress, and developmental factors. Monkeys were raised under different conditions—for example, some were raised by their mothers for the first 6 months and then with their peers, some were raised by their peers with many separations and some with few, while still others were raised by their mothers but then placed alone in a single cage at the age of 6 months, and so on. The monkeys then were tested under different psychosocial situations, such as in a single cage alone, in a group situation, or in a playroom with other monkeys. The dependent variable in the experiment was the dosage of AMPT (which depletes brain norepinephrine and dopamine) necessary to cause in each group of monkeys significant changes in huddling behaviors and decreases in locomotion. By their reasoning, the more AMPT required to produce these "depressive equivalents," the less vulnerable to depression, or depression-prone, were the monkeys. They found that mother-reared

TABLE V. Role of Neurotransmitters in Major Biological Theories of Affective
Disorders[a]

Norepinephrine (NE) theory of affective disease
  Depression = low NE
  Mania   = high NE

Serotonin theory of depression
  Depression = low serotonin
  Mania   = high serotonin

Permissive theory
  Depression low NE, low serotonin
  Mania high NE, low serotonin

Two-disease theory
  NE type   Serotonin type
  Depression—low NE, normal serotonin; no   Depression—low serotonin, normal
    specific theory of mania   NE; no specificity theory of
                                                     mania

[a]Adapted from Davis (1977).

monkeys required 4–8 times the dose of AMPT than peer-reared monkeys did to produce comparable effects on either social or separation
behaviors. Also, peer-reared monkeys with many previous separations
were more susceptible to the effects of AMPT than peer-reared monkeys
with few separations. Most strikingly, very large doses of AMPT (20–40
times as high as doses found to have behavioral effects in other groups
and situations) were required to alter the social behavior of animals
placed in a playroom environment, given that they normally lived alone.
These findings, although preliminary, are exciting because they attempt
to integrate the roles of biological, psychosocial, and developmental factors in depression.

The tendency for depression and mania to occur much more frequently in some families than in others has been observed by scientists
and physicians over the centuries. Kraepelin, using the limited scientific
techniques available to a 19th-century psychiatrist, was the first to study
the problem systematically. He found an affective "taint" in the parents,
grandparents, or siblings of one-third of his patients with mood disorders. When he examined the family histories of only those patients who
had *repeated* episodes of mania and/or depression, he discovered that
almost one-half of his patients had a significant family history of affective disorder. Biologists and psychiatrists have continued to investigate
the role of genetics in the etiology of depression and manic-depressive
illness. In fact, family histories are routinely obtained from patients sus-

pected of having an affective disorder in most clinical settings, particularly clinics specializing in mood disorders.

There are problems with the genetic approach. For example, the exact mode of genetic transmission in affective disorders is unknown but, of course, is assumed to be highly complex. Likewise, there can be many clinical expressions of the disorder, which reflects the confusing biological heterogeneity of the affective disorders. Too, depression and mania can range in age of onset from childhood to old age, which makes it difficult to rule out the possibility that a seemingly "normal" family member might in fact have a mood disorder but not yet have experienced its clinical symptomatology.

Virtually all of the genetic studies done to date indicate that bipolar illness has a very large genetic component and unipolar illness a much lesser one. Estimates of concordance for bipolar illness range from 70 to 100% for monozygotic twins, and 15 to 25% for dizygotic twins (Fieve, 1978; Klerman, 1978). The risk of developing manic-depressive illness is 15% in first-degree relatives, in comparison to the general population's risk of 1 to 2% for the same illness (Klerman, 1978).

One of the most exciting theoretical advances in the study of mood disorders centers on the hallmark of the cyclic psychoses—their periodicities and recurrent nature. Recent work by Wehr and Goodwin (1978) and others has focused on the biological rhythms of the affective illnesses. Because of its intrinsic fascination, and the relationship that the biological rhythm research has to the topic at hand, we present below extensive excerpts from Wehr and Goodwin (1978).

> Biological rhythms are involved in affective disorder in two ways. First, disturbances in 24-hour (circadian) rhythms of activity, sleep, mood, and neuroendocrine function play an integral role in the pathophysiology of mania and depression. Second, the long-term cyclicity of the illness per se is a pathological example of a biological rhythm. More specifically, some cases of recurrent affective disorder appear to be pathological expressions of normal menstrual, seasonal, or annual rhythms.
>
> The Hypothalamic Clock—It is now well established that all forms of life, including single cells, exhibit 24-hour patterns of variation in most aspects of functioning and that these daily oscillations are driven by endogenous, self-sustained clocklike mechanisms which persist in the absence of any environmental input. In multicellular organisms, the central nervous system provides the control and integration of circadian rhythms. In several mammals, probably including man, a hierarchically dominant central circadian pacemaker is located in the suprachiasmatic nucleus of the hypothalamus and drives daily rhythms in activity and rest, as well as rhythms in certain neuroendocrine and physiological parameters (Stetson and Watson-Whitmyre, 1976). When animals are kept in constant conditions and follow their own schedules ("free run"), the intrinsic periodicity of the central pacemaker is expressed. Under these conditions, each species demonstrates its own characteristic periodicity, deviating slightly from 24 hours. "Circa-

dian," which is derived from "circa" (about) and "dian" (daily), is used to describe these self-sustained biological rhythms with near 24-hour periodicity.

Pharmacology of the Circadian Clock—In general, hypothalamic circadian clock mechanisms are remarkably resistant to manipulation by pharmacological or physical agents. It is notable that the few drugs which can alter the behavior of biological clocks are quite familiar to psychopharmacologists. Lithium and ethanol markedly slow the intrinsic rhythm of the circadian pacemaker in experimental animals; that is, these drugs lengthen the period of the circadian rhythm in free-running conditions by as much as one-half (Engelmann, 1973). Estrogen, on the other hand, accelerates the rhythm (Morin *et al.*, 1977).

Tricyclic antidepressants have been shown to shorten the amount of time experimental animals require to resynchronize their rhythms with a changed environmental schedule; in other words, they accelerate the process of reentrainment after a phase shift (Baltzer and Weiskrantz, 1975).

Finally, chlorpromazine has recently been shown, in schizophrenic patients, to greatly increase daytime plasma levels of maletonin, a secretory product of the pineal gland which plays an important role in the genesis of circadian activity rhythms in animals (Smith *et al.*, 1977).

Long-Term Biological Rhythms and Affective Illness—Recent epidemiological findings (Grof *et al.*, 1974) emphasize that affective illness is recurrent. Some patients appear to have no particular pattern or periodicity in their recurrences, while others remit and relapse with clockwork regularity. As a group, affective patients tend to experience recurrences with increasing frequency as they grow older (Grof *et al.*, 1974). In those patients who do demonstrate some periodicity in their recurrences, it is unclear whether the illness is cyclic in its very nature, or if it has become linked with some normal long-term biological rhythm. In the former case, the illness would itself be a type of biological rhythm, albeit an abnormal one. In the latter case, the illness process would not be intrinsically cyclic but would be driven by a normal process which is intrinsically cyclic. Associations between recurring affective disorder and other long-term biological rhythms are familiar to clinicians. Occurrence of mania and depression in relation to the menstrual cycle has been described by several investigators, and as many as one-third of patients with frequent episodes may show an annual or seasonal pattern (Grof *et al.*, 1978; Faust, 1976). Psychiatric hospitalization for mania (Walter, 1977), use of electroconvulsive therapy (ECT), and incidence of suicide (Eastwood and Peacocke, 1976) have also been shown to exhibit seasonal patterns. These patterns in affective illness may bear some relation to seasonal and annual neuroendocrine and neurochemical rhythms recently reported to exist in normal humans. For example, thyroid hormones (Smals *et al.*, 1977), norepinephrine (Descovitch *et al.*, 1974), serum melatonin, and platelet serotonin (Arendt *et al.*, 1978) exhibit characteristic changes through the year. The role of the circadian clock in the genesis of seasonal and annual rhythms has been referred to previously. Thus, dysregulation of such a clock, already implicated in the pathophysiology of manic and depressive episodes, may also contribute to their seasonality.

The Circadian Activity–Rest Cycle—Continuous monitoring of the 24-hour activity–rest cycle has provided data for most of the basic research into the mechanisms which regulate circadian rhythms in animals. Recent technological developments have made it possible to continuously monitor motor activity–rest cycles in ambulatory human subjects (Colburn et al., 1976). We have studied 10 manic-depressive patients for periods of one to two years through both phases of their illness. Not surprisingly, activity levels and the duration of the active phase are greatly increased in mania compared to depression. Of more importance to our discussion of biological rhythms, however, was the finding that the phase or timing of the activity–rest cycle was advanced (shifted earlier) in the first one to two weeks of mania. Thus patients' daily activity phase began progressively earlier after the switch into mania. Some patients, two weeks into a manic episode, were arising shortly after midnight. Because of the progressive phase shift in early mania, the period of the circadian activity cycle was as much as one-half hour shorter than 24.0 hours; in other words, the circadian clock was running fast during the first week of mania.

Foster and Kupfer (1975) studied 24-hour activity patterns in unipolar and bipolar depressed patients and found abnormal increases in evening activity, which could be interpreted as a phase delay (later peak) in the circadian activity rhythm.

Neuroendocrine Rhythms—The 24-hour patterns of secretion of growth hormone, thyroid-stimulating hormone (TSH), adrenocorticotropic hormones (ACTH), melatonin, testosterone, and prolactin are each quite distinctive and have characteristic temporal relationships to sleep and time of day. There is an intricate sequence in which each hormone reaches its maximum levels, then gives way to another. The functional significance of this sequence and the mechanism by which it is orchestrated are poorly understood at the present time.

In summary, several lines of evidence support the clinical impression that disturbances in timing of circadian rhythms play an important role in the pathophysiology of affective disorder. The most salient feature of the sleep EEG in depression—decreased REM latency and early occurrence of the longest REM period—can be interpreted as evidence of a phase advance (earlier maximum) of REM sleep pressure relative to the time of day in which subjects are studied. Furthermore, activity–rest cycle monitoring indicates that sudden acceleration of the circadian clock to frequencies faster than one cycle per 24 hours is a characteristic of the first week of mania and results in progressively earlier morning awakening; interestingly, lithium might be expected to counteract this change by virtue of its ability to dramatically slow the rate of oscillation of circadian clocks. Neuroendocrine and neurotransmitter circadian rhythms also are disturbed in depression.

These and other findings suggest that the mechanisms which synchronize circadian rhythms with one another (internal synchronization) and/or with the environment (external synchronization) are impaired in affective illness and that some psychopharmacologic agents may act by means of their effects on these mechanisms.

TREATMENT

Given the wide variety of mood disorders—typical or atypical—it is not surprising that many different treatment methods have evolved for people with affective disorders. With the cycloid mood psychoses, problems still remain with the notion of "typical" and "atypical," although, as we have seen in earlier sections, this problem has been mitigated somewhat by more refined diagnostic systems. These systems, while allowing for a wide variation of clinical signs and symptoms within a given diagnostic class, require a specificity and homogeneity that make modern diagnosis of affective illness more reliable, valid, and prognostic. Lithium has affected diagnostic practice, and we shall spend most of the time in the treatment section discussing the tremendous impact of lithium on the treatment and diagnosis of recurrent psychotic mood disorders. The clinical use of the trycyclic antidepressants and the MAO inhibitors are well covered in the literature, as is the use of psychotherapeutic interventions.

Lithium, an alkali metal found in mineral rocks and water in its salt form, was used as a mineral water cure for mental problems at least as early as the second century. In the fifth century the physician Aurealianus used alkaline springs, now known to contain high concentrations of lithium, to treat both mania and melancholia (Fieve, 1977); however, it was not until 1949 that John Cade, an Australian psychiatrist, discovered and systematically described the antimanic effects of lithium. Evidence of its considerable effectiveness in the treatment of acute manic episodes (often in conjunction with the temporary use of phenothiazines and hospitalization), and especially as a prophylactic measure against recurrent manic and depressive episodes in bipolar manic-depressive illness, is quite convincing.

More than 60 studies in the scientific literature report the success of lithium in the treatment of ongoing manic episodes, with an estimated success rate of 70–80%. In acute mania and hypomania marked clinical improvement is seen within 3–14 days. Chlorpromazine, while sometimes useful in the temporary management of mania, has no overall effect on the actual course of bipolar illness (that is, it cannot prevent future episodes of mania or hypomania) and produces a more sedated and "drugged" response in most people. Controlled clinical trials indicate that lithium is particularly useful in treating the core affective and ideational symptoms of bipolar manic-depression, and that chlorpromazine is slightly more useful in treating the psychomotor symptoms of acute mania (Goodwin and Zis, 1979); haloperidol and pimozide, both dopamine receptor blockers, also have been shown to be useful in the rapid control of manic behavior and symptomatology (Shopsin et al., 1975; Goodwin and Zis, 1979).

The use of lithium as a prophylactic agent has been even more thoroughly documented than its use in the treatment of acute manic episodes. Prophylaxis, in this sense, refers to both the actual prevention of affective episodes (manic and depressive) and the early treatment of an episode resulting in a decrease in duration and intensity of symptoms. Methodological problems in this kind of clinical research are substantial, including the adequate definition of "prevention," the amount of time involved to determine whether or not prevention of episodes (highly variable in their onset and time course) has taken place, and ethical problems inherent in withholding a demonstrated effective medication from a control group at high risk for suicide.

Fieve (1977) and many other investigators have concluded that lithium is unquestionably highly effective in preventing recurrent mania or hypomania, quite effective (although less demonstrably so) in preventing and treating severe depressions in bipolar patients, and possibly effective in preventing and treating depressive episodes in some unipolar patients (particularly those who have no personal history of mania or hypomania but who do have a family history of bipolar illness). In a recent review of the literature, Mendels et al. (1979) found that 9 of 12 well-controlled studies concluded that lithium was an effective antidepressant, and that it was much more effective in bipolar patients but still effective in a significant percentage of unipolar depressives.

Lithium's effectiveness in other periodic disorders (such as severe premenstrual tension, periodic catatonias, recurrent aggression, and schizoaffective disorders) is still unclear (Kline and Simpson, 1975), but there are many ongoing research programs looking at lithium and other periodic processes. One of the most famous recent atypical cycloid psychosis patients (Jenner et al., 1967)—a man with 48-hour cycles of elation and depression, essentially uninterrupted and impervious to treatment— responded well to lithium therapy. This "atypical" manic-depressive, in fact, responded in a "typical" manner to lithium. Too, his symptoms were consistent with a diagnosis of bipolar illness; only the frequency and regularity of his cycles were atypical, again raising the issue of what defines "atypicality."

Despite the impressive ability of lithium to prevent recurrences of affective episodes in most bipolar patients, a significant proportion of patients appears to be resistant to lithium treatment. Studies of lithium failure indicate that 20–50% of patients relapse while taking lithium. For example, Angst et al. (1970) found a failure rate ranging from 31 to 64%, and Prien et al. (1973) found a rate of 31%. Stallone et al. (1973), in a large-scale placebo-controlled study, concluded that 50% of manic-depressive patients treated with lithium relapsed over a 2-year period compared with 90% of those on placebo. Methodological and interpretative problems make generalizations or conclusions difficult about failure rates across investigations. For example, a significant interpretative problem is the definition of "lithium failure," which can refer to failures in the treatment of acute mania, hypomania, or depression. Likewise, failure can reflect an inability to entirely prevent or, instead, to simply diminish the intensity, frequency, and duration of depressive or manic episodes. Studies vary in their success criteria from demanding no recurrences at all, to a set criterion of less than x number of episodes per unit time, to highly sophisticated criteria that measure decreases in severity, intensity, and duration and/or a significant improvement in functioning and relapse rate over prelithium treatment levels. For example, a patient who experiences eight episodes of depression and/or mania per year may, on lithium, experience only four. By some research standards he would be considered a lithium failure, by others a success.

Other problems of rate comparison include nonstandardization, or uncontrolled heterogeneity, of diagnostic subgroups. Further, in some investigations maintenance of a minimal lithium blood level or the systematic measurement of blood samples has not been required. Thus, undoubtedly, many patients categorized as lithium failures may well have been either noncompliant with the treatment regimen or medicated at a suboptimal dosage level. The probable overlap between lithium-nonresponsive patients and noncompliant ones has not been satisfactorily examined.

As noted earlier, several possible physiological and clinical correlates of lithium responsiveness have been posited. Studies of average event-related potentials (ERP) suggest that bipolar patients tend to have an augmenting response to visual stimuli and that such a pattern correlates with good lithium responsiveness (Borge et al., 1971; Buchsbaum et al., 1971; Baron et al., 1975). Low platelet MAO activity partially predicts lithium response in unipolar patients at a rate greater than chance, and possibly in bipolar patients as well (Goodwin et al., 1978). A few authors have attempted to relate diagnostic or clinical subgroups of affective patients to lithium response. For example, Murphy and Beigel (1974) studied response to treatment in 30 bipolar patients who had been categorized as "elated-grandiose" (75%) or "paranoid-destructive" and found that the elated-grandiose patients were significantly ($p < .01$) more likely to respond well to lithium. Johnson et al. (1971) found that paranoid thinking was related to lithium resistance, although Forssman and Welinder (1969) did not confirm these findings. A recent study by Krishna et al. (1978) did not find that paranoid thinking predicted nonresponsiveness to lithium. These authors suggest that such thinking may be associated with greater genetic penetrance and that, with this group, if lithium treatment is pursued, it is usually successful.

The majority of studies have found that the more clearly a patient fits the diagnostic criteria for bipolar illness, the more likely he/she is to respond well to lithium. Generally, the more schizoaffective features a patient exhibits, the less lithium responsiveness will be demonstrated

(Schou *et al.*, 1954; Schou, 1968; Grof *et al.*, 1970; Prien *et al.*, 1972). Other clinical factors that appear to correlate with poor lithium response include recent history of frequent affective episodes requiring hospitalization, a clinical history of rapid cycling often defined as four or more affective episodes per year (Grof *et al.*, 1970; Dunner and Fieve, 1974; Prien *et al.*, 1974), a positive family history of bipolar illness (Mendlewicj *et al.*, 1973), although this was not confirmed by Prien *et al.* (1974), and a previous history of lithium failure (Prien *et al.*, 1974). Both Prien *et al.* (1974) and Dunner and Fieve (1974) found that most lithium failures occur within the first year of treatment. Reviewing a sample of 200 patients in a 9-year study, Grof *et al.* (1978) reported that the clinical criteria of (1) diagnostic subtype, (2) quality of symptom-free interval, and (3) frequency of episodes preceding lithium treatment predicted lithium response at a better rate than did laboratory studies.

Nonresponsiveness to lithium treatment often extends to other pharmacological agents (e.g., tricyclics), and estimates of recurrence rates (a recurrence of symptoms within 6–9 months following initial symptoms) range from 12 to 79% (see Klerman, 1978, for a recent review). Recent studies of tricyclics either have not been conclusive or have appeared to cause additional clinical problems, e.g., inducing manic episodes through the use of tricyclics alone. More recent interventions have combined tricyclics and lithium, but the overall clinical outcome of this combination remains to be tested (Klerman, 1978).

To summarize, a number of clinical and laboratory studies over the past 10 years have increased the specificity with which response to lithium can be predicted, at least when relatively large samples of patients are investigated. These studies may be contrasted to the usual clinical method of treating individual patients, which is to prescribe lithium and observe a patient's response. Nonresponders are important primarily for related reasons: (1) Do they represent meaningful subgroups within this diagnostic category? (2) Can the nonresponders who are compliers be more precisely characterized so as to facilitate the early choice of the most appropriate treatment interventions? (3) How useful is lithium among patients who suffer manic and depressive relapses (sometimes classified as nonresponders)?

Lithium noncompliance is also a substantial problem; estimates of the extent of temporary or permanent rejection of lithium treatment range from 25 to 50% of patients on a maintenance regimen (Van Putten, 1975; Van Putten and Jamison, 1979; Jamison *et al.*, 1979). A wide range of explanations for lithium noncompliance (intrapsychic, interpersonal, and medical) have been proposed (Fitzgerald, 1972; Polatin and Fieve, 1971; Jamison *et al.*, 1979, 1970; Van Putten, 1975).

The mechanism of action of lithium is still not clear, although several hypotheses have been suggested. Lithium is thought to inhibit the release of norepinephrine and dopamine and to markedly influence the electrolyte balance across membranes, including neurons (Baldessarini, 1978), to stabilize the sensitivity of dopamine receptors (Bunney et al., 1979), and to slow circadian oscillators (Atkinson et al., 1975; Wehr and Goodwin, 1978). The latter phenomenon has been demonstrated in some rodent and plant species that have particularly pronounced biological rhythms (Engelmann, 1973).

Many patients with mood disorders receive several kinds of treatment at the same time; e.g., probably the most widely used treatment for depression is a combination of medication and psychotherapy (Klerman, 1978). In this section we shall examine this combined use of drugs and psychotherapy.

Large numbers of patients are treated with both drugs and psychotherapy for their mood disorders. Many individuals who are on lithium and/or tricyclic antidepressants are also seen in individual or group psychotherapy. The types of psychotherapy vary, as do the frequency (from once a month to those patients undergoing psychoanalysis four to five times a week) and the rationales for combined treatment (which range from well-thought-out scientific criteria to less rigorous, less rational, and more pragmatic reasons). The potential positive and negative effects of combined therapies have been discussed by Klerman (1975) and Weismann (1978):

Positive Effects of Combined Treatment. (1) A combination of drugs and psychotherapy may increase the effects of psychotherapy by making the patient more able to concentrate through the drug's capacity to reduce anxiety, improve memory, and restore normal sleep patterns. (2) Drugs can aid in increasing a depressed person's energy level, thus making him more amenable to interacting with other people and more fully able to participate in the psychotherapeutic process. (3) Psychotherapy may facilitate the patient's compliance with the drug regimen. For example, patients' refusal to take lithium is a common and important therapeutic problem.

Negative Effects of Combined Treatment. A combined treatment program may (1) lead to a focus on symptoms and drug side effects, rather than on a patient's behavior patterns; (2) encourage the physician to take the "easy way out" (drugs) and to become more of an authority figure, thus undermining the patient's motivation for active participation in the treatment program; (3) lead to increased anxiety and depression brought about by psychotherapy, thus counteracting the beneficial symptom reduction brought about by medication.

Advances in the diagnosis of recurrent affective disorders, coupled with the highly effective treatments available to people having such disorders, have made it possible to treat unipolar and bipolar disorders on an outpatient basis (Fieve, 1977; Daily, 1978). In the past several years clinics specializing in the treatment of mood disorders have been set up all over the world, particularly in Western Europe, Great Britain, and the United States. These clinics provide diagnostic and treatment services for people with primary affective disorders; they are often research and teaching facilities as well. Such clinics usually provide a wide range of treatments, including medication; individual and group psychotherapy; patient education about the nature of the disorder, prognosis, and information about medication; crisis intervention; family therapy; and referral to the hospital when it is felt that the patient needs closer supervision than can be provided on an outpatient basis.

REFERENCES

Abraham, K., 1942, Notes on the psychoanalytic investigation of manic-depressive insanity and allied conditions (1911), in "Selected Papers on Psychoanalysis," pp. 137–156, Hogarth Press, London.

Akiskal, H. S., and McKinney, W. T., 1975, Overview of recent research in depression: Integration of ten conceptual models into a comprehensive clinical frame, Arch. Gen. Psychiatry 32:285.

Akiskal, H. S., and Webb, W. L. (Eds.), 1978, "Psychiatric Diagnosis: Exploration of Biological Predicators," Spectrum, New York.

Angst, J., Weiss, P., Grof, P., Baastrup, P.C., and Schou, M. 1970, Prophylaxis in recurrent affective disorder. Br. J. Psychiatry 116:604–614.

Angst, J., and Grof, P., 1976, The course of monopolar depression and bipolar psychoses, in "Lithium in Psychiatry: A Synopsis" (Villeneauve, A., ed.), Les Presses de L'Université Laval, Quebec.

Arendt, J., Wirz-Justice, A., and Bradtke, J., 1978, Annual Rhythm of Serum Melatonin in Man, Neuro-Sci. Lett.

Asberg, M., Thoren, P., Traskman, L., Petrilsson, L., and Ringberger, V., 1976, Serotonin depression—A biochemical subgroup within the affective disorders? Science 191:478.

Atkinson, M., Kripke, D. F., and Wolf, S. R., 1975, Authorrhythmometry in Manic-Depressives, Chronobiologia 2:325.

Baldessarini, F. J., 1978, Chemotherapy, in "The Harvard Guide to Modern Psychiatry" (Micholi, A. M., ed.), Belknap Press, Cambridge, Massachusetts.

Baltzer, V., and Weiskrantz, I., 1975, Antidepressant Agents and Reversal of Diurnal Activity Cycles in the Rat, Biol. Psychiatry 10:199.

Baron, N., Gershon, E., Rudy, V., Buchsbaum, M., and Jonas, Z., 1975, Lithium carbonate response in depression, Arch. Can. Psychiatry, 32:1107.

Beck, A. T., 1967, "Depression: Causes and Treatment," University of Pennsylvania Press, Philadelphia.

Beck, A. T., 1970, Cognitive therapy: Nature and relation to behavior therapy, Behav. Ther. 1:184.

Borge, G. D., Buchsbaum, M., Goodwin, F., Murphy, D. L., and Silverman, J., 1971, Neuropsychological correlates of affective disorders, Arch. Gen. Psychiatry 24:501.

Buchsbaum, M., Goodwin, F., Murphy, D., and Borge, G., 1971, AER in affective disorders, *Am. J. Psychiatry* 128:19.

Bunney, W. E., Jr., and Hartmann, E. L., 1965, Study of a patient with 48-hour manic-depressive cycles, *Arch. Gen. Psychiatry* 12:611.

Bunney, W. E., Jr., Pert, A., Rosenblatt, J., Pert, C. B., and Gallaper, D., 1979, Mode of action of Lithium: Some biological considerations, *Arch. Gen. Psychiatry* 36:898.

Carlson, G. A., and Goodwin, F. K., 1973, The stages of mania, *Arch. Gen. Psychiatry* 34:1087.

Chodoff, P., 1974, The Depressive Personality: A critical review, in "The Psychology of Depression: Contemporary Theory and Research" (Friedman, R. J., and Katz, M. M., eds.) pp. 55–70, John Wiley & Sons, New York.

Colburn, T. R., Smith, B. M., Guarini, J. J., et al., 1976, "An Ambulatory Activity Monitor with Solid-State Memory," paper presented at the 13th Annual Rocky Mountain Bioengineering Symposium and 13th International Biomedical Sciences Instrumentation Symposium, Laramie, Wyoming (May, 1976).

Coyne, J. C., 1976, Toward an interactional description of depression, *Psychiatry* 39:28.

Daly, R. M., 1978, Lithium-responsive affective disorders: Model comprehensive plan for treatment. *N.Y. St. J. Med.* (1978):594–601.

Davis, J. M., 1977, Central biogenic amines and theories of depression and mania, in "Phenomenology and Treatment of Depression" (Fann, W. F., Karacan, I., Pokorny, A. D., and Williams, R. L., eds.) Spectrum Publications, New York.

Descovitch, G. C., Montalbetti, N., Kuhl, J. F. W., Rimondi, S., Halberg, F., and Ceredit, C., 1974, Age and catecholamine rhythms, *Chronobiologia* 1:163.

Dömling, W., 1804, Vermischte medizinisch-praktische Beobachtungen: Geschichte und Heilung einer sehr langwierigen periodischen und zwar dreitagigen Melancholie, *Arch. Med. Erfahr* 5:1.

Dunner, D. L., and Fieve, R. R., 1974, Clinical factors in lithium carbonate prophylaxis failure, *Arch. Gen. Psychiatry* 30:229.

Dunner, D. L., and Fieve, R. R., 1978, The lithium ion: Its impact on diagnostic practice, in "Psychiatric Diagnosis: Exploration of Biological Predictors" (Akiskal, H. S., and Webb, W. L., eds.), Spectrum Publications, New York.

Eastwood, M. R., and Peacocke, J., 1976, Seasonal patterns of suicide, depression and electroconvulsive therapy, *Br. J. Psychiatry* 129:472.

Engelmann, W., 1973, A slowing down of circadian rhythms by lithium ions, *Z. Naturforsch* 29:733.

Faust, V., 1976, "Biometeorologie: Der Fintluss von Wetter und Klima auf Gesunde und Kranke," Hippokrates Verlag, Stuttgart, pp. 118–145.

Ferster, C. B., 1966, Animal behavior and mental illness, *Psychol. Rec.* 16:345.

Fieve, R. R., 1977, Lithium: An overview, in "Handbook of Studies in Depression" (Burrows, G. D., ed.), *Excerpta Med.*, Amsterdam.

Fitzgerald, R. G., 1972, Mania as a message. *Am. J. of Psychoth.*, 26:547.

Forssman, H., and Welinder, J., 1969, Lithium treatment on atypical indication. *Acta Psychiatr. Scand.*, 207:34–40.

Foster, F. G., and Kupfer, D. J., 1975, Psychomotor activity as a correlate of depression and sleep in acutely disturbed psychiatric inpatients, *Am. J. Psychiatry* 132:928.

Freud, S., 1917, "Mourning and Melancholia," pp. 237–260, Hogarth Press, London.

Glowinski, J., and Axelrod, J., 1964, Inhibition of uptake of tritiated noradrenaline in the intact rat brain by imipramine and related compounds, *Nature* 204:1318.

Goodwin, F. K., 1977, Diagnosis of affective disorders, in "Psychopharmacology in the practice of medicine" (Jarvik, M. E., ed.) pp. 219–228, Appleton-Century-Crofts, New York.

Goodwin, F. K., Cowdry, R. W., and Webster, M. H., 1978, Predictors of drug response in the affective disorders: Toward an integrated approach *in* "Psychopharmacology: A Generation of Progress" (Upton, M. A., DiMarcio, A., and Killam, K. P., eds.), Raven Press, New York.

Goodwin, F. K., and Zis, A. P., 1979, Lithium in the treatment of mania, *Arch. Gen. Psychiatry* 36:840.

Grof, P., Schou, M., Angst, J., Baastrup, P. C., and Weiss, P. 1970, Methodological problems of prophylactic trails in recurrent affective disorders, *Brit. J. Psychiatry* 116:599.

Grof, P., Angst, J., and Haines, T., 1974, The clinical course of depression: Practical issues, in "Symposia Medica Hoescht 8: Classification and Prediction of Outcome of Depression" (Angst, J., ed.) Schattauer Verlag, New York.

Grof, P., Zis, A. P., Goodwin, F. K., and Wehr, J. A., Patterns of recurrence in bipolar affective illness," Paper presented at the Annual Meeting of the American Psychiatric Association, Atlanta, Georgia, May, 1978.

Grof, P., MacCrimmon, D., Raab, E., Saxana, B., Daigle, L., Varma, B. A., Werstierk, E., Blagchman, M., Fritze, K., and Murphy, D., 1978. Paper presented at the American Psychiatric Assn., Atlanta, Georgia, May, 1978.

Hammen, C., and Peters, S., 1978, Interpersonal consequences of depression: Responses to men and women enacting a depressed role, *J. of Abnorm. Psychol.* 87:322.

Hirschfeld, R. M., and Klerman, G. L., 1979, Personality attributes and affective disorders, *Am. J. Psychiatry* 136:67.

Jamison, K. R., Gerner, R. H., and Goodwin, F. K., 1979, Patient and physician attitude about lithium: Relationship to compliance, *Arch. Gen. Psychiatry* 36:866.

Jamison, K. R., Gerner, R. H., Hammen, C., and Padesky, C., 1980, Clouds and silver linings: Positive experiences associated with the primary affective disorders. *Am. J. Psychiatry* 137:195.

Jenner, F. A., Gjessing, L. R., Cox, J. R., et al., 1967, A manic depressive psychotic with a persistent forty-eight hour cycle, *Brit. J. Psychiatry* 113:895.

Johnson, G., Kershon, S., Beerdock, B. I., et al., 1971, Comparative effects of lithium and chlorpromazine in the treatment of acute manic states, *Brit. J. Psychiatry* 119:267.

Kety, S. S., 1971, Commentary, *J. Nerv. Ment. Dis.* 153:323.

Kleist, K., *Fortschritte der Psychiatrie* 1947. Frankfurt-am-Main: Kramer.

Klerman, G. L., 1975, *in* "Drugs in Combination with Other Therapies," (Greenblatt, M., ed.) pp. 67–81, Grune and Stratton, New York.

Klerman, G. L., 1978, Long-term treatment of affective disorders, *in* "Psychopharmacology: A Generation of Progress" (Lipton, M. A., DiMascio, A., and Killam, K. F., eds.) Raven Press, New York.

Kline, N. S., 1958, Clinical experience with iproniazid (marsilid), *J. Clin. Exp. Psychopathology* 19: Suppl. 1.

Kline, N. S., and Simpson, G. M., 1975, Lithium in the treatment of conditions other than the affective disorders, *in* "Lithium Research and Therapy" (Johnson, F. N., ed.), Academic Press, London.

Kramer, G. W., and McKinney, W. T., 1979, Interactions of pharmacological agents which alter biogenic amine metabolism and depression, *J. of Affective Disorders* 1:33.

Kraepelin, E., 1921, "Manic-Depressive Insanity and Paranoia," Churchill Livingstone, London.

Krishna, U. R., Taylor, M. A., and Abrams, R. N., 1978, Response to lithium carbonate, *Biol. Psychol.* 13:601.

Leonhard, K., 1961, Cycloid psychoses—endogenous psychoses which are neither schizophrenic nor manic-depressive, *J. of Mental Science* 107:633.

Leonhard, K., Korff, I., and Shulz, H., 1962, Die Temperamente in den famillien der monopolaren und bipolaren phasischen psychosen, *Psychiat. Neurol.* 143:416.

Lewin, B. D., 1950, "The Psychoanalysis of Elation," W. W. Norton, New York.

Lewin, B. D., 1965, Reflections on affect, in "Drives, Affects, Behavior," (Schur, M., ed.), Vol. 2. International Universities Press, New York.

Lewinsohn, P. H., 1974, A behavioral approach to depression, in "The Psychology of Depression: Contemporary Theory and Research," (Friedman, R. J., and Katz, M. M., eds.), Wiley, Washington, D.C.

Maas, J. W., 1978, Clinical implications of pharmacological differences among antidepressants, in "Psychopharmacology: A Generation of Progress" (Lipton, M. A., DiMascio, A., and Killam, K. F., eds.), Raven Press, New York.

Mendels, J., Stern, S., and Frazer, A., 1976, Biochemistry of depression, Dis. of the Nerv. Syst. 37:3.

Mendels, J., Ramsey, A., Dyson, W., and Frazer, A., 1979, Lithium as an antidepressant, Arch. Gen. Psychiatry 36:845.

Mendlewicj, J., Fieve, R. R., and Stallone, F., 1973, Relationship between the effectiveness of lithium therapy and family history, Am. J. Psychiatry 130:1011.

Morin, L. P., Fitzgerald, K. M., and Zucker, I., 1977, Estradiol shortens the period of hamster circadian rhythms, Science 196:305.

Murphy, D. L., and Biegel, A., 1974, Depression, elation, and lithium carbonate responses in manic patient subgroups, Arch. Gen. Psychiatry 31:643.

Polatin, P., and Fieve, R. R., 1971, Patient rejection of lithium carbonate prophylaxis, J. Am. Med. Assoc. 218:864.

Prange, A. J., Wilson, I. C., Knox, A., et al., 1970, Enhancement of imipramine by thyroid stimulating hormone: Clinical and theoretical implications, Am. J. Psychiatry 127:191.

Prien, R. F., Caffey, E. M., Jr., Klett, C. J., 1972, Comparison of lithium carbonate and chlorpromazine in the treatment of mania, Arch. Gen. Psychiatry 26:146.

Prien, R. F., Caffey, E. M., and Klett, J., 1974, Factors associated with treatment success in lithium carbonate prophylaxis, Arch. Gen. Psychiatry 31:189.

Prien, R. F., Klett, C. J., and Caffey, E. M., Jr., 1973, Lithium carbonate and imipramine in prevention of affective episodes, Arch. Gen. Psychiatry 29:420.

Schildkraut, J. J., 1965, The catacholamine hypothesis of affective disorders: A review of supporting evidence, Am. J. Psychiat. 122:509.

Schmale, A. H., 1973, Giving up as a final common pathway to changes in health, Adv. Psychosom. Med. 8:20.

Schou, M., Juel-Nielson, N., Stromgren, E., and Voldby, H., 1954, The treatment of manic psychoses by the administration of lithium salts, Neurol. Neurosurg. Psychiat. 17:250–260.

Schou, M., 1968, Lithium in psychiatric therapy and prophylaxis, J. Psychiatr. Res. 6:67.

Seligman, M. E. P., 1974, Depression and Learned Helplessness, in "The Psychology of Depression: Contemporary Theory and Research," (Friedman, R. J., and Katz, M. M., eds.) pp. 83–113, John Wiley and Sons, New York.

Shopsin, B., Gershon, S., Thompson, H., and Collins, P., 1975, Psychoactive drugs in mania: A controlled comparison of lithium carbonate, chlorpromazine, and haloperidol, Arch. Gen. Psychiatry 32:32.

Skinner, B. F., 1953, "Science and Human Behavior," Macmillan, New York.

Smals, A. G. H., Ross, H. A., and Kloppenborg, P. W. C., 1977, Seasonal variation in serum I and II levels in man, J. Clin. Endocrinol. Metab. 44:993.

Smith, J. A., Mee, T. J. X., and Barnes, J. D., 1977, Increased serum melatonin levels in chlorpromazine treated psychiatric patients, in "Abstracts of the International Symposium on the Pineal Gland," (Jerusalem), p. 75.

Spitzer, R. L., Endicott, J., and Robins, E., 1978, Research diagnostic criteria: Rationale and reliability, Arch. Gen. Psychiatry 35:773.

Stallone, F., Shelley, E., Mendlewicz, J., and Fieve, R., 1973, The use of lithium in affective disorders: II. A double-blind study of prophylaxis on bipolar illness, *Am. J. Psychiatry* 130:1006.

Stetson, M. H., and Watson-Whitmyre, M., 1976, Nucleus suprachiasmaticus: The biological clock in the hamster? *Science* 191:197.

Van Putten, T., 1975, Why do patients with manic depressive illness stop their lithium? *Compr. Psychiatry* 16:179.

Van Putten, T., Jamison, K. R., 1979, Rejection of lithium therapy by the patient. To appear *in* "Handbook of Lithium Therapy" (Johnson, F. N., ed.), NTP Press, Lancaster, England.

Walter, S. D., 1977, Seasonality of mania: A reappraisal, *Br. J. Psychiatry* 131:345–350.

Wehr, T. A., and Goodwin, P. K., 1978, Biological rhythms and affective illness, *Weekly Psychiatry Update Series*, 2:2.

Weismann, M. M., 1978, Psychotherapy and its relevance to the pharmacotherapy of affective disorders: From ideology to evidence, *in* "Psychopharmacology: A Generation of Progress" (Lipton, M. A., DiMascio, A., and Killam, K. F., eds.), Raven Press, New York.

Winokur, G., 1978, Mania, depression: Family studies, genetics, and relation to treatment, *in* "Psychopharmacology: A Generation of Progress" (Lipton, M., DiMascio, A., and Killam, K., eds.), Raven Press, New York.

Zis, A. P., and Goodwin, F. K., 1979, Lithium in the treatment of mania, *Arch. Gen. Psychiatry* 36:840.

16

Unusual Presentations of Schizophrenia

IRA M. LESSER

Through the years, the diagnostic criteria for schizophrenia have undergone many revisions, with the syndrome being classified in myriad ways. A listing of some proposed subtypes of schizophrenia illustrates this diversity: hebephrenic, catatonic, simple, paranoid, chronic undifferentiated, latent, process, reactive, schizoaffective, atypical, affect-laden paraphrenia, cataphasia, schizophasia, good prognosis, poor prognosis, systematic, nonsystematic, and oneirophrenia. At the other extreme, one is also confronted with a group of psychiatrists who deny the very existence of the entity called "schizophrenia" (Szasz, 1974).

Despite this, most clinicians would probably agree upon a typical presentation of schizophrenia, such as the following: an insidiously appearing illness, beginning in adolescence or young adulthood, featuring interpersonal withdrawal, poor social and work habits, a thought disorder with primarily auditory (not visual) hallucinations, and a gradual and progressive deterioration in all spheres of the personality, seen in an individual with a clear sensorium. The illness is chronic, the prognosis poor.

The situation, however, is far from this simple, and many varied clinical presentations are subsumed under the schizophrenic spectrum. Indeed, the history of medicine is replete with examples of illnesses that have been classified together on the basis of clinical symptoms but that over time have proved to be vastly different entities. In psychiatry, this may be the case with schizophrenia. The following disorders, while currently considered to be schizophrenic, may, with newer diagnostic methods, ultimately represent different categories of illness. These unusual

IRA M. LESSER • Department of Psychiatry, University of California at Los Angeles, Harbor General UCLA Medical Center, Torrance, California.

presentations need to be identified and studied because their treatment and prognosis can be significantly different from those of the classic syndrome.

Atypical schizophrenia (schizoaffective), *late paraphrenia, periodic catatonia,* and *oneirophrenia* are entities currently considered unusual subtypes of schizophrenia. They are of interest not only because they all differ from classic schizophrenia in significant ways but because they raise intriguing questions about the very nature of schizophrenic illness.

ATYPICAL SCHIZOPHRENIA

Atypical schizophrenia, also called "schizoaffective schizophrenia," "good prognosis schizophrenia," and "acute schizophrenic reaction," has a number of characteristics that differentiate it from classic schizophrenia: good premorbid functioning, acute or subacute mode of onset, presence of external precipitants, high degree of affective symptoms, good response to treatment, favorable prognosis, and family history of affective illness. When one looks at these various parameters, the similarity to affective illness becomes apparent, and thus the confusion as to the proper place along the diagnostic spectrum.

Typically, the affected individuals are floridly psychotic, manifest a thought disorder, seem to be responding to an external stress, and have a history of good premorbid functioning. Often, the psychosis has a marked affective component. The illness tends to remit rather quickly, and there may not be a second episode. If there is, the gross deterioration in personality noted in other schizophrenics is seldom seen. These patients may respond to treatment with lithium carbonate (Procci, 1976), whereas classic schizophrenics show a less positive response, if any. Studying their family history, one notes an increased incidence of affective disease, rather than of schizophrenia. The following case highlights some of these features.

Case 1. A., a 23-year-old single male, was brought to the hospital emergency room after 3 days of bizarre talking and difficulty sleeping. His chief complaint was that "the species cannot evolve fast enough and will die out." He manifested vagueness, thought control, ideas of influence, and looseness of associations. There were no disturbances in memory functions, and drug screens were negative. There was no prior history of any psychotic behavior. His family history was positive for depression in his mother. His father was an alcoholic. Several days prior to this episode, he had broken off a relationship with a girl friend. While in the hospital, he exhibited periods of depression alternating with mild hypomanic behavior. Psychological testing showed him to be highly intelligent, and to be using intellectualizing and obsessional defenses; there were no responses indicating a thought disorder. His hospital course was marked by rapid reconstitution with moderate doses of neuroleptics. Follow-up for 3 years revealed no further psychotic episodes, but periods of marked depression were present.

Comment

The diagnosis of atypical or schizoaffective schizophrenia is not as rare as it once was. This is, in large part, due to the proliferating literature that addresses (1) family and genetic histories, (2) a longitudinal view of the patient, (3) the course of the psychosis and patterns of remission or chronicity, and (4) a willingness to examine the strict manic-depressive/ schizophrenia dichotomy that was presented by Kraepelin (1919).

Procci (1976) reviewed the concept of schizoaffective psychosis and found solid grounds for distinguishing it from classic schizophrenia. However, he was less clear about the nature of its relationship to affective disorders, although he did note the many points of similarity. Others (Pope and Lipinski, 1978; Cerrolaza and Cleghorn, 1971) have noted that, as diagnostic acumen improves, some of the disorders that have historically been seen as schizophrenia, especially "atypical schizophrenia," may be reclassified as belonging to the class of affective disorders.

Therapeutic and prognostic considerations make it important to differentiate this entity from the more classic schizophrenias. Continuing to refer to this clinical picture as "atypical" schizophrenia adds to the confusion regarding diagnosis. The use of "schizoaffective disorder," as in the DSM-III (APA, 1978), is a step toward the clarification of this issue.

LATE PARAPHRENIA

It is generally accepted that schizophrenia affects younger people and rarely, if at all, makes its initial appearance beyond the age of 40. In fact, some research groups insist that, to make the diagnosis of schizophrenia, the symptoms *must* appear prior to age 40 (Feighner et al., 1972). Illness in the later decades that manifests psychotic symptoms is usually considered to be part of the affective disease spectrum or belonging to the psychoses of organic brain disease. However, since the time of Kraepelin, there have been various writings that describe the late onset of a psychosis resembling classic schizophrenia in all aspects except for its late appearance. In most cases, there is a definite paranoid flavor to the disorder. This has led to much debate regarding diagnosis, i.e., are such cases manifestations of paranoid schizophrenia, affective disease with paranoid symptoms (involutional paranoia), paranoid state, true paranoia, or psychoses of senility?

In 1919, Kraepelin described 1000 cases of schizophrenic illness and noted that somewhat greater than 10% presented after the age of 40. He acknowledged the difficulty in noting the exact age of onset in this insidiously appearing illness, but felt confident that there was a late-appearing subtype, most cases of which had predominantly paranoid symptoms. He attempted to divide paranoid illness into three distinct types: paranoid schizophrenia, which followed the deteriorating course typical of other schizophrenias; paraphrenia, which shared some symptoms with paranoid schizophrenia but showed less disorder of volition and emotion, and which did not demonstrate progressive personality or intellectual deterioration; and paranoia, which presented without hallucinations. He felt that, in the elderly, the illness was likely to take the form of paraphrenia.

Since Kraepelin's historic formulations, several workers have disagreed that the entities he described are, in fact, separate. Mayer (1921) and Roth (1955) have shown that, with long follow-up, paraphrenic patients become virtually indistinguishable from paranoid schizophrenics. However, they do not dispute the existence of a schizophrenic illness that presents in later life.

Roth (1955) studied mental disorders in the aged and has been a strong proponent of the concept of late-appearing schizophrenia, which he termed "late paraphrenia." He defined this group as presenting with "a well-organized system of paranoid delusions with or without auditory hallucinations existing in the setting of a well-preserved personality and affective response." He felt that the majority of such cases presented after the age of 60. Fish (1960) reported on a study of 111 female chronic schizophrenics and noted that 23 exhibited their initial psychotic symptom after the age of 40, with one woman presenting after age 60. He also cited the work of Manfred Bleuler who, in 1943, found that 15% of a chronic hospital population had onset after age 40, symptoms similar to earlier presentations of schizophrenia, and no evidence of organic brain disease.

Roth (1955) did a retrospective study of 472 patients, aged 60 and over, who were hospitalized prior to 1949. He divided them into five groups by using history and clinical presentation: late paraphrenia (as defined above), affective psychosis (admission based on depressive or manic-depressive symptom complex), senile psychosis (a gradual and progressive failure in everyday life with memory and intellectual deficits), arteriosclerotic psychosis (dementia associated with focal signs and symptoms of cerebrovascular disease), and acute confusion (rapidly evolving clouding of consciousness without definite dementia). On this basis, more than 50% were accounted for by the affective psychoses and about 10% by late paraphrenia. What lends credence to the separation of the late paraphrenic group from the others are the follow-up data. Between 30% and 50% of the senile, arteriosclerotic, and confusional groups had died within 6 months of admission, while only 2 of 46 late paraphrenic patients had died. Furthermore, a much greater percentage of late paraphrenic patients remained hospitalized, as opposed to patients with affective psychoses, who showed a high discharge rate.

The descriptive studies of late paraphrenia are in general agreement regarding the clinical presentation of these patients. The incidence of late paraphrenia among first psychiatric inpatient admissions over the age of 65 is reported to be around 8–10% (Slater and Roth, 1969; Kay and Roth, 1961; Roth, 1955). There is a striking preponderance of women patients, reported to be as high as 10:1 (Kay, 1963). There is a higher percentage of nonmarried women than is seen in other schizophrenias (controlled for age), and there also seems to be a large number of childless women even among those married (Herbert and Jacobson, 1967; Kay and Roth, 1961). A consistent finding has been the high degree of isolation, both social (i.e., from people) and sensory (i.e., secondary to deafness and/or decreased visual acuity). The hearing deficits seemed overrepresented in comparison to other physical ailments and occurred with greater frequency than in age-matched nonparaphrenics. Family history of schizophrenia has been estimated to be about 15–20% (Slater and Roth, 1969). Premorbidly, the great majority of people displayed characteristics of a schizoid, paranoid, querulous, and suspicious nature.

Clinically, the predominant findings are paranoid delusions of varying systematic organization, auditory hallucinations, some degree of irritability and excitability, preserved memory and intellectual functioning, and maintenance of orientation and lucid speech. The patients usually progress to some degree of affective blunting. The delusions quite often take the form of being spied upon, being listened to through walls or floors, and having devices implanted into one's ears for the purposes of control. The frequency with which such delusions occur in a population with marked hearing deficits is striking. It seems that the paucity of sensory and object-relationship input results in the delusions acquiring this specific form. This finding may have important treatment implications.

The course is usually a chronic and progressive one, with poor outcome in terms of the patient being able to live independently again. There is clearly a lower rate of medical hospitalization and a longer life expectancy than for patients with evidence of senile and arteriosclerotic changes. The preexisting sensory and social isolation contributes to the poor prognosis. The judicious use of neuroleptics and attention to the community treatment of these patients can increase the possibility of discharging them from the hospital (Herbert and Jacobson, 1967).

Case 2. B., a 61-year-old woman, presented with the chief complaint of "having a voice machine on my throat that causes me to hear voices of Frank Sinatra, Danny Thomas, and Jackie Onassis." These voices "tell me what to do and I have to constantly fight with them." They had begun 2 years earlier, and she obtained relief after treatment with neuroleptics. About 30 years earlier she had had heavy alcohol use, but she denied any current substance abuse. In addition to her auditory hallucinations and delusions, she appeared to be mildly depressed (but had no vegetative signs of depression) and had a blunted affect. She displayed no memory or cognitive defects. Her daughters reported that she had always been a difficult person to live with and had trouble keeping friends. She was divorced about 15 years prior to admission and, after the divorce, lived with her mother in an isolated manner. She remained aloof on the ward, often presenting an air of haughty indifference. She was treated with neuroleptics, which markedly decreased the auditory hallucinations, but the delusional system about the voice machine remained intact. Five years later she continued to live an isolated, lonely life and manifested symptoms of a thought disorder.

Comment

Most workers consider late paraphrenia to be a type of schizophrenia and distinguish it from the affective and organic disorders seen in the elderly. There is controversy, however, between the "lumpers" and the "splitters." Fish (1960) rejected the unitary concept of late paraphrenia and viewed this group of patients as displaying much heterogeneity, with only some of the patients being schizophrenic. Tanna (1974), on the other hand, felt that a case could be made for a distinct entity of late paraphrenia, apart from schizophrenia. The majority of writers, however (Slater and Roth, 1969; Bucci, 1965; Kay and Roth, 1961), felt that late paraphrenia was the late-occurring form of schizophrenia proper.

Upon reviewing the literature, one is struck by the virtual lack of research interest in late paraphrenia among American investigators. Only recently have geriatric problems received serious attention in this country, and one wonders whether late paraphrenia will soon come under more careful clinical scrutiny. The tendency to view psychiatric illness in the elderly as solely a manifestation of coarse brain disease, and thus essentially untreatable, must be reevaluated. More discriminating diagnostic criteria need to be established, and treatment plans tailored to meet the needs of the individual.

PERIODIC CATATONIA

Among the most thoroughly and carefully researched syndromes in psychiatry is the entity called periodic catatonia. Much of this work is the result of a family effort begun by Rolv Gjessing in 1929 and continued to the present by his son, Liev R. Gjessing, and his collaborators. The disease is not common and, particularly since the advent of neuroleptic drugs, it is only rarely diagnosed. As will be seen, recognition of the cyclic nature of the illness, and its response in some cases to lithium carbonate, has led some investigators to reclassify periodic catatonia as an affective disease. For historical reasons, and until more definitive closure is reached regarding its place in the nosology, it is included here with the atypical types of schizophrenia. For a fascinating glimpse at the painstaking clinical and research protocols employed by R. Gjessing, the reader is referred to a recently translated collection of his group's work (R. Gjessing, 1976).

Clinically, periodic catatonia is characterized by the abrupt appearance and abrupt cessation of periods of catatonic excitement and stupor. Between attacks, the patients appear normal, though on closer scrutiny there are deficits in their judgment and insight. Along with the clinical manifestations, there are a host of metabolic shifts that occur with remarkable regularity.

The *excited form of periodic catatonia* was described by Kraepelin and included the characteristic features of the illness: abrupt onset of confused states of excitement occurring perhaps every few weeks or even every few years, abrupt switch to periods of calm, sudden weight loss, in some instances delusions and hallucinations, dullness and indifference, and little or no insight into what had occurred. He considered that the illness might represent manic-depressive insanity, but decided against this. Acknowledging the similarities, he concluded, "Formerly, I regarded these forms [periodic dementias] as belonging to manic-depressive insanity. . . . The states of excitement described here which are repeated in short periods of time form only an episode in the course of a disease which otherwise is undoubtedly dementia praecox . . ." (Kraepelin, 1919).

In the early 1930s R. Gjessing described the syndrome of *periodic catatonic stupor*. He found that these cases occurred much less frequently than the excited types. The abrupt onset and recovery were similar to those for the excited type, but the clinical manifestations were vastly different. According to Kraepelin and R. Gjessing, the combined frequency of the two types is 2–3% of all schizophrenias (Gjessing, 1969).

Most of the research on periodic catatonia has been conducted on wards where patients were hospitalized for prolonged periods of time under controlled circumstances. Numerous behavioral and physiologic observations were made on these patients (Gjessing, 1976). Over a span of 30 years, 32 patients were studied with an intensity that is unparalleled today.

The majority of cases are classified as *"ss-type"* (synchronous-syntony), which indicates that the excitement or stupor begins suddenly and the pathophysiological changes are in synchrony with the clinical state. Other subgroups, showing increasingly little correlation between physiological and clinical parameters, are classified as *dys-synchronous-dys-syntony (dd)* and *a-synchronous-a-syntony (aa)*.

During the intervals between attacks, the patients are lucid, oriented, and able to perform tasks on the ward. Their judgment is somewhat impaired, and they have little or no insight into their condition. Physiologically, they demonstrate a slow pulse (50–60 per minute), low basal metabolic rate (BMR), low protein-bound iodine (PBI), leukopenia, lymphocytosis, and low fasting blood sugar.

The transition phase into psychosis may last only hours when ushering in a stupor, or take a day or two when leading to the excitement phase. Physiologically, this period is one of lability, with widely varying pulse rate and changing pupil size. The excitement phase of the psychosis consists of increased psychomotor activity, which may progress to stereotypic excitement and may show marked regression to primitive states. The excitement reaches a maximum early in the psychosis, then gradually decreases. Throughout the episode, orientation is maintained. In stupor, the patient lies immobile, is mute, displays negativism, and seems out of contact with his surroundings. Interestingly, both types manifest a similar physiologic response. There is increased pulse, blood pressure, temperature, BMR, PBI, blood sugar, and saliva; decreased urinary output; weight loss and mydriasis. The following case illustrates much of the clinical picture (excerpted from Gjessing, 1976).

Case 3. The patient first presented with psychotic symptoms at the age of 22, after 5 years of increasing isolation. He had the acute onset of auditory and visual hallucinations, uncontrolled psychomotor unrest, and catastrophic feelings of anxiety and terror. He did not recover to his premorbid condition and during the ensuing 5 years had several periods of catatonic restlessness and was autistic, but at times made attempts to show some initiative. Around age 27, the periods of catatonic stupor became more pronounced, lasting 12–27 days and occurring with increasing frequency. They would usually start at night. He would go to bed in his usual state, then in the morning be found half sitting up, pale, and motionless, with widely dilated pupils and showing no reaction to others. He would remain in this state for from 3 to 5 days, then begin to care more for himself by the 8th day. This phase would end dramatically when he awoke, asked what day it was, looked for letters he might have received during his stupor, and promptly began answering them. During the interval phase, he was alert, talkative, friendly, and at times hyperactive with a flight of ideas. His metabolic studies showed a baseline oxygen consumption and pulse rate during the interval, with a marked rise in both during stupor. His nitrogen excretion would begin to rise on day 2 and peak around day 6. It would fall around the 8th day of his interval phase. This pattern was constant for all his attacks. Treatment with thyroxine ameliorated the course of the episodes, but did not "cure the disorder."

Comment

Studies of nitrogen balance have occupied center stage in attempts to assess the etiology and pathophysiology of periodic catatonia. In the stuporous type, positive nitrogen balance continues to rise higher and higher during the interval phase until, by some mechanism, nitrogen excretion begins, and the stupor concomitantly appears. This can be viewed as a means of reestablishing equilibrium. In the excited type, however, the retention of nitrogen and low excretion rate occur simultaneously, rather than prior to the psychotic state. The swings in the nitrogen balance are of the same duration as the swings in the autonomic functions, but there may be substantial time lags between them. There seem to be (an) as yet unknown factor(s) that govern(s) both the nitrogen balance and autonomic functions, which in turn profoundly affect metabolism. A possible explanation may reside in the functioning of the thyroid gland. The phasic swings in the ss-type of periodic catatonia (either excited or stuporous) may be abolished with the administration of large doses of thyroxine at the proper time. Cessation of thyroxine treatment results in recurrence of catatonic periods. This suggests that, in some manner, thyroid function is crucial to the chain of metabolic changes that occurs (Gjessing, 1976).

Urinary catecholamines are excreted normally during the interval phase but in increased amounts during the psychosis. Studies of corticosteroids have yielded conflicting results (Vestergaard, 1969). There are also marked changes in cholesterol: total cholesterol drops during the psychotic phase, rises during the interval, and reaches its highest value just prior to the onset of psychosis (Maeda *et al.*, 1969).

As one might expect, there is a dramatic disruption of sleep during the course of the illness. During the interval phase, until about 1 to 3 days prior to the appearance of symptoms, sleep architecture is normal. Then, abrupt changes occur, resulting in a marked decrease in REM sleep and total sleep time and an increase in REM latency time (Gjessing, 1974; Takahashi and Gjessing, 1972). The sleep changes described also occur in other cases of acute schizophrenia and do not seem to be specific to periodic catatonia.

The physiologic changes described repeat themselves with little variation as each patient cycles between psychotic and interval phases. Current knowledge of neurophysiology leads to the hypothesis that there is involvement of the hypothalamic–pituitary axis. It seems clear that there is a "switch" from a primarily cholinergic (hypoarousal) state to an adrenergic (hyperarousal) state. R. Gjessing sums up this idea as follows: "It is as if an unseen hand were playing on the keyboard of the vegetative nuclei in the hypothalamus: First, as the prelude, single notes or two-note chords are played softly and from time to time fuller chords are coming from the cholinergic base register. Then the composition moves toward the adrenergic atonal . . . the two contrasting autonomic registers sound together or alternate until finally the individual melody of the reaction phase is established. It may all stem from stimulation of the autonomic centers, it may be hormonal in nature, but from where remains an open question . . ." (quoted in Gjessing, 1969).

Various treatments have been successful in attenuating the psychotic episodes and, to a lesser degree, in preventing them. The phenothiazines and butyrophenones suppress the psychotic behavior, as do disulfiram, reserpine, and α-methyldopa (Gjessing, 1967). As noted above, large doses of thyroxine have abolished the periodicity of the pathophysiological changes, enabling patients to recover completely. More recently, a number of reports (Wald and Lerner, 1978; Petursson, 1976; Sovner and McHugh, 1974) have described the use of lithium carbonate in treating patients who fulfilled the criteria for periodic catatonia. The results of treatment with lithium have been encouraging, but this area needs further investigation.

With the early and rapid neuroleptic treatment of psychoses, the diagnosis of periodic catatonia is difficult to make. A longitudinal view of the individual is needed, with careful attention paid to the biological parameters of the illness. In recurring psychotic episodes displaying signs of catatonic stupor or excitement, the clinician should be alert to the diagnosis of periodic catatonia. The treatment and prognosis may differ from that of other schizophrenias.

ONEIROPHRENIA

When Bleuler (1950) defined criteria for schizophrenia, he specified that the illness must take place in a person with a clear sensorium, that is, unimpaired orientation, memory, and level of consciousness. A clear sensorium is usually seen as the primary distinguishing factor in so-called functional versus organic illness. However, one can see episodes of confusion and what appear as disturbances of consciousness in the setting of an otherwise typical functional psychosis, with no overt evidence of disordered central nervous system function. This has often been called "schizophreniform states" (Langfeldt, 1939), "oneiroid experience" of Mayer-Gross (Slater and Roth, 1969), or "oneirophrenia" (Meduna, 1950).

The root *oneiro* is derived from the Greek word meaning "dream." Oneirophrenia, as defined by Meduna, is a disorder of acute or subacute onset characterized by perceptual disorganization, which alienates the individual from his/her environment. The perceptual difficulties are referred to by patients as changes in their own bodies, in the world, or in both. The degree of perceptual alteration can be so severe as to resemble a waking, terrifying nightmare. Disorientation and memory disturbance may occur during an acute episode.

Meduna stressed that the basic symptom in oneirophrenia was the disordered perception. This could affect any of the sensory modalities, with visual disturbances observed most frequently. The patients he described often complained of trouble with their vision, of seeing things through a "fog," and of misinterpreting existing visual stimuli. Another common disturbance involved the proprioceptive senses. Patients would be overattentive to sensations arising from their own bodies and these would serve as the nidus for somatic delusions. The result of these alterations was extreme fear and confusion. He noted that these episodes were relatively short-lived, often did not recur, and were not followed by personality deterioration.

Meduna (1950) felt that an integral part of oneirophrenia was a disorder of glucose metabolism. He found that the patients they studied, as compared to normals, had glucose tolerance curves that showed a delayed return to baseline after a glucose load, a diabetic-like response, and a resistance to insulin. These findings were true during the acute episode and reverted to normal during remission. However, further study along these lines has failed to replicate the findings (Langfeldt, 1953; Mayer-Gross, 1952). These later investigators felt that there may, indeed, be abnormal carbohydrate and endocrinological responses in acute states of psychosis and confusion. However, they found no relationship between glucose metabolism and specific diagnostic entities.

Rather, they felt that the responses seen were secondary to the generalized increased stress, motor activity, etc., that acute psychotics display.
Since Meduna had used the findings of abnormal glucose metabolism to
support his contention that oneirophrenia was a separate entity, one cannot easily accept his conclusions. The following case (excerpted from
Meduna, 1950) covers the salient features of the disorder.

Case 4. A 23-year-old male was in his usual state of health until he
returned home from a movie in an anxious state, telling his parents that
a character in the movie "came out after him." He did not recognize his
father and, at that moment, attacked him. Later that night he appeared
confused, did not recognize his home, and was very frightened. He complained of seeing animals in his room. At times, he was not sure if he
was dreaming or if he was awake; at other times, he was convinced of
their reality. He also heard the voice of an "invisible man." On formal
testing, he was oriented to place and time, but he manifested distortions
of his time sense. During the next 2 weeks, his mood, despite these
frightening episodes, remained cheerful. A few weeks later, his sensorium began to clear and he "recognized" his past strange experiences as
dream states. During the psychotic phase, he responded to a glucose load
with a highly abnormal, diabetic-like curve. This normalized as he
became less confused.

Comment

How can we understand these disturbances in perception, memory,
orientation, and level of consciousness—are they part of a schizophrenic
process, or are they not schizophrenia and thus a separate category? (In
the above case, Meduna stressed that the diagnosis had to be oneirophrenia.) Chapman (1966) studied patients diagnosed on admission as
schizophrenic, with the diagnosis confirmed at follow-up. He was interested in the early manifestations of their illness and interviewed patients
within 1–33 months after onset of symptoms. He found that 40% of the
patients reported experiencing changes in visual perception: changes in
the size and shape of objects, alterations in color, illusions of moving
objects, and loss of stereoscopic vision. In addition, 95% experienced
blocking phenomena that they characterized as "trances," "blank spells,"
or "dazes"; at times, these progressed to stages of increasing distractabil-
became less confused.
image. The symptoms described by Chapman were very similar to those
described in the case reports by Meduna (1950). Meduna felt that,
because of the confusion and the disorders of memory and level of
awareness, the illness was not part of the schizophrenic process. Chap-

man, however, viewed the schizophrenic process (in part, at least) as a response to the alteration in perceptual and psychomotor functions, resulting in a flooding of consciousness with sensory data that the person was unable to integrate. He saw the blocking phenomena as manifestations of a transient alteration of consciousness related to the failure to exclude irrelevant stimuli that arise from internal and external sources. Thus, the disordered perception (and its sequelae) were an integral part of the pathology of schizophrenia, rather than excluding criteria.

Meduna's distinction of oneirophrenia as an illness apart from schizophrenia does not seem tenable. Careful review of his case histories reveals descriptions of early psychotic decompensations, but no substantial follow-up was done. The symptoms described as being unique to oneirophrenia (severe perceptual distortions and abnormal glucose metabolism) have been shown to be common in patients who were diagnosed as schizophrenic when studied for a longer period of time. Patients whose illness presents in the manner described above may, on the other hand, very well be a group that can be separated from the more classic schizophrenias. Some patients showing confusion amid other symptoms of schizophrenia may be part of the schizoaffective group described earlier and may therefore have a more favorable prognosis (Procci, 1976).

CONCLUSIONS

A number of schizophrenic subtypes have been described that differ from the classical syndrome in significant ways. Some are considered quite rare, while others are now being recognized more frequently. Good diagnostic evaluation is imperative if appropriate treatment is to follow. To some research groups "diagnosis is prognosis" (Woodruff et al., 1974).

We are entering a phase of psychiatry where objective criteria and biological markers are becoming a more integral part of the diagnostic process. The unusual syndromes described here offer the opportunity to examine the nature of our classification system and to question some long-held beliefs that may no longer be valid. They also serve to remind us of the diversity of human behavior and the uniqueness that each individual manifests in trying to cope with his/her life's stresses.

REFERENCES

American Psychiatric Association, 1978, "Diagnostic and Statistical Manual of Mental Disorders, DSM III Draft," American Psychiatric Association, Washington, D.C.
Bleuler, E., 1950, "Dementia Praecox or the Group of Schizophrenias," International Universities Press, New York.

Bucci, L., 1965, Senile psychosis and paraphrenia—Some theoretical and practical considerations, *Int. J. Neuropsychiatry* 1:561.

Cerroloza, M., and Cleghorn, R., 1971, Atypical psychosis: A search for certainty in this ambiguous borderland, *Can. Psychiatr. Assoc. J.* 16:507.

Chapman, J., 1966, The early symptoms of schizophrenia, *Br. J. Psychiatry* 112:225.

Feighner, J. P., Robins, E., Guze, S. B., Woodruff, R. A., Winokur, G., and Munoz, R., 1972, Diagnostic criteria for use in psychiatric research, *Arch. Gen. Psychiatry* 26:57.

Fish, F., 1960, Senile schizophrenia, *J. Ment. Sci.* 106:938.

Gjessing, L. R., 1967, Effect of thyroxine, pyridoxine, orphenadrine-HCl, reserpine and disulfiram in periodic catatonia, *Acta Psychiatr. Scand.* 43:376.

Gjessing, L. R., 1969, Longitudinal studies of periodic catatonia, in "Schizophrenia: Current Concepts and Research" (D. V. Siva Sankar, ed.), pp. 638–644, PJD Publications, Hicksville, N.Y.

Gjessing, L. R., 1974, A review of periodic catatonia, *Biol. Pychiatry* 8:23.

Gjessing, R., 1976, "Contributions to the Somatology of Periodic Catatonia," Pergamon Press, Oxford.

Herbert, M. E., and Jacobson, S., 1967, Late paraphrenia, *Br. J. Psychiatry* 113:461.

Kay, D. W. K., 1963, Late paraphrenia and its bearing on the aetiology of schizophrenia, *Acta Psychiatr. Scand.* 39:159.

Kay, D. W. K., and Roth, M., 1961, Environmental and hereditary factors in schizophrenias of old age ("late paraphrenia") and their bearing on the general problem of causation in schizophrenia, *J. Ment. Sci.* 107:649.

Kraepelin, E., 1919, "Dementia Praecox and Paraphrenia," E. & S. Livingstone, Edinburgh.

Langfeldt, G., 1939, "The Schizophreniform States," Oxford University Press, London.

Langfeldt, G., 1953, The insulin tolerance test in mental disorders, *Acta Psychiatr. Neurol. Scand. (Suppl.)* 80:189.

Maeda, M., Borud, O., and Gjessing, L. R., 1969, Investigation of cholesterol and fatty acids in periodic catatonia, *Br. J. Psychiatry* 115:81.

Mayer, W., 1921, Ueber paraphrena Psychosen, *Z. Gesamte Neurol. Psychiatr.* 71:187.

Mayer-Gross, W., 1952, The diagnostic significance of certain tests of carbohydrate metabolism in psychiatric patients and the question of "oneirophrenia," *J. Ment. Sci.* 98:683.

Meduna, L. J., 1950, "Oneirophrenia," University of Illinois Press, Urbana.

Petursson, H., 1976, Lithium treatment of a patient with periodic catatonia, *Acta Psychiatr. Scand.* 54:248.

Pope, H. G., and Lipinski, J. F., 1978, Diagnosis in schizophrenic and manic-depressive illness, *Arch. Gen. Psychiatry* 35:811.

Procci, W., 1976, Schizo-affective psychosis: Fact or fiction? *Arch. Gen. Psychiatry* 33:1167.

Roth, M., 1955, The natural history of mental disorder in old age, *J. Ment. Sci.* 101:281.

Slater, E., and Roth, M., 1969, "Clinical Psychiatry," Williams and Wilkins, Baltimore.

Sovner, R. D., and McHugh, P. R., 1974, Lithium in the treatment of periodic catatonia: A case report, *J. Nerv. Ment. Dis.* 158:214.

Szasz, T. S., 1974, "The Myth of Mental Illness," Harper & Row, New York.

Takahashi, S., and Gjessing, L. R., 1972, Studies of periodic catatonia III: Longitudinal sleep study with urinary excretion of catecholamines, *J. Psychiatr. Res.* 9:123.

Tanna, V. L., 1974, Paranoid states: A selected review, *Comp. Psychiatry* 15:453.

Vestergaard, P., 1969, Periodic catatonia—Some endocrine studies, in "Schizophrenia: Current Concepts and Research" (D. V. Siva Sankar, ed.), pp. 645–688, PJD Publications, Hicksville, N.Y.

Wald, D., and Lerner, J., 1978, Lithium treatment of periodic catatonia: A case report, *Am. J. Psychiatry* 135:751.

Woodruff, R. A., Goodwin, D. W., and Guze, S. B., 1974, "Psychiatric Diagnosis," Oxford University Press, New York.

Index